Register Now for Online Access to Your Book!

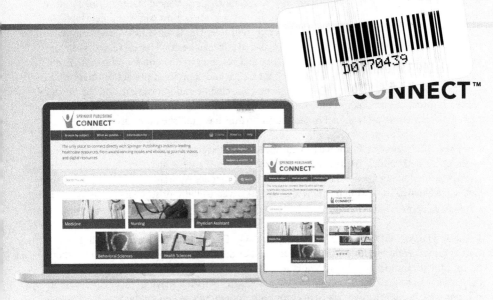

CONNECT™

Your print purchase of *Data-Driven Quality Improvement and Sustainability in Healthcare* **includes online access to the contents of your book**—increasing accessibility, portability, and searchability!

Access today at:
http://connect.springerpub.com/content/book/978-0-8261-3944-3
or scan the QR code at the right with your smartphone and enter the access code below.

Y3EV5RLM

Scan here for quick access.

If you are experiencing problems accessing the digital component of this product, please contact our customer service department at cs@springerpub.com

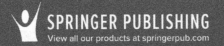

SPRINGER PUBLISHING
View all our products at springerpub.com

Patricia L. Thomas, PhD, RN, NEA-BC, ACNS-BC, CNL, FAAN, FNAP, FACHE, is Associate Dean Nursing Faculty Affairs and Associate Dean at Wayne State University. As a member of the executive team, she is responsible for operational oversight and development faculty in the college of nursing. Prior to her current role, Dr. Thomas held leadership positions in practice and academe in local, regional, and national health. Having served as a chief nursing officer and director of nursing practice and research in a national health system and as an academic leader, she recognizes the importance and significant impact of interprofessional practice, the use of data in sustainable practice change and innovation, and the impact academic–practice partnerships have on patient and organizational outcomes. Dr. Thomas has served on numerous professional organization boards, has published and disseminated outcomes widely, and serves as an academic and practice consultant nationally and internationally. She holds board certification as an advanced nurse executive, in healthcare management, as an adult health clinical nurse specialist, and as a clinical nurse leader. Dr. Thomas serves as an American Nursing Credentialing Center (ANCC) Magnet Appraiser and Commission on Collegiate Nursing Education (CCNE) Visitor and is a consultant for strategic planning, leadership development, and evaluation.

James L. Harris, PhD, PMHCNS-BC, MBA, CNL, FAAN, is Professor of Nursing in the Community/Mental Health Nursing Department at the University of South Alabama where he coordinates online masters and doctoral level courses. Prior to his current role, he was the Department Chair for Community/Mental Health Nursing, playing an integral part in redesigning clinical learning experiences for both undergraduate and graduate students, thus facilitating new academic–service partnerships in community mental health systems in rural communities. Dr. Harris has held numerous administrative positions for the Department of Veterans Affairs (VA) on local, regional, and national levels, and has an extensive background in professional scholarship. He remains active as a board-certified advanced practice nurse and consultant to healthcare organizations, developing and evaluating improvement projects.

Brian Collins, BS, is Director of Decision Support at Lawrence General Hospital in Lawrence, Massachusetts, a community hospital with 186 licensed inpatient beds and 70,000 emergency room visits annually. In this role he has leveraged past experiences in operations, business development, information systems, data analysis, and performance improvement. Previously, Mr. Collins helped create clinical decision support practices that were part of Tufts Medical Center being recognized as the 6th Best Academic Medical Center by the University HealthSystem Consortiums annual rankings. Using data analytics and outreach to establish core business processes centered on safety, timeliness, effectiveness, efficiency, equity, and patient-centered care (STEEEP), Tufts was elevated from the bottom half of national performance. In his tenure at ProHealth, Mr. Collins helped create a physician practice with more than 200 providers in 75 sites and management services that were later acquired by OptumCare and United Healthcare Group. In addition to growing the clinical and financial performance of the organization, the independent ambulatory practice was among the first to write electronic prescriptions, conduct web-based patient visits with copays and insurance reimbursement, and enter outcomes-based population health contracts. Mr. Collins has presented at local and national conferences on quality improvement and clinical practice cost analysis and has published in peer-reviewed journals.

DATA-DRIVEN QUALITY IMPROVEMENT AND SUSTAINABILITY IN HEALTHCARE

An Interprofessional Approach

Patricia L. Thomas, PhD, RN, NEA-BC, ACNS-BC, CNL, FAAN, FNAP, FACHE

James L. Harris, PhD, PMHCNS-BC, MBA, CNL, FAAN

Brian Collins, BS

EDITORS

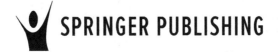 SPRINGER PUBLISHING

Springer Publishing Company, LLC
11 West 42nd Street, New York, NY 10036
www.springerpub.com
connect.springerpub.com/

Acquisitions Editor: Adrianne Brigido
Compositor: Exeter Premedia Services Private Ltd.

ISBN: 978-0-8261-3943-6
ebook ISBN: 978-0-8261-3944-3
DOI: 10.1891/9780826139443

20 21 22 23 24 / 5 4 3 2 1

The author and the publisher of this Work have made every effort to use sources believed to be reliable to provide information that is accurate and compatible with the standards generally accepted at the time of publication. Because medical science is continually advancing, our knowledge base continues to expand. Therefore, as new information becomes available, changes in procedures become necessary. We recommend that the reader always consult current research and specific institutional policies before performing any clinical procedure or delivering any medication. The author and publisher shall not be liable for any special, consequential, or exemplary damages resulting, in whole or in part, from the readers' use of, or reliance on, the information contained in this book. The publisher has no responsibility for the persistence or accuracy of URLs for external or third-party Internet websites referred to in this publication and does not guarantee that any content on such websites is, or will remain, accurate or appropriate.

Library of Congress Cataloging-in-Publication Data

Names: Thomas, Patricia L., 1961- editor. | Harris, James L. (James
   Leonard), 1956- editor. | Collins, Brian (Brian J.), editor.
Title: Data-driven quality improvement and sustainability in healthcare :
   an interprofessional approach / Patricia L. Thomas, James L. Harris,
   Brian Collins, editors.
Description: New York, NY : Springer Publishing Company, LLC, [2021] |
   Includes bibliographical references and index.
Identifiers: LCCN 2020038083 (print) | LCCN 2020038084 (ebook) | ISBN
   9780826139436 (paperback) | ISBN 9780826139443 (ebook)
Subjects: MESH: Data Mining--methods | Quality Improvement--organization &
   administration | Datasets as Topic | Sustainable Development | Health
   Services Administration--standards
Classification: LCC R859.7.D35 (print) | LCC R859.7.D35 (ebook) | NLM W
   26.55.I4 | DDC 610.285--dc23
LC record available at https://lccn.loc.gov/2020038083
LC ebook record available at https://lccn.loc.gov/2020038084

Contact us to receive discount rates on bulk purchases.
We can also customize our books to meet your needs.
For more information please contact: sales@springerpub.com

Printed in the United States of America.

To our families, partners, and colleagues who supported us in the creation of this work, we are grateful for the encouragement and understanding as this endeavor progressed. Equally, we appreciate Springer Publishing Company for their support and guidance in bringing our shared vision for this textbook to reality.

Contents

Chapter Contributors

Michael R. Bleich, PhD, RN, NEA-BC, FNAP, FAAN, President and CEO, NursDynamics, LLC, Senior Professor and Director, Virginia Commonwealth University School of Nursing, Langston Center for Innovation in Quality and Safety, Richmond, Virginia

Clista Clanton, MSLS, Senior Librarian, University of South Alabama, Mobile, Alabama

Brian Collins, BS, Health Systems Management, Director of Decision Support, Lawrence General Hospital, Lawrence, Massachusetts

Lauran Hardin, MSN, RN-BC, CNL, FNAP, FAAN, Senior Advisor Partnerships and Technical Assistance, National Center for Complex Health and Social Needs, Camden Coalition of Healthcare Providers, Camden, New Jersey

James L. Harris, PhD, PMHCNS-BC, MBA, CNL, FAAN, Professor of Nursing, University of South Alabama, Mobile, Alabama

Niranjani Radhakrishnan, Director for the Center for Information and Analytics, Regional One Health, Center for Information and Analytics, Memphis, Tennessee

Kathryn Sapnas, PhD, RN-BC, Office of Nursing Services, Policy and Strategic Planning, Washington, District of Columbia

Patricia L. Thomas, PhD, RN, NEA-BC, ACNS-BC, CNL, FAAN, FNAP, FACHE, Associate Dean, Nursing Faculty Affairs & Associate Professor, Cohn College of Nursing, Wayne State University, Detroit, Michigan

Megan Williams, MSN, RN, CNL, Manager, Complex Care, Regional One Health, Memphis, Tennessee

Exemplar Contributors

Kiyoko Abe, PhD, CNL, Japanese Red Cross College of Nursing, Professor, Nursing Management

Cyrus Batheja, EdD, MBA, BSN, PHN, RN, National Vice President Policy and Clinical Solutions, UnitedHealthcare Community & State, Minnetonka, Minnesota

Brianne Burke, BA, Patient Services Manager/Medical Biller, Family Health Center, Grand Rapids, Michigan

Beth Carson, EdD, RN CEN, OSF Saint Anthony College of Nursing, Dean, Undergraduate Affairs & Professor, Rockford, Illinois

Brian Collins, BS, Health Systems Management, Director of Decision Support, Lawrence General Hospital, Lawrence, Massachusetts

Sean Collins, ScD, Physical Therapy Program Director, Plymouth State University, Plymouth, New Hampshire

Mark Contreras, DNP, NP-C, Affiliate Clinical Faculty, Adult Gerontology Nurse Practitioner, Grand Valley State University, Kirkhof College of Nursing, Family Health Center, Grand Rapids, Michigan

John Deckro, DNP, RN-BC, CPHIMS, RN Clinical Information Systems, Coordinator/Educator, Providence VA Medical Center, VA Nursing Academic Partnership (VANAP) Faculty, Providence VAMC & Rhode Island School of Nursing, Providence, Rhode Island

Erika DeMartinis, MSN, RN-BC, Associate Chief Nurse, Medical Center Education & Designated Learning Officer, Corporal Michael J. Crescenz, VA Medical Center, Philadelphia, Pennsylvania

Gordana Dermody, PhD, RN, CNL, Instructor, Edith Cowan University School of Nursing and Midwifery, Centre for Nursing, Midwifery and Health Services Research, Edith Cowan University, Perth, Australia

Heather R. Hall, PhD, RN, NNP-BC, Dean and Professor, University of South Alabama, College of Nursing, Mobile, Alabama

Lauran Hardin, MSN, CNL, Senior Advisor National Center for Complex Health and Social Needs, Maysville, Kentucky

Nancy J. Hauff, PhD, RNC-OB, Clinical Instructor, Cohn College of Nursing, Wayne State University, Detroit, Michigan

Minami Kakuta, MSN, RN, CNL, OSF Saint Anthony College of Nursing, Instructor, Rockford, Illinois

Asako Katsumata, PhD, RN, Professor, Faculty of Medicine, University of Tsukuba

Shannon Lizer, PhD, FNP-BC, FAANP, Dean, Graduate Affairs & Research, Professor, OSF Saint Anthony College of Nursing, Rockford, Illinois

Brandie Messer, DNP, RN, PCOE, OSF Saint Anthony College of Nursing, Assistant Professor, DNP Coordinator, Rockford, Illinois

Mark Morreo, Senior Programmer, Information Services, Lawrence General Hospital, Lawrence, Massachusetts

Charlene M. Myers, DNP, CNS, ACNP-BC, Associate Professor of Nursing, University of South Alabama, College of Nursing, Mobile, Alabama

John Nelson, PhD, CEO, Healthcare Environment, St. Paul, Minnesota

Kazuko Nin, PhD, RN, Department of Human Health Sciences, Graduate School of Medicine, Professor, Kyoto University, Kyoto, Japan

K. Ninomiya, MSN, RN, Japanese Red Cross Society, Tokyo, Japan

Debra Novak, PhD, National Personal Protective Technology Laboratory, National Institute for Occupational Safety Health (Retired), Lexington, Kentucky

Teresa Pazdral, MD, FACEP, Medical Director of Quality and System Improvement, Lawrence General Hospital, Lawrence, Massachusetts

Niranjani Radhakrishnan, Director for the Center for Information and Analytics, Regional One Health Center for Information and Analytics, Memphis, Tennessee

Alison M. Scarry, MS, H, BB (ASCP), Administrative Laboratory Director, Lawrence General Hospital, Lawrence, Massachusetts

Shanda Scott, DNP, CRNP, ANP-BC, Assistant Professor of Nursing, University of South Alabama, College of Nursing, Mobile, Alabama

Raja Senguttuvan, MD, Director, Neonatology, and Neonatologist, Lawrence General Hospital, Assistant Professor, Tufts University School of Medicine, Boston, Massachusetts

Michael Sims, LPC-MHSP, Jail Diversion Coordinator, Alliance Healthcare Services, Memphis, Tennessee

Coy L. Smith, ND, RN, MSN, NEA-BC, FACHE, CPHQ, Associate Director Patient Care Services/Nurse Executive, Corporal Michael J. Crescenz, VA Medical Center, Assistant Dean Clinical Practice-PENN School of Nursing, Philadelphia, Pennsylvania

Karen L. Spada, DNP, FNP, MPH, MHA, Health Administration Consultant, Las Vegas, Nevada

Peter Sylvester, Systems Architect, Information Services, Lawrence General Hospital, Lawrence, Massachusetts

Patricia L. Thomas, PhD, RN, NEA-BC, ACNS-BC, CNL, FAAN, FNAP, FACHE, Associate Dean, Nursing Faculty Affairs & Associate Professor, Cohn College of Nursing, Wayne State University, Detroit, Michigan

Tamara VanKampen, DNP, RN, Practice Manager, Family Health Center, Grand Rapids, Michigan

Lonnie K. Williams, MSN, RN, Education Consultant, Washington, District of Columbia

Megan Williams, MSN, RN, CNL, Manager, Complex Care, Regional One Health, Memphis, Tennessee

Christina Wolf, MS, RN, Director of Population Health, Lawrence General Hospital, Lawrence, Massachusetts

Preface

Ideas are generated constantly as individuals interact with one another, attend and participate in improvement activities, and experience life. Ideas can remain stagnant or become innovative opportunities that change the future. As ideas are developed, transformation occurs. Prevailing practices and processes are challenged. When challenged, organizations must respond proactively and utilize the talents of others to create pathways to manage impending situations. Data and evidence are the primary drivers in these situations. Understanding and managing data is requisite for organizational change and sustainability in contemporary society.

This textbook, originating from an idea, was developed using information from the literature, experiences as educators and managers, and contributions from others in various health and allied disciplines. We contend that the textbook is not all-inclusive. Rather, the textbook provides a snapshot to:

- Improve decision-making
- Meet consumer demands
- Develop business cases
- Influence policy and regulation
- Understand the value of data collection, analysis, use, and diffusion that will inform quality, safety, and operational efficiency

Unique attributes of this textbook include "real-world" exemplars and reflection questions for each chapter that demonstrate how data and evidence inform the application of improvement tools, data analysis techniques, and concepts across interprofessional disciplines. We anticipate that the information provided will assist improvement teams to improve healthcare processes, guide educators to provide tools and techniques germane to education development, and help students glean knowledge necessary to lead improvement as future healthcare professionals and leaders.

Patricia L. Thomas
James L. Harris
Brian Collins

Acknowledgments

People working in healthcare who are committed to achieving exceptional outcomes generate a palpable energy. When engaged in meaningful work, a synergy is generated and acts as a catalyst for innovation and improvement. In this complex and interconnected biosphere, creativity and commitment propel us to new heights. My colleagues and I are unable to identify all the clinicians and leaders who provided purposeful insights about improvement, data use, and management, or how future health professionals could best be educated, but we identified themes that formed the genesis of this book. First, there is an appreciation that data will continue to be generated and we need to learn how to be disciplined in its use. Second, the need for innovation and creative expression is essential to bring about positive change. Last, we are on the cusp of transformation as unimaginable possibilities are being brought forward through technological advances. The expanse of data will change the healthcare landscape and influence the ways we value, use, analyze, and incorporate it into our work.

The Footprint of Data Across Healthcare Organizations

James L. Harris

CHAPTER OBJECTIVES

1. Examine the drivers affecting the current healthcare landscape.
2. Explain how healthcare technology has advanced during the past decade to create infinite databases.
3. Determine how healthcare data are being used to meet policy, regulatory, and consumer demands.

CORE COMPETENCIES

- Knowledge of the healthcare environment and current trends
- Information technology knowledge and future trends
- Management and use of evidence-based healthcare data
- Knowledge of healthcare care policy, regulations, and consumer demands

INTRODUCTION

The healthcare industry is constantly experiencing change. How the industry responds will be determined by numerous influences. The influences include data and platforms, digital therapeutics, healthcare reform, consumer-centric products, care communities, and a shift from healthcare to health and wellness (DeloitteHealth, 2019; Siwicki, 2019). As with other industries, healthcare organizations must be business savvy, risk averse, and persist in the use of meaningful evidence-based data to achieve quality, safety, and sustainable value-based outcomes. This chapter will focus on the drivers affecting the current and future healthcare landscape and how technology will continue to generate databases that are essential for sustainability, policy development, and meeting regulatory requirements and consumer demands.

The chapters that follow will include information necessary to accelerate knowledge, improve decision-making, and enable healthcare professionals, students, and educators to use data to achieve quality, safety, and value-based outcomes. Specifically, Chapter 2 focuses on a new age of imperatives that will impact quality, safety, and value-based outcomes within the context of new rules, leadership skills, and a competitive healthcare market. Chapter 3 concentrates on different quality improvement tools, methods, and selecting the right tool for interprofessional projects. Tools that are pivotal to planning data collection and analysis will be explored. Chapter 4 provides information on the value of data to inform administrative and clinical decisions to achieve peak performance, anchor strategic initiatives, and improve operational thinking. Chapter 5 is an overview to understand how data science accelerates discovery, improves decisions, and creates a data-driven economy for healthcare success. Chapter 6 discusses the advantage of collecting, managing, and analyzing big data and how the 5Vs (volume, velocity, veracity, variety, and value) are central to mapping and designing interprofessional strategies to promote organization-wide improvement. Chapter 7 provides information on how data influences and guides the development, implementation, and interpretation of policy and regulations by interprofessional teams. Chapter 8 is a discussion of the importance of innovation, data diffusion, and dissemination necessary for interprofessional teams who participate in data improvement processes. Chapter 9 presents information needed by interprofessional teams when developing a business case for change and practice innovation. Chapter 10 is an introduction on how consumer demands and data are driving change by consumers and leveraging interprofessional team power. Chapter 11 provides an introduction to data mining tools and techniques beneficial to interprofessional teams. Chapter 12 discusses how interprofessional teams use evidence to guide quality and safety initiatives. Chapter 13 focuses on how interprofessional teams extract and use data effectively. Chapter 14 provides a futuristic perspective of data and charting a course for care in the 21st and beyond.

Each of the chapters is central to understanding how data frames quality, safety, innovation, and sustainability in interprofessional practice as consumers become more engaged in their care. Adding value to each chapter are case exemplars for application authored by experts from practice, management, and education.

CURRENT AND FUTURE HEALTHCARE INFLUENCES AND DRIVERS

On a daily basis, leaders in healthcare organizations are confronted with the rising costs of care, shortfalls of quality and efficiency of care, and how interprofessional teams can collaboratively use evidence-based data to achieve improved results, satisfy patients, and create data rich infrastructures. Healthcare of the future will be driven by innumerable data connectivity and consumer engagement. Archetypes that create strategic initiatives and improved business models will be commonplace in order to develop a "culture of health, reduce disparities, and improve well-being of the U.S. population in the 21st century" (DeloitteHealth, 2019; National Academy of Medicine, 2019, para. 2).

Data and platforms are the cornerstone of a health ecosystem that generates decision-making insights fundamental to invest in new and improved healthcare technology (DeloitteHealth, 2019). With the increasing cost burden generated by chronic health conditions and an aging demographic, the use of data is a beneficial investment in the digital health technology market. This investment will offer individuals across the care continuum expanded opportunities to manage well-being. Favorable reimbursement policy development and efficacy research are possible as digital technology expands.

Digital therapeutics has increasingly become a debated and discussed topic in order to establish a comprehensive network of options for disorders and diseases. According to the Digital Therapeutics Alliance, "digital therapeutics deliver evidence-based therapeutic interventions to patients that are driven by high-quality software programs to prevent, manage, or treat a broad spectrum of physical, mental, and behavioral conditions" (Digital Therapeutics Alliance, 2019, p.1). Digital therapeutics produces a broader product from others available in the digital health landscape (Comstock, 2018). The benefits in this field are infinite for all stakeholders as it evolves.

Nationally, healthcare reform continues to remain an agenda item as prices escalate, mandates for quality and safety outcomes increase, and prevention services expand (Centers for Medicare and Medicaid Services [CMS], 2011a, 2011b). While the Patient Protection and Affordable Care Act of 2010 remains law, parts have been restructured with actions that create positive and negative outcomes (Office of Legislative Council, 2010). Regardless of the changes, meaningful use, collection, and analysis of data remain central to healthcare organizations survival. Understanding the value of data, selecting various digital platforms and devices, and analysis of information will continue to be markers for success as future reforms occur and interprofessional teams collectively engage in improvement activities.

The growth of consumer engagement in healthcare continues to expand and consumer-centric products are continuously being introduced into the market. In 2016, 46% of U.S. consumers were active users of digital health devices (Adams et al., 2016). The demand will continue as healthcare consumers become more knowledgeable about the benefits of preventive health and digital products that are unique to their behavior, lifestyle, genetics, and the environment. While healthcare products are marketed daily, developers must consider that each consumer is structurally, emotionally, and chemically different (Babalola, 2017). Consider for example the healthcare consumer who has the option to trial and purchase a phone application to measure pulse rates during walking. Based upon market demand, the product margin is predictable based on volume. Unlike the phone application, cardiac bypass surgery does not offer a trial period before the procedure is performed (Babalola, 2017; Mwachofi & Al-Assaf, 2011). This presents developers of new products with many challenges. Future research and development departments will require large quantities of data collection and analysis as new consumer-centric health products are marketed in order to personalize services.

The U.S. population continues to age at a rapid rate. As Americans age, the number of continuing care communities (CCCs) continue to grow contributing to a demographic who are active, use digital technologies to manage health status for a productive and meaningful life, and seek care communities for continuum of care options (Szlauderbach, 2020). As the popularity of CCCs increase, multiple markets will be tasked to develop new technologies that promote preventive health dedicated to health and well-being. Metrics will guide data collection and analysis that focus on outcomes important to individuals, families, and care providers (Rowe et al., 2016).

The shift from health to health and wellness will continue to be a significant influence in contemporary society as life expectancy anddemands for new technologies and wellness-focused commodities increase (Alder et al., 2016). Influencing the shift is data coupled with personalized health coaching in order to create a pathway that optimizes individual healthy outcomes. As data from genetic testing are collected and analyzed, research opportunities that focus on prevention and care for illnesses will transpire (Mann, 2019).

HEALTHCARE TECHNOLOGY ADVANCEMENTS DURING THE PAST DECADE

In the past decade, the healthcare industry has experienced an information revolution similar to the industrial revolution. The information revolution is credited with a variety of technology advancements in an era where the electronic medical record was adopted. As healthcare organizations leverage technology to improve outcomes, the technology advances of the past decade provide roadmaps for developing a future landscape for transforming quality, while ensuring safe and affordable care. As outcome-driven markets increase, digital health markets will continue to soar. In 2018, the digital health market represented a funding investment increase by 230% with predictions to continuing rising (Zweig et al., 2018).

Change in healthcare is constant and how data are obtained and disseminated impacts daily operations. Quantum leaps in efficiency and effectiveness have and will continue to occur with the diffusion of technology and availability of electronic networks that provide instant access across all points of care (Geibert, 2017). Technology has evolved with a shift from power to value as evidenced by greater throughput and efficiency in emergency departments and clinics with the use of protocol automation.

The previous example is only one of the many advances where value, both human and financial, is attributed to technology advances during the past decade. The following technological advances are further examples that will transform healthcare and the importance of data, as individuals remain the centrality of care delivery beyond the 21st century.

Telemedicine has gained much popularity since its introduction, offering opportunities to treat chronic diseases without traditional visits to providers and expanded accessibility to care in remote areas. One of the most documented uses of telepresence is in mental health. Patients receive prevention, treatment, and reduced stigma associated with office visits using this technology (Newman, 2017).

Patient-centric devices that are wearable have continuously entered the market. Patients are able to transmit cardiac, weight, pulse, and oxygen level information without visiting a provider's office. Future advancements will offer opportunities where biochips will aid in the treatment and management of chronic disorders such as diabetes, cardiac disease, and dosing requirements required from many chronic conditions (Shah, 2015).

Traditional software of the past decade is incapable of providing seamless data to consumers and providers. Cloud-based technologies offer new advances for rapid capture and transmission of electronic medical records (Shah, 2015). This advancement does however raise red flags related to patient privacy and data security. Healthcare organizations are therefore confronted with the question, "is the data value greater than financial gains"? (Newman, 2017). The answer remains a significant challenge nationally and globally in healthcare organizations and information technology circles.

Maximizing technology and use of data management systems during the past decade has offered multiple opportunities in healthcare. The value of big and small data remains a valuable source of information when analyzed and integrated into strategic and financial planning. Big data that are generated from multiple sources offer a snapshot of what is occurring without answering why. The data are used to describe, interpret, and predict (Henley, 2014). Small data on the other hand provides material to answer a specific question or address a problem. Small data can support big data by generating new knowledge and has potential for change in care, operational efficiency, and satisfaction (McCartney, 2015). Future healthcare demands will require shifts from big and small data to meaningful specialty-specific analytics. The prominence of specialty-specific analytics will intensify as healthcare organizations access, share, and analyze evidence that will include population health management and efficient treatment pathways (Das, 2018).

These are only a few of the many advances in the past decade that will benefit the healthcare industry. Future developments remain promising and offer opportunities for entrepreneurs to capture segments of healthcare technology markets.

MEETING HEALTHCARE POLICY, REGULATIONS, AND CONSUMER DEMANDS

Meeting policy, regulations, and consumer demands require continuous actions by any healthcare organization due to the volumes of data generated daily. The best-case scenario of how data influences each of these demands is characteristic of the activities related to each demand.

Policy in healthcare establishes a general plan of action to guide desired outcomes and make decisions. For example, policies guide how data are collected, analyzed, and used to improve healthcare quality, safety, and efficiency. Policy changes occur often due to provisions within healthcare reforms, federal and state requirements, the Centers of Medicare and Medicaid provisions, the Joint Commission Standards, and other accrediting requirements. Therefore, communication of health policies to employees and use of technologies that regularly update them based on evidence are foundational to success, consistent practice, and avoidance of deficiencies and penalties (Leahy, 2019).

The exponential number of federal regulations that affect the healthcare industry requires significant resources in order to meet the demands. According to the American Hospital Association (AHA) (2017), there are 629 regulatory requirements mandated by four agencies that promulgate the requirements. The agencies include the Centers for Medicare and Medicaid, the Office of Civil Rights, the Office of Inspector General, and the Office of the National Coordinator for Health Information Technology. While regulatory frameworks are necessary for ensuring basic standards compliance, it is estimated that $39 billion per year is dedicated to comply with the administrative aspects of compliance. While the requirements are steeped in a foundation aimed at ensuring patients receive quality and safe care, the results evidence less time spent in patient care and spiraling healthcare costs (AHA, 2017; Singh, 2018).

How the healthcare industry continues to respond to the regulatory challenges is unclear. However, there is current evidence that the challenges have resulted in fines for data breaches, increased information technology infrastructure costs, lowering of reimbursements, and fraudulent claims to identify a few (Singh, 2018). One thing remains constant, regulatory demands will continue. Capturing meaningful data and thorough analysis remains a key ingredient for the vitality of healthcare organizations and dealing with human lives.

Healthcare organizations depend on patients in order to generate revenues. Understanding patient needs and demands is requisite to remain competitive and maintain loyalty. Using data from a variety of sources such as satisfaction scores, type and frequency of services used, and health data create a data-centric culture where patient-centrality becomes central to strategic decisions and actions (Betts & Korenda, 2018). More patients are reviewing quality ratings and prices when making decisions regarding care and providers. Engaging patients to become active consumers of health and well-being can result in improved outcomes, improve the patient experience, lower healthcare costs, and ultimately meet patient demands.

SUMMARY

- The healthcare industry is constantly changing based on internal and external influences. Change will be driven by data connectivity and consumer engagement.
- Healthcare is experiencing an information revolution similar to the industrial revolution.

- Data and platforms, digital therapeutics, health reform, consumer-centric products, care communities, and a shift from health and wellness are influencing the healthcare industry.
- Healthcare organizations must use meaningful evidence-based data to achieve, quality, safety, and sustainable outcomes.
- Interprofessional practice teams use evidence-based data to improve results, satisfy patient demands, and create data rich infrastructures.
- Comprehensive strategy and new business models are requisite in order to develop a culture of health, reduce disparities, and improve health.
- Data and data platforms generate decision-making insights fundamental to improving technology.
- Digital therapeutics delivery evidence-based interventions necessary to prevent and manage physical, mental, and behavioral conditions.
- Healthcare reform remains an ongoing agenda item in order to meet the challenges demands confronting healthcare.
- Consumer engagement is driving digital product introduction that are unique to one's behavior, lifestyle, genetics, and the environment.
- Data coupled with health coaching create pathways for optimal health.
- Technology has shifted from power to value that generates new efficiencies and value in healthcare.
- Cloud-based technologies offer rapid advances to capture and transmit electronic medical records.
- Big data offers a snapshot of what is occurring without answering why; whereas, small data provides information to answer a specific question or address a problem.
- Health policy establishes a plan of action to guide desired outcomes and make decisions.
- Federal regulations are affecting the healthcare industry by requiring significant resources for compliance.
- Meeting consumer and patient demands will continue to be an essential activity for the ongoing development of technology and survival of a healthcare organization.

REFLECTION QUESTIONS

1. Select an internal influence affecting healthcare delivery in an organization. What data should be collected to assist in managing the identified influence in order to achieve quality, safety, and sustainable outcomes?
2. Access a business model to use when introducing a new digital product in a healthcare organization. What steps will you take to introduce the product based on the business model selected?
3. Why is it essential to identify and synthesize data before introducing a new idea or product in healthcare?

4. Review the list of federal regulations required for compliance by health-care organizations. Which of the regulations do you recommend for elimination and why?

REFERENCES

Adams, A., Shankar, M., & Tecco, H. (2016). *50 things we now know about digital health consumers: 2016 digital health consumer adoption survey results.* https://rockhealth.com/reports/digital-health-consumer-adoption-2016

Alder, N. E., Cutler, D. M., Fielding, J. E., Galea, S., Glymour, M. M., Koh, H. K., & Satcher, D. (2016). *Addressing social determinants of health and health disparities: A vital direction for health and health care.* National Academy of Medicine. Discussion Paper.

American Hospital Association. (2017). *Regulatory overload report. Assessing the regulatory burden on health systems, hospitals, and post-acute care providers.* https://www.aha.org/guidesreports/2017-11-03-regulatory-overload-report

Babalola, O. (2017). Consumers and their demand for healthcare. *Journal of Health & Medical Economics, 3*(1), 6.

Betts, D., & Korenda, L. (2018). *Inside the patient journey: Three key touch points for consumer engagement strategies. Findings from the Deloitte 2018 health care consumer survey.* https://www2.deloitte.com/us/en/insights/industry/health-care/patient-engagement-health-care-consumer-survey.html

Centers for Medicare and Medicaid Services. (2011a). *CMS issues final rule for first year of hospital value-based purchasing program.* Fact sheets. https://www.cms.gov/Newsroom/MediaReleaseDatabase/Fact-sheets/2011-Fact-sheets-items/2011-04-29.html

Centers for Medicare and Medicaid Services. (2011b). Medicare program: Hospital inpatient value-based purchasing program. Final rule. *Federal Register, 76*(88), 26490–26547.

Comstock, J. (2018). *Digital Therapeutics Alliance releases definition, best practices for burgeoning space.* https://www.mobihealthnews.com/content/digital-therapeutics-alliance-releases-definition-best-practices-burgeoning-space

Das, R. (2018). Top 8 healthcare predictions for 2019. *Forbes.* https://www.forbes.com/sites/reenitadas/2018/11/13/top-8-healthcare-predictions-for-2019/#61e59bbf700e

DeloitteHealth. (2019). *The future of health. Looking ahead to 2040.* https://www2.deloitte.com/us/en/pages/life-sciences-and-health-care/articles/future-of-health.html

Digital Therapeutics Alliance. (2019). *What are digital therapeutics?* https://www.dtxalliance.org/dtx-solutions

Geibert, R. C. (2017). The information revolution: Using data and technology to support patient care. In S. Davidson, D. Weberg, T. Porter-O'Grady, & K. Malloch (Eds.), *Leadership for evidence-based innovation in nursing and health Professions* (pp. 241–262). Jones & Bartlett Learning.

Henley, S. J. (2014). Mother load and mining tools: Big data for science. *Nursing Research, 63*(3), 155. https://doi.org/10.1097/nnr.0000000000000041

Leahy, T. (2019). *The importance of healthcare policy and procedures.* https://www.policymedical.com/importance-healthcare-policy-and-procedures

Mann, D. (2019). *This is what being healthy will look and feel like in 2020.* The Healthy. https://www.thehealthy.com/habits/being-healthy-look-feel-like-2020/

McCartney, P. R. (2015). Big data science. *The American Journal of Maternal/Child Nursing, 40*(2), 130. https://doi.org/10.1097/nmc.0000000000000118

Mwachofi, A., & Al-Assaf, A. F. (2011). Health care market deviation from the ideal market. *Sultan Qaboos University Medical Journal, 11*(3): 328–337. https://www.ncbi.nlm.nih.gov/pmc/articles/PMC3210041/

National Academy of Medicine. (2019). *The future of nursing 2020-2030.* https://nam.edu/publications/the-future-of-nursing-2020-2030

Newman, D. (2017). Top five digital transformation trends in health care. *Forbes.* https://www.forbes.com/sites/danielnewman/2017/03/07/top-five-digital-transformation-trends-in-healthcare/#5bb8c6692561

Office of Legislative Council. (2010). *Patient protection and affordable care act (as amended through May 1, 2010, including patient protection and affordable care act health related portions of the health care and education reconciliation act of 2010).* U.S. Government Printing Office.

Rowe, J., Berkman, L., Fried, L., Fulmer, T., Jackson, J., Naylor, M., Novelli, W., Olshansky, J., & Stone, R. (2016). *Preparing for better health and health care for an aging population. Discussion paper, vital directions for health and health care series.* National Academy of Medicine.

Shah, M. (2015). 3 technology trends transforming health care. *Forbes.* https://www.forbes.com/sites/athenahealth/2015/04/13/3-technology-trends-transforming-health-care/#1caeb1441a5b

Singh, R. (2018). *Top ten regulatory challenges in the healthcare environment.* https://www.navexglobal.com/blog/article/top-10-regulatory-challenges-in-the-healthcare-environment/

Siwicki, B. (2019). *Here are 6 major issues facing healthcare in 2019, according to PwC.* https://www.healthcareitnews.com/news/here-are-6-major-issues-facing-healthcare-2019-according-pwc

Szlauderbach, D. (2020, June 24). *Continuing care retirement communities (CCRCs): An all-in-one senior living option.* A Place for Mom. http://www.aplaceformom.com/blog/continuing-care-retirement-communities/

Zweig, M., Tecco, H., Huang, M. (2018). *2018 midyear funding review: Digital health déjà vu in yet another recording breaking half.* Rock Health. https://rockhealth.com/reports/2018-midyear-funding-review-digital-health-deja-vu-in-yet-another-record-breaking-half/

CASE EXEMPLARS FOR APPLICATION

A Lean Lab

Alison M. Scarry

A change in the process to order lab tests led to a significant increase in duplicate orders at our 186-bed community hospital, prompting immediate action. The efforts to address duplicate orders reduced the duplications by 50% and represented a significant cost savings. The laboratory processes over 100,000 tests for 15,000 patients each month with daily volume reaching as high as 4,000 tests in inpatient, observation, surgical, and emergency settings. Given the size and volume of our lab service, it is not uncommon to have duplicate tests ordered as a subset of unnecessary lab tests (Salisbury et al., 2011) and overuse of diagnostic tests are in fact identified as medical errors (Levick et al., 2013).

Payment for lab services are most often bundled into the overall payment for a given inpatient, surgical encounter, emergency room visit, or observation stay. Additionally, our service is a stand-alone outpatient and central processing facility for physician office labs (POL's), which is mostly fee for service (FFS). This provides high-quality lab services and incredible economies of scale for our community. The balance of services means that overuse for inpatients, for example, consumes the capacity for providing outpatient FFS lab work.

Given "Duplicate Lab Orders" are defined as the same patient, test, and start date for nine of the most common labs, over four and a half years or 54 months between January 2012 and June 2016 charted in Figure 1.1 (Scarry et al., 2017), the following patterns emerged. The overall average rate of duplicate orders over the 54 months is 6.5%, indicated by the straight gray horizontal line in the middle of Figure 1.1. The duplicate rate was between 6.5% to 7.5% for 22 months (January 2012 to October 2013), then rose sharply in November 2013 for six months through April 2014, above 7.5% and more than one standard deviation from the mean indicated by the top horizontal dotted line. This was among 10 straight months above the mean rate of 6.5%, from November 2013 to August 2014 including two straight months (January and February 2014) more than 8.5% and two standard deviations above the mean indicated by the top horizontal line.

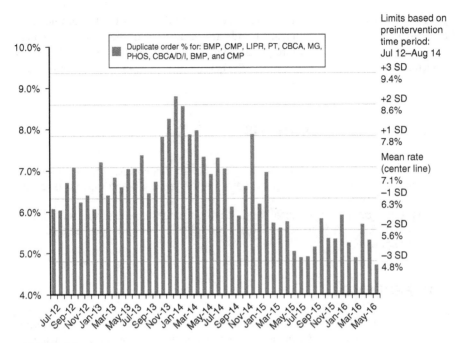

FIGURE 1.1 Duplicate lab orders: same patient and same test start date.

Source: Data from Scarry, A., Eamranond, P., Joshi, M., Haque, I., Geary, S., & Collins, B. (2017). A system-wide movement to improve patient care and reduce unnecessary laboratory testing. *Medical Lab Observer, Mar 21, 2017.*

All of these anomalies are beyond the signals of statistical significance and system change. In fact, the hospital had changed the lab ordering process in November 2013 moving from a laboratory information system (LIS) to a hospital information system (HIS). The LIS had clinical decision support (CDS) builtin that alerted providers of duplicate orders. Despite the possibly perceived nuisance of such alerts, the absence certainly presented in significant terms. During this time, over 500 complaints were made through the hospital incident reporting system about this patient safety issue mainly by phlebotomists worried they were being asked to needlessly draw blood from a patient. Instead, they questioned the order and escalated to lab managers who researched and likely cancelled the order, then made the formal complaint with details. That process was more time intensive and therefore more costly than performing the test but it was much better for the patient and drove systemic improvement.

In short time, a multidisciplinary team was formed between the laboratory utilization committee and medical administration. Within months, systemic, cultural, and significant results were achieved (Scarry et al., 2017). By September 2014 the duplicate order rate was below the mean rate 6.5% for the first time in a year and a half. For the last 16 months in Figure 1.1 (March 2015 to June 2016) the duplicate percent has been below the mean rate. Including four consecutive months below 5.5%

or one standard deviation (June-September 2015) indicated by the bottom horizontal dotted line. Both are significant trends and indication of major system change. Duplicate results are now a more predictable 4% to 5% versus 6.5% to 9.5% and we continue to improve and model these efforts for MRI, CT scans, and other ancillary services.

REFLECTION QUESTIONS

1. Examine the care you deliver for gaps or redundancies. What steps could you take to ensure the gaps in care were filled or to eliminate the redundant practice?
2. As you consider the data required to address the issues identified in number 1, what first step could you take to bring awareness to your colleagues?

REFERENCES

Levick, D. L., Stern G., Meyerhoefer, C. D., Levick, A., & Pucklavage, D. (2013). Reducing unnecessary testing a CPOE system through implementation of a targeted CDS intervention. *BMC Medical Informatics and Decision Making, 13*, 43.

Salisbury, A. C., Reid, K. J., Alexander, K. P., Masoudi, F. A., Lai, S. M., Chan, P. S., Bach, R. G., Wang, T. Y., Spertus, J. A., & Kosiborod, M. (2011). Diagnostic blood loss from phlebotomy and hospital-acquired anemia during acute myocardial infarction. *Archives of Internal Medicine, 171*(18), 1646–1653.

Scarry, A., Eamranond, P., Joshi, M., Haque, I., Geary, S., Collins, B. (2017). A system-wide movement to improve patient care and reduce unnecessary laboratory testing. *Medical Lab Observer, Mar 21, 2017.* https://www.mlo-online.com/information-technology/lis/article/13009046/a-systemwide-movement-to-improve-patient-care-and-reduce-unnecessary-laboratory-testing.

Higher Education Outcomes

Heather R. Hall

The well-documented need for faculty and administration to collaborate requires processes to collect, analyze and use data to inform programs, curriculum development, and evaluation (Kezar et al., 2007). The need for increased clinical placement settings, faculty, student enrollment and outcomes presents increased challenges for nursing programs. These challenges provide the need for additional administrative requirements and faculty collaborations to ensure successful higher education outcomes.

A committee of graduate track coordinators and administrators of a nursing program was appointed to review the competencies for specialty tracks, clinical placement processes, policies and procedures. The committee continuously used data to enhance the student documentation used for clinical placement. These processes included management of clinical affiliations, documentation requirements, clinical paperwork, faculty certifications, and licensure to ensure completion of program learning outcomes. The administrators serving on the committee reviewed the policies and procedures recommended by the committee and made sure the appropriate committees within the college were included in the discussion and implementation. The faculty and administrators collaborated to ensure compliance with updated specialty competencies, criteria for nurse practitioner programs, and standards for accreditation for Master of Science in Nursing, Doctor of Nursing Practice and Post-Graduate APRN Certificate programs (Commission on Collegiate Nursing Education Accreditation, 2020; The National Organization of Nurse Practitioner Faculties, 2020).

The implementation of the committee's recommended changes improved the specialty track curricula, clinical placement processes, and student outcomes. In addition, positive feedback has been received from students, faculty, and administrators. The committee meets on a regular basis to discuss current challenges that may be improved by processes developed and recommended by the committee. The curriculum and operations within the graduate specialty tracks and clinical placement processes are more efficient. Student satisfaction has increased upon graduation from all programs. The faculty and administrators have identified the committee outcomes as successful and has led to greater efficiency in the use of data and resources.

REFERENCES

Commission on Collegiate Nursing Education Accreditation. (2020). *Standards, procedures and guidelines.* https://www.aacnnursing.org/CCNE-Accreditation/Accreditation-Resources/Standards-Procedures-Guidelines

Kezar, A., Lester, J., Carducci, R., Gallant, T. B., & McGavin, M. C. (2007). Where are the faculty leaders? *Liberal Education, 93*(4), 14–21.

The National Organization of Nurse Practitioner Faculties. (2020). *Criteria for evaluation of NP programs.* https://www.nonpf.org/page/15

Imperatives for Quality, Safety, and Value-Based Outcomes in a Data-Driven Healthcare Environment

Patricia L. Thomas and Brian Collins

OBJECTIVES

1. Describe regulatory, payer, and accreditation pressures that influence healthcare delivery.
2. Examine the history of healthcare payment systems in the United States.
3. Define value-based outcomes in the U.S. delivery system.
4. Highlight leadership skills necessary for quality, safety, and fiscally responsible care.

CORE COMPETENCIES

- Understanding of healthcare delivery
- Appreciation for the influence of healthcare regulation and policy on care delivery
- Differentiating between episodic- and population-focused payment systems
- Leaders using a systems thinking lens to guide strategic initiatives and decision-making

INTRODUCTION

In the last decade, significant time, attention, and resources have been allocated to quality, safety, and clinical and financial outcomes. Influenced by the Institute of Medicine's (IOM) landmark reports, *To Err is Human: Building a Safer Health System* (1999) and *Crossing the Quality Chasm: A New Health System for the 21st Century* (2001), principles of quality improvement, safety, evidence-based practices, and outcomes have become a primary focal point for providers and organizations. These seminal publications provided a disciplined and systematic review of the U.S. health system. The publications underscored that while elements of the U.S. delivery system were envied across the globe, there were significant concerns about quality, safety, and cost. They provided a professional and ethical mandate for critical examination of often unspoken and less than desirable outcomes to catalyze purposeful and needed improvement. Embedded in the publications was an acknowledgement that gaps and deficits of the current system could be addressed by a series of systematic, deliberate, and disciplined improvement processes, innovation, and measurement of clinical interventions and outcomes.

Recognizing the cost of care in the United States was not sustainable, emphasis was placed on reimbursement structures and costs of care, access, and the translation and replicability of preeminent practices through innovative care redesign (IOM, 2001). As a result, consistent, sustainable, and favorable clinical and financial outcomes were possible. The call for profound care redesign, improvement in outcomes, and long-term sustainability of healthcare were established as guideposts. The six aims for patient safety (safe, patient-centered, timely, efficient, effective, and equitable care) were coupled with principles for rules for redesign. Regulatory agencies and accrediting bodies followed with an increased focus on leadership, measurement, and self-assessment demonstrating deliberate and disciplined improvement (IOM, 2001; Joint Commission, 2019; Moran et al., 2016; NCQA, 2019).

In the early 1990s, many payors had initiated cost control models and attempted to shift the paradigm from treatment of disease to promoting wellness. Despite these efforts, the expected cost reductions were not actualized (Langabeer, 2018; Lighter, 2011; NCQA, 2019). Whereas healthcare services had historically been linked to community service or a care-driven enterprise, the financial viability of many hospitals was in question. The description of health services was viewed as two poles; one with quality care at any cost and the other as care at low cost. A visual depiction of this would be a pendulum swung between extremes. Rather than a wildly swinging pendulum, today this might be visualized as a metronome finding balance and rhythm with equal attention to quality and costs paced to accommodate different situations.

Over time, advances in technology, electronic health records, wearable devices, data science, and consumerism have further defined and refined the health delivery system. Building on the foundation established in Chapter 1, this chapter focuses on how regulation, accreditation, and consumerism have influenced care delivery initiatives and shaped the requisite leadership capabilities to forge a strategic path forward.

ACCREDITATION, REGULATION, AND PAYOR INFLUENCES

While accreditation and regulation are often spoken of in a single sentence, they are distinct entities that warrant definition and discussion. Simply stated, regulation is mandatory and accreditation is voluntary (Dunham-Taylor, 2015; Johnson & Sollecito, 2020; Landry & Erwin, 2019). Both offer direction to the work of healthcare but the differences are important particularly in the realm of patient safety, care redesign, and practice change. Within the context of reimbursement and payor defined requirements, the expectation is full compliance with regulatory statutes and explicitly stated expectations in accreditation standards.

Accreditation is voluntary and as such, typically denotes meeting or exceeding defined standards. Accreditation typically includes self-assessment and peer review related to predetermined standards that evidence high quality care. Continuous improvement and organizational learning are common foundations (Accreditation Commission for Health Care [ACHC], 2019; Joint Commission, 2019). Examples of accrediting bodies include the Joint Commission (TJC), the National Committee for Quality Assurance (NCQA), the American Medical Accreditation Program, the Accreditation Commission for Health Care (ACHC), Utilization Review Accreditation Commission (URAC), and the Accreditation Association for Ambulatory Healthcare (AAAHC). Each of these accrediting bodies has unique missions, activities, board composition and history. While they differ in accreditation processes and practice settings, what they hold in common are specified standards that must be demonstrated in processes and outcomess for specific programs (AAAHC, 2020; Ambulatory Health Care [AHC], 2020; Joint Commission, 2019; NCQA, 2019; URAC, 2020). It is important to consider that limitations in the accreditation process have been identified. Analysis of accredited versus nonaccredited health systems demonstrates inconsistent findings related to quality outcomes and implies the cost of accreditation may not be justified (Lam et al., 2018; Mumford et al., 2013).

Regulation

Regulation, as a process, defines what is expected and required through parameters and minimum obligations. In the United States, there is no single regulatory authority. This is a unique attribute compared to countries with single-payor national healthcare. Agencies create regulations (also known as "rules") under the authority of Congress to assist the government to carry out public policy (Dunham-Taylor, 2015; Department of Health and Human Services [HHS], 2019a). Regulatory stipulations provide protection to the public by ensuring care processes meet clinical, quality, and safety standards derived from evidence-based practices that demonstrate positive care outcomes.

The Department of Health and Human Services, Centers for Disease Control and Prevention, Centers for Medicare and Medicaid Services, the Food and Drug Administration, and National Institutes of Health provide national direction and frameworks for regulation. Generally speaking, the Department of Health and

Human Services (HHS) is the national entity that administers and oversees regulations in the United States and is responsible for protecting all Americans in the provision of essential human services (HHS, 2019b). Table 2.1 lists the major HHS divisions and responsibilities.

Each of the HHS entities generates and relies on data, big data, and complex analysis of data in healthcare service delivery that cross professional disciplines, service delivery settings, and extends beyond traditional health service entities. Research, quality improvement, program evaluation, and rigorous analysis of complex data are inherent to the decision-making for health systems, payors, regulators, and providers.

The scope of work for HHS is broad; however, the five focal areas to improve health and well-being for Americans have been defined. The priorities include: 1) bringing an end to the opioid crisis of addiction and overdose; 2) improving availability and affordability of health insurance; 3) lowering prescription drug costs for

TABLE 2.1 Department of Health and Human Services Divisions and Responsibilities

HHS DIVISION	RESPONSIBILITIES
Centers for Medicare and Medicaid Services (CMS)	• Oversight and related quality assurance activities for the federal health insurance for the elderly and disabled in conjunction with state services, the Children's Health Insurance Program (CHIP), the Health Insurance Portability and Accountability Act, and key portions of the 2015 Medicare Access and CHIP Reauthorization Act (MACRA) law. • CMS also has financial, quality, safety, regulatory, and programmatic elements that impact and influence care for consumers of all ages and across care settings, is responsible for the Health Insurance Marketplace and is the payor and reimbursement arm for seniors enrolled in the Medicare program and provides support to states in Medicaid. • www.cms.gov
Agency for Healthcare Research and Quality (AHRQ)	• Create evidence for care quality and safety by offering guidance for accessible, equitable, and affordable care. • Partners with member organizations within and outside the HHS to make evidence understandable and usable. • In addition to clinical guidelines and best practices for quality care, AHRQ has recently proposed strategic initiatives aligned with value-based care and the use of data and analytics that informs clinicians and policy makers through integrated data analytics and information platforms to provide a 360° view of the health care system (AHRQ, n.d. a; AHRQ Office & Programs, n.d. b; AHRQ Views, 2019). • www.ahrq.gov/ • www.ahrq.gov/cpi/index.html

(continued)

TABLE 2.1 Department of Health and Human Services Divisions and Responsibilities (continued)

HHS DIVISION	RESPONSIBILITIES
Centers for Disease Control and Prevention (CDC)	• Part of the Public Health Service, the CDC is responsible for the protection of the public by providing direction and leadership in the control and prevention of disease and responding to public health emergencies. • While considered to be a national organization, the CDC has international influence and engages globally to stop health threats oversees before they spread to the United States. • Currently, global programs address more than 400 diseases and health threats through programs run by the CDC partnering with foreign governments and ministries of health, the World Health Organization, academic institutions, foundations, faith-based organizations, and businesses and private organizations. • In addition to clinicians across many disciplines, the CDC works closely with experts in epidemiology, surveillance, informatics, and laboratory systems (CDC, 2019a). • Recent examples of CDC influence include HIV prevention and treatment, the spread of tuberculosis, malaria, and food, water, and sanitation efforts. • www.cdc.gov
Office of Inspector General (OIG) Within HHS	• Investigates complaints or allegations of fraud and abuse in Medicare, Medicaid, and health and human service programs. • Responsible for investigating wrongdoing or misconduct aimed to combat fraud, waste, and abuse. Part of this responsibility includes also includes improving efficiency. • The OIG oversees the Centers for Disease Control and Prevention, National Institutes of Health, and the Food and Drug Administration (OIG, n.d., 2019). • oig.hhs.gov • oig.hhs.gov/about-oig/about-us/index.asp
Food and Drug Administration (FDA)	• Responsible for ensuring food is safe, pure, and wholesome; human and animal drugs, biological products, and medical devices are safe and effective; and electronic products that emit radiation are safe. • Also supervises the safety of tobacco products, dietary supplements, prescriptions, over-the-counter medications, vaccines, biopharmaceuticals, blood transfusions, and veterinary products, food, and feed. • As part of the Public Health Service Act, they regulate lasers, cellular phones, and condoms. • In support of quality and safety, the FDA issues recalls, alerts, and market withdrawals (FDA, n.d., 2019). • www.fda.gov • www.fda.gov/about-fda/what-we-do

(continued)

TABLE 2.1 Department of Health and Human Services Divisions and Responsibilities (continued)	
HHS DIVISION	**RESPONSIBILITIES**
Health Resources and Services Administration (HRSA)	• Part of the Public Health Service, HRSA is the federal agency responsible for improving care to people who are geographically isolated, or economically or medically vulnerable through 90 programs and 3,000 grantees. • Four overarching goals guide their work: 1. to improve access to quality health services; 2. foster a healthcare workforce able to address current and emerging needs; 3. to achieve health equity and enhance population health; 4. optimize HRSA operations and strengthen program management (HRSA, 2019). • HRSAs mission is to improve health outcomes and address health disparities through access to quality services and a skilled workforce. • HRSA supports the training of health professionals and the distribution of providers to areas where they are most needed to improve healthcare delivery (HRSA, n.d., 2019). • www.hrsa.gov • www.hrsa.gov/about/index.html
Indian Health Service (IHS)	• Part of the Public Health Service, IHS provides American Indians and Alaska Natives with comprehensive health services by developing and managing programs to meet their health needs. • Committed to improving the physical, mental, social, and spiritual health of American Indians and Alaska Natives through strong partnerships and culturally responsive practices in communities and healthcare systems. • Grew out of government-to-government relationships between the federal government and Indian tribes in 1787 that includes treaties, laws, Supreme Court decisions, and Executive Orders. • Provides care in 36 states to 2.2 million of the 3.7 million American Indian and Alaskan Natives in 573 recognized tribes. • In 2017 there were 26 hospitals, 59 health centers, and 32 health stations. There are 12 regional offices that oversee the clinical operations for individual facilities that encompass inpatient, outpatient, primary care, pharmacy, dental, behavioral health, physical rehabilitation, and optometry services. • www.ihs.gov/ • www.ihs.gov/aboutihs/ • www.ihs.gov/newsroom/factsheets/

(continued)

TABLE 2.1 Department of Health and Human Services Divisions and Responsibilities (continued)	
HHS DIVISION	**RESPONSIBILITIES**
National Institutes of Health (NIH)	• Part of the Public Health Service • Their mission is to conduct research for the acquisition of new knowledge to present, detect, diagnose, and treat disease and disability. • The Office of the Director (OD) is responsible for setting NIH policy and coordinating and managing the 27 NIH Institutes that transverse clinical, disciplinary, and lifespan foci. • Supports biomedical and behavioral research in the United States and abroad. • Trains researchers and promotes the collection and sharing of medical knowledge (NIH, n.d. a, n.d. b). • www.nih.gov • www.nih.gov/about-nih/what-we-do

Administration for Children & Families (ACF)	• Promotes the economic and social well-being of families, children, individuals, and communities through education and support programs in partnership with states, tribes, and community organizations (Administration for Children & Families [ACF], n.d. a).
	• Goals of ACF are to:
	  1. mpower individuals and families toward economic independence and productivity;
	  2. encourage healthy communities that will have a positive impact on the development and quality of life of children;
	  3. create partnerships with service providers, states, localities and tribal communities to identify and implement solutions that transcend traditional program boundaries;
	  4. improve access to services, and
	  5. address the needs of vulnerable populations including people with developmental disabilities, refugees, and migrants (ACF, n.d. b).
	• www.acf.hhs.gov
	• www.acf.hhs.gov/about/what-we-do

HHS, Department of Health and Human Services.

all Americans without discouraging innovation; 4) transforming the health system to pay for value; and 5) continuing efforts directed at data security and integrity. Noteworthy about these priorities given the regulatory role of HHS are attention to both care quality and cost (HHS, n.d. c). Each of these priorities spans multiple disciplines and municipalities that bring attention to entities within governmental or regulatory agencies and the public-private sector. In each priority, disciplined and systematic measurement, standardization of metrics and definitions, new partnerships, and innovation are aimed toward. Table 2.2 summarizes the HHS priorities and the value-based care strategies and initiatives to accomplish this work.

In each of the priorities established by HHS the use of data, analytics, and data mining capabilities are foundational to success. For example, the FDA has been granted the authority to launch data analytic capabilities using large-scale data warehouses to evaluate social and clinical trends contributing to the opioid crisis. Using machine learning algorithms and predictive analytics, it is hoped that trends will be identified so points of vulnerability can be remedied through policy and regulatory changes (Barlas, 2017; Gottlieb, 2017; Kent, 2019). Initiatives like prescription data monitoring programs (PDMPs) in state Medicaid programs have leveraged big

TABLE 2.2 Department of Health and Human Services Priorities and Strategies

HHS PRIORITY	STRATEGIES TO ACCOMPLISH
End opioid crisis of addition and overdose	• Five-Point Strategy to reduce opioid misuse, prevalence, and deaths across all disciplines. 1. Strengthen data collection and reporting 2. Increase access to overdose reversing drugs 3. Improve pain management approaches 4. Improve access to addiction prevention and treatment 5. Increase research focus on pain management and opioid use disorders (HHS, n.d. c; Johnson et al., 2018) • The FDA was given the authority to limit access to certain drugs associated with illicit use and use big data to help combat opioid use and misuse. • Thirteen states and the District of Columbia were awarded funds to improve data collection and analysis, develop strategies in prescribing opioids, and to develop prevention programs under the CDCs Data-driven Prevention Initiative (DDPI) (CDC, 2017, 2018). • www.hhs.gov/about/leadership/secretary/priorities/index.html#opioids
Improve availability and affordability of health insurance	• Continue support of the Affordable Care Act of 2010 to ensure access, lower costs, and quality outcomes • The goal is for all Americans to have access to personalized healthcare that meets their individual needs and fits their budget • Establish coordination across HHS departments focused on the cost and availability of insurance • www.hhs.gov/about/leadership/secretary/priorities/index.html#health-insurance-reform

(continued)

TABLE 2.2 Department of Health and Human Services
Priorities and Strategies (continued)

HHS PRIORITY	STRATEGIES TO ACCOMPLISH
Lower prescription drug costs for all Americans without discouraging innovation	Continuous efforts to identify generic alternatives to prescribed medications and cost savings programs • May 2018 the comprehensive American Patients First blueprint, a comprehensive plan to bring down prescription drug prices and out-of-pocket costs was released. • The four challenges in the U.S. drug market are identified as: 1. High list price for drugs 2. Seniors and government programs overpaying for drugs due to a lack of negotiation tools 3. High and rising out-of-pocket costs for consumers 4. Foreign governments free-riding off American investment in innovation • The four key Blueprint strategies for reform are: 1. Improved competition 2. Better negotiation 3. Incentives for lower list prices 4. Power out-of-pocket costs • www.hhs.gov/sites/default/files/AmericanPatientsFirst.pdf • www.hhs.gov/about/leadership/secretary/priorities/drug-prices/index.html
Transform the health system to pay for value	Acknowledgement that lower cost, higher quality, and sustainability are essential to care delivery and data is a cornerstone • Adopt that the definition of value will be health outcomes that matter to patients per healthcare dollar spent being delivered through a treatment plan that is tailored to patient preferences (Keswani et al., 2016). • Three cross-cutting platforms regardless of how care is financed have been identified by the HHS Secretary: 1. Reforming how care is financed 2. Deriving better value from care 3. Improving health in specific impactable areas • www.hhs.gov/about/leadership/secretary/index.html • www.hhs.gov/about/leadership/secretary/speeches/2019-speeches/remarks-at-the-2019-learning-and-action-network-summit.html • www.hhs.gov/about/leadership/secretary/priorities/value-based-healthcare/index.html

(continued)

TABLE 2.2 Department of Health and Human Services Priorities and Strategies (continued)

HHS PRIORITY	STRATEGIES TO ACCOMPLISH
Data security, integrity, and privacy	• Introduce national legislation programs, incentives, and initiatives to support standardization of data, data definitions, interoperability, and reporting. • Continue to support the Health Insurance Portability and Accountability Act of 1996 and modifications to ensure health plans, clearinghouses, researchers, and providers obtain authorization for the use of patient data before sharing protected data. • Ensure that EHR data has interoperability across practice settings for data exchange. • Support MU to expand HIT standardization with financial incentives as part of the Merit-based Incentive Payment program to advance care information performance. • www.healthit.gov/topic/about-onc/health-it-strategic-planning

EHR, Electronic Health Record; FDA, Food and Drug Administration; HHS, Department of Health and Human Services; HIT, Health Information Technology; MU, meaningful use.

data to identify prescribing patterns and "doctor shopping" to curtail the number of providers visited by patients identified with opioid abuse. In addition to training employees on the use of PDMP and the available real-time reports, PMPDs have been incorporated into electronic health records and made available on mobile devices to encourage use (Barlas, 2017; Gottlieb, 2017; Johnson et al., 2018).

Shifting from a disease-focused volume-dependent system to a health- and value-focused system is complex. In recent years, CMS has initiated several proactive initiatives dependent on strategies to remove obstacles frequently identified as limiting factors in value-based care. These include deliberate consensus-building strategies to establish measures and outcomes that matter to patients, increasing transparency around clinical and financial outcomes, and addressing care coordination across settings and providers to decrease fragmentation (Keswani et al., 2016). Bundled payment for care improvement (BPCI), reimbursement for documentation of advanced directives and end-of-life wishes, and websites to compare cost and quality outcomes in hospitals, skilled nursing facilities, and home care agencies to name a few initiatives (Centers for Medicare and Medicaid Services [CMS], n.d.; Knickman & Elbel, 2019). While there have been unintended consequences and mixed reviews related to these initiatives, they signal change aimed to bring lower costs, greater transparency, and awareness to the public.

Data security, integrity, and safety will continue to be a national focal point that requires policies, procedures, physical safeguards, and technical intervention at the individual, organizational, and governmental levels (Davis, 2020; Office for Civil Rights, 2020). The HHS's authority from the Recovery and Reinvestment Act to improve healthcare quality, safety, and efficacy through health data is actualized when data is leveraged to its full potential. New ways of interacting with patients through kiosks, mobile devices and applications, and patient portals necessitates new approaches to data warehousing and brings unique challenges to any health system accustomed to managing and controlling data security. These distinct opportunities also raise new challenges in security that have not been faced before. Finally, improvements in the flow and exchange of electronic health data will be essential and significant resources will need to be mobilized around standardization and end-user access to fulfill the anticipated potential in support of patients, providers, payors, and policy makers (Davis, 2020).

TRAJECTORY OF HEALTHCARE PAYMENT SYSTEMS IN THE UNITED STATES

One consistent message about healthcare delivery in the United States is that the current delivery system and costs are unsustainable. While we hear about this regularly in the press and in our organizations, this concern has been with us for several decades and different approaches to address it have come in the form of regulatory changes, financial incentives, and disruptive innovations (Dunham-Taylor & Pinczuk, 2015; Elbel, 2019; Knickman & Elbel, 2019; Leger & Dunham-Taylor, 2018).

One of the most notable changes came with the implementation of Diagnostic Related Groups (DRGs) and the paradigm shift that resulted when DRGs were tied to reimbursement. In years before DRGs, organizations and providers were paid retrospectively using fee for service and line item billing. In this scenario, volume generated revenue and reimbursement and more services or interventions brought greater reimbursement (Dunham-Taylor, 2015).

With the implementation of DRGs, prospective assignment of reimbursement ensued based on a classification system that grouped similar use of resources for diagnoses or procedures into an assigned DRG. Hospitals would be reimbursed prospectively based on a classification system that considered the resources typically used for a given diagnosis or service. For the first time, organizations were rewarded for efficiency and quality but felt the loss financially if they were unable to provide the care using similar resources to those expected by the DRG. For the first time, healthcare delivery was viewed as a product industry rather than a community service and costs and quality of care delivery became part of the vernacular. Volume could offset some of the financial pressure but if the processes within the organization were ineffective, redundant, or had processes and care delivery systems laden with gaps, volume alone would not be enough to offset the costs (Dunham-Taylor & Pinczuk, 2015; Kimberly et al., 2008; Mayes, 2007).

DRGs were the first large-scale regulatory reimbursement initiative that forever changed how providers and organizations viewed care delivery. Initially implemented with state and private payors, when adopted by CMS for Medicare and Medicaid service reimbursement, there was no turning back to retrospective reimbursement. DRGs also brought to the forefront an awareness of efficiency and effectiveness, the need to measure and monitor cost and quality, and the interdependence of providers, team members, and organizations in systems of care. With the implementation of prospective payment, the foundation was laid for future cost reduction initiatives like the CMS Bundled Payment approach to address rising costs walking a parallel path with quality improvement strategies for greater efficiency and performance sustainability (Knickman, 2019; Radley & Marchica, 2019).

As health delivery systems made adjustments to how care was delivered and engaged in quality and process improvements, other financial incentives were introduced through health policy and regulatory activities. Providers and organizations were incentivized through payments or penalties to implement change based on the adoption of electronic health records, readmission rates, hospital-acquired infections, and fulfillment of best-practice guidelines (Dunham-Taylor, 2015; Radley & Marchica, 2019). Significant national efforts have been undertaken to promote technology and standardized reporting but there is still significant work to be done.

Defining value, measuring it, and linking payment to value-based delivery has gained acceptance yet the definitions for value and value-based care are not agreed upon (Radley & Marchica, 2019; Tsevat & Moriates, 2018). A widely cited definition of value offered by Porter (2010) is health outcomes achieved per dollar spent (Porter, 2010; Tsevat & Moriates, 2018). A key challenge in value-based care is the ability to measure patient-centered outcomes and the lack of consistency in definitions. (Radley & Marchica, 2019). Failures and gaps in care delivery and care coordination in a highly complex system compounds this issue. Value-based payment models like the CMS bundled payments for care improvement (BPCI) initiative enabled providers to voluntarily enter payment arrangements that had both financial and performance accountability but the results have been inconsistent.

In 2016, CMS released the final rule for Quality Payment Program under the Medicare Access and CHIP Reauthorization Act (MACRA). This program offers new payment options from one of two tracks; the Merit-based Incentive Payment System (MIPS) for providers participating in traditional Medicare Part B or the Advanced Alternative Payment Model (APMs) for those in value-based models (CMS, 2019; Radley & Marchica, 2019). MIPS participants earn payment adjustments based on quality of care, cost of care, clinical practice improvements, ad advancing care information extending work from meaningful use. Those participating in APMs can earn a 5% lump sum incentive for use of certified electronic health record technology and quality measures similar to MIPs with providers having more financial risk (CMS, 2019; Radley & Marchica, 2019).

As individuals grapple with challenges related to access to care, costs, and variation in clinical care outcomes, population health has become a popular framework to guide care delivery redesign. The CDC defines population health as an interdisciplinary customizable approach that links practice and policy together. It uses nontraditional partnerships in different sectors of a community like community and public health, industry, academe, healthcare systems, and governmental agencies to address the gaps and barriers in the current system (CDC, n.d.) The goal of population health is "the systematic and transparent delivery of services to improve the health status of a given population at a prospective price, ultimately delivering better outcomes at lower cost" (Becker's Hospital Review, 2015, para 1). An emphasis is placed on wellness and health promotion rather than high cost interventions. If healthcare is needed, getting patients to the right care at the right setting is part of the goal of population health which is expected to reduce costs and severity of disease because the system of care delivery puts patient centered considerations and access in the forefront (CDC, 2019b). Inherent in a population health focus is awareness that new infrastructures will be required, reimbursement strategies will need revision, and a culture change will need to take place that puts an emphasis on health and wellness care rather than sick care.

As population health is implemented, the social determinants of health and their influence on health outcomes become more obvious. Social determinants are defined as the conditions and places people live, work, learn, and play. As such, they represent the complex interrelated social structures and economic systems that shape these conditions. Discrimination, income, education level, marital status, the physical environment including transportation, buildings, place of residence, crowding, and availability of health services become important variables for consideration related to health outcomes. The lack of opportunity and resources to protect, improve, or maintain health are tied directly to these social determinants of health and collectively generate health inequities (CDC, 2010; World Health Organization [WHO], 2020).

Whether redesigning existing health delivery systems or redesigning care with a population health lens, the ability to access data, analyze it, and attribute outcomes or costs to services undergirds success. While significant attention in terms of regulation and financial incentives have been directed to health systems as they are known today with related data infrastructure, data exchange, and interoperability, the same cannot be said for the social and economic systems that shape social determinants of health.

DATA, MEASUREMENT, AND MONITORING IMPLICATIONS

The intertwined relationship between cost, quality, and policy have been highlighted but the foundation to any discussion brings the requisite ability to define, describe, and demonstrate outcomes using data. A tension between what we do and what we know often brings about a dialogue or debate about the data that often becomes a misdirected centerpiece. It is incumbent on those in healthcare to widen the discussion so issues of standardization, exchange, and sophisticated analysis of existing data paves the way to actionable knowledge.

Whether provider, payor, clinician, regulator, or patient it is evident that acceleration of the sophistication and science in data management and analysis is essential (Bates & Singh, 2018; Masica & Escarce, 2019; O'Connor, 2018). Disciplined and replicable approaches to data management, mining, and analysis is key to decision-making and monitoring as it is the basis upon which policy makers and payors make determinations about initiating and discontinuing programs or services and funding.

As the pressures to validate how scarce human and fiscal resources are allocated, the requirements to standardize data definitions, data management, and methods for analysis, and implementation of evidence-based interventions mount.

REQUISITE LEADERSHIP SKILLS FOR QUALITY, SAFETY, AND FISCALLY RESPONSIBLE CARE DELIVERY

Much has been written about leadership, attributes, and skills needed for success in the 21st century. Central to leadership is the ability to plan and predict so actions taken achieve desired clinical or organizational results. What is emerging as a new leadership competency is the ability to innovate and manage change (Porter-O'Grady & Malloch, 2015; Weberg & Davidson, 2021).

Innovation is often viewed as "risky" because there is no guarantee of success. Stated differently, innovation has winners and losers. Not every innovation will achieve the desired result. While based on best evidence, the crux of innovation is future orientation and vision, creativity, and bringing together unique nontraditional teams that are willing to cocreate solutions to many longstanding problems by not relying on current practices. Innovators see beyond the barriers and obstacles to envision revolutionary changes in care delivery models, team composition, technological applications, and new processes to spawn solutions. Innovation differs from leading change because there is a radical departure from the status quo. There is no roadmap for implementation and the ambiguity during the change brings detractors uneasy with the possibility that success will require large-scale change (Johnson & Sollecito, 2020; Weberg & Davidson, 2021).

Porter-O'Grady and Malloch (2015) highlight that in the post-digital and post-reform era, to achieve the healthcare transformation desired, leaders must create both strategic and structural imperatives that embrace technology and innovation that become the "way we do business." Creating a culture of innovation requires that healthcare and healthcare delivery will need to be replaced with new organizational cultures. Historically driven by hierarchy, rigidly controlled order, and physician dominated decisions, health services will need to be reconceptualized to integrate technology, interdisciplinary and transdisciplinary team members, new infrastructure, and revised reimbursement mechanisms. The historic reliance on fictionalism and process-fixed work make innovation difficult. Revision and transformation of the care delivery system will require harnessing the shared knowledge and motivation of varied disciplines and teams seeking sustainable impact and outcomes. A key shift in thinking will be the establishment of equity in groups whereby each contributing team member with a stake in the results holds value and shares equally in problem identification, solutions, and implementation of change. Likewise, it implies the collective professional community can only be represented by the sum of the contribution of each member that includes both traditional and nontraditional contributors.

Leaders need to find ways to embrace some uncertainty if they want to create or generate the care delivery systems and processes of the future. Advances in automation, technology, and artificial intelligence have propelled healthcare organizations and leaders into new territory. Given this, leaders have had to expand the ways they encourage and support the creative members of their teams and cultivate partnerships with community, industry, technology, and payors to reconceptualize healthcare of the future. This includes partnering with those who were once viewed as competitors, inviting people from outside healthcare to participate as full team members in an innovation, and trusting those engaged in the work are fully committed to the groups success (Porter-O'Grady & Malloch, 2015). Given this, the ability to innovate is emerging as a new leadership competency to support the volume and pace of change in healthcare.

Another 21st century leadership competency resides in team composition and team management. As a point of how business has been done in healthcare, team members have typically been viewed as either clinical or administrative. Recently, team composition has expanded to include technology, community partners, and support staff. In recognition of patient perspective and the need for patient engagement and activation, many organizations are adding patients to governing committees and quality- or process-improvement teams to ensure the consumer's perspective is embedded in the decision-making process.

As efforts to co-create, co-design, and innovate for effectiveness, efficiency, timeliness, and patient-centeredness solidify, healthcare leaders are embracing adding nontraditional healthcare participants and partners. Engineers, architects, data scientists, hospitality leaders, technology leaders, and community partners and a variety of health providers are included in healthcare delivery redesign teams (Bhavnani et al., 2016; Masica & Escare, 2019; Massie et al., 2020; Weberg & Davidson, 2021).

SUMMARY

- Data will continue to drive decisions pertaining to value, cost, and quality for administrators and policy makers.
- Decisions about services provided, reimbursement, and incentivizing research and performance rely on data and data analytics.
- The HHS guides health policy, reimbursement, and health quality through regulation of health services.

REFLECTION QUESTIONS

1. You have been asked to develop a proposal for how to improve an environment of care standard identified as deficient in a recent accreditation visit. Identify two key elements of your proposal that demonstrate distinctions between regulation and accreditation.
2. Given the accreditation deficiency identified in question one, what recommendations would you make to the executive team?
3. You are having lunch with a colleague from an ambulatory care clinic. They ask you to describe the leadership attributes you think are most important for innovations in care redesign. What is your answer?

4. Pick a health professional discipline and list three regulatory bodies that oversee that practice. What attributes does each of the regulatory bodies hold in common and what distinctive attributes do each hold?

REFERENCES

Accreditation Association for Ambulatory Healthcare. (2020). *Why AAAHC?* https://www.aaahc.org/should-my-organization-seek-accreditation

Administration for Children & Families. (n.d. a). *About ACF.* https://www.acf.hhs.gov/about

Administration for Children & Families. (n.d. b). *What we do.* https://www.acf.hhs.gov/about/what-we-do

Accreditation Commission for Health Care. (2019). *What is accreditation.* ACHC.org

Agency for Healthcare Research and Quality. (n.d. a). *Agency for Healthcare Research and Quality.* https://www.ahrq.gov

Agency for Healthcare Research and Quality. (n.d. b). *Offices and programs.* https://www.ahrq.gov/cpi/index.html

AHRQ Views. (2019). *AHRQ's Road ahead: Seizing opportunities in three essential areas to improve patient care.* https://www.ahrq.gov/news/blog/ahrqviews/ahrqs-road-ahead.html

Ambulatory Health Care. (2020). *Ambulatory Care Accreditation Survey Activity Guide.* The Joint Commission. https://www.jointcommission.org/-/media/tjc/documents/accred-and-cert/ahc/ambulatory-care-organization-sag.pdf

Barlas, S. (2017). U.S. and States ramp up response to opioid crisis: Regulatory, legislative, and legal tools brought to bear. *Pharmacy & Therapeutics, 42*(9), 569–571,592.

Bates, D., & Singh, H. (2018). *Two decades after to Err is Human: An assessment of progress and emerging priorities in patient safety.* https://www.healthaffairs.org/doi/pdf/10.1377/hlthaff.2018.0738

Becker's Hospital Review. (2015). *Key considerations for population health management.* https://www.beckershospitalreview.com/population-health/key-considerations-for-population-health-management.html

Bhavnani, S., Munoz, D., & Bagai, A. (2016). Data science in healthcare: Implications for early career investigators. *Circulation: Cardiovascular Quality Outcomes, 9,* 683–687. https://doi.org/10.1161/circoutcomes.116.003081

Centers for Disease Control and Prevention. (n.d.). *Centers for Disease Control and Prevention.* https://www.cdc.gov

Centers for Disease Control and Prevention. (2010). *Establishing a holistic framework to reduce inequities in HIV, Vvral hepatitis, STDs, and tuberculosis in the United States: An NCHHSTP white paper on social determinants of health.* https://www.cdc.gov/nchhstp/socialdeterminants/docs/SDH-White-Paper-2010.pdf

Centers for Disease Control and Prevention. (2017). *Data-Driven Prevention Initiative (DDPI).* https://www.cdc.gov/drugoverdose/foa/ddpi.html

Centers for Disease Control and Prevention. (2018). *Understanding the epidemic.* https://www.cdc.gov/drugoverdose/epidemic/index.html

Centers for Disease Control and Prevention. (2019a). *Global health: Our partnerships.* CDC.gov

Centers for Disease Control and Prevention. (2019b). *Population health training.* https://www.cdc.gov/pophealthtraining/whatis.html

Centers for Medicare and Medicaid Services. (n.d.). *Centers for Medicare and Medicaid Services.* https://www.cms.gov

Centers for Medicare and Medicaid Services. (2019). *MACRA: What is MACRA*. https://www.cms.gov/Medicare/Quality-Initiatives-Patient-Assessment-Instruments/Value-Based-Programs/MACRA-MIPS-and-APMs/MACRA-MIPS-and-APMs

Chilingerian, J. (2008). Origins of DRGs in the United States: A technical, political, and cultural story. In J. R. Kimberly, G. de Pouvourville, & T. D'Aunno (Eds.), *The globalization of managerial Iinnovation in health care* (pp. 4–33). Cambridge University Press.

Davis, J. (2020). *ONC draft federal health IT strategy puts privacy, security in focus*. https://healthitsecurity.com/news/onc-draft-federal-health-it-strategy-puts-privacy-security-in-focus

Department of Health and Human Services. (2019a). *Programs and Services*. https://www.hhs.gov/programs/index.html

Department of Health and Human Services. (2019b). *Secretary priorities*. https://www.hhs.gov/about/leadership/secretary/priorities/index.html

Dunham-Taylor, J. (2015). Healthcare stakeholders: Consumers, providers, payors, suppliers, and regulators. In J. Dunham-Taylor & J. Pinczuk (Eds.), *Financial management for nurse managers: Merging the heart with the dollar* (3rd ed.). Jones & Bartlett Learning.

Dunham-Taylor, J., & Pinczuk, J. (Eds.). (2015). *Financial management for nurse managers: Merging the heart with the dollar* (3rd ed.). Jones & Bartlett Learning.

Elbel, B. (2019). The challenge of health care delivery and health policy. In J. Knickman & B. Elbel (Eds.), *Jonas & Kovners's health care delivery in the United States* (12th ed.). Springer Publishing Company.

Food and Drug Administration. (n.d.). *Food and Drug Administration*. https://www.fda.gov

Food and Drug Administration. (2019). *About FDA. What we do*. https://www.fda.gov/about-fda/what-we-do

Gottlieb, S. (2017). *Dr. Gottlieb's remarks delivered before FDA's scientific meeting on opioids*. Food and Drug Administration. www.fda.gov/NewsEvents/Speeches/ucm566189.htm

Health and Human Services. (n.d. a). *Laws and Regulation*. https://www.hhs.gov/regulations/index.html

Health and Human Services. (n.d. b). *HHS agencies & Ooffices*. https://www.hhs.gov/about/agencies/hhs-agencies-and-offices/index.html

Health and Human Services. (n.d. c). *Priorities*. https://www.hhs.gov/about/leadership/secretary/priorities/index.html

Health Resources & Services Administration. (n.d.). https://www.hrsa.gov

Health Resources & Services Administration. (2019). *About HRSA*. https://www.hrsa.gov/about/index.html

Indian Health Service. (n.d. a). *Indian Health Service*. https://www.ihs.gov

Indian Health Service. (n.d. b). *Factsheets*. https://www.ihs.gov/newsroom/factsheets

Indian Health Service. (n.d. c). *About IHS*. https://www.ihs.gov/aboutihs

Institute of Medicine. (1999). *To err is human: Building a safer health system*. National Academy Press.

Institute of Medicine. (2001). *Crossing the chasm: A new health system for the 21st century*. National Academy Press.

Johnson, J., & Sollecito, W. (2020). *McLaughlin & Kaluzny's continuous quality improvement in health care* (5th ed.). Jones & Bartlett Learning.

Johnson, K., Jones, C., Compton, W. Baldwin, G., Fan, J., Mermin, J., & Bennett, J. (2018). Federal response to the opioid crisis. *Current HIV/AIDs Reports, 15*(4), 293–301. https://doi.org/10.1007/s11904-018-0398-8

Joint Commission. (2019). *Benefits of accreditation.* jointcommission.org

Kent, J. (2019). *FDA: Data analytics, new policies will curb opioid abuse in 2019.* https://healthitanalytics.com/news/fda-data-analytics-new-policies-will-curb-opioid-abuse-in-2019

Keswani, A., Koenig, K.M., Ward, L. et al. (2016). Value-based healthcare: Part 2—Addressing the obstacles to implementing integrated practice units for the management of musculoskeletal disease. *Clinical Orthopaedics and Related Research, 474,* 2344–2348. https://doi.org/10.1007/s11999-016-5064-0

Knickman, J. (2019). Health care financing. In Knickman, J., & Elbel, B (Eds.), *Jonas & Kovner's health care delivery in the United States* (12th ed.). Springer Publishing Company.

Knickman, J., & Elbel, B. (2019). *Jonas & Kovner's health care delivery in the united states* (12th ed.), Springer Publishing Company.

Landry, A., & Erwin, C. (2019). Organization of Care. In J. Knickman & B. Elbel (Eds.), *Jonas & Kovner's Health Care Delivery in the United States* (12th ed.; pp. 15–50). Springer Publishing Company.

Lam, M., Figueroa, J., Feyman, Y., Rimold, K., Oray, E., & Jha, A., (2018). Association between patient outcomes and accreditation in US hospitals: observational study. *BMJ, 363,* k4011. https://doi.org/10.1136/bmj.k4011

Langabeer, J. (2018). *Performance improvement in hospitals and health systems: Managing analytics and quality in healthcare* (2nd ed.). CRC Press.

Leger, M., & Dunham-Taylor, J. (2018). *Financial management for nurse managers: Merging the heart with the dollar* (4th ed.). Jones & Bartlett Publishing.

Lighter, D. (2011). *Advanced performance improvement in healthcare: Principles and methods.* Jones and Bartlett Publishers.

Masica, A., & Escarce, J. (2019). Innovative data science to transform health care: All the pieces matter. *Generating Evidence & Methods to Improve Patient Centered Outcomes, 7*(1), 47. https://doi.org/10.5334/egems.314

Massie, S., Randolph, C., & Randolph, G. (2020). Continuous quality improvement in U.S. Public Health Organizations: Widespread adoption and institutionalization. In J. Johnson, & W. Sollecito (Eds.), *McLaughlin & Kaluzny's continuous quality improvement in healthcare* (5th ed.). Jones & Bartlett Learning.

Mayes, R. (2007). The origins, development, and passage of medicare's revolutionary prospective payment system. *Journal of the History of Medicine and Allied Sciences, 62*(1), 21–55. https://doi.org/10.1093/jhmas/jrj038

Moran, K., Harris, I., & Valenta, A., (2016). Quality improvement: A synthesis of recommendations in influential position papers. *The Joint Commission Journal on Quality and Patient Safety, 42*(4), 162–169. https://doi.org/10.1016/S1553-7250(16)42020-9

Mumford, V., Forde, K., Greenfield, D., Hinchcliff, R., & Braithwaite, J. (2013). Health services accreditation: what is the evidence that the benefits justify the costs? *International Journal of Quality Healthcare, 25*(5), 606–620. https://doi.org/10.1093/intqhc/mzt059

National Committee for Quality Assurance. (2019). *Latest Evidence: Benefits of NCQA Patient-Centered Medical Home Recognition.* https://www.ncqa.org/programs/health-care-providers-practices/patient-centered-medical-home-pcmh/benefits-support/pcmh-evidence

National Institutes of Health. (n.d. a). *National Institutes of Health.* https://www.nih.gov

National Institutes of Health. (n.d. b). *About NIH: What We Do.* https://www.nih.gov/about-nih/what-we-do

O'Connor, S. (2018). Big data and data science in health care: What nurses and midwives need to know. *Journal of Clinical Nursing, 27,* 2921–2922. https://doi.org/10.1111/jocn.14164

Office for Civil Rights. (2020). *Summary of the HIPAA security rule.* https://www.hhs.gov/hipaa/for-professionals/security/laws-regulations/index.html

Office of the Inspector General. (n.d.). *Office of the Inspector General.* https://oig.hhs.gov

Office of the Inspector General. (2019). *About OIG.* https://oig.hhs.gov/about-oig/about-us/index.asp

Porter, M. (2010). What is value in healthcare?, *New England Journal of Medicine, 363,* 2477–2281. https://doi.org/10.1056/NEJMp1011024

Porter-O'Grady, T., & Malloch, K. (2015). *Quantum leadership: Building better partnership for sustainable health.* Jones & Bartlett Learning.

Radley, D., & Marchica, J. (2019). Health care costs and value. In J. R. Knickman & B. Elbel (Eds.), *Jonas & Kovner's Health Care Delivery in the United States* (12th ed.). Springer Publishing Company.

Tsevat, J., & Moriates, C. (2018). Value-based healthcare meets cost-effectiveness analysis. *Annals of Internal Medicine, 169*(5), 329–333.

Utilization Review Accreditation Commission. (2019). *Accreditation process.* https://www.urac.org/accreditation-process

Weberg, D., & Davidson, S., (2021). *Future of evidence, innovation, and leadership in healthcare: A model for change in leadership for evidence-based innovation in nursing and health professions* (2nd ed.). Jones & Bartlett Learning.

World Health Organization. (2020). *Social determinants of health.* https://www.who.int/social_determinants/sdh_definition/en

CASE EXEMPLAR FOR APPLICATION

Closing Documentation Gaps: Increasing CMI in a Community Special Care Nursery

Raja Senguttuvan

Case mix index (CMI) is the relative value of a diagnosis related group (DRG) assigned to patient discharges from a hospital. There are ways to improve a hospital's CMI to more accurately reflect the acuity and resources required to care for a patient. Improving documentation practices of physicians is one such activity. Coders can only report what the physician documents in the patient's record. As a community level 2A Special Care Nursery (SCN), seeking to close the documentation gaps to improve the CMI, our methods and results are presented below.

The identified hospital specific to this exemplar averages 1,450 deliveries a year with close to 250 infants being admitted to the Special Care Nursery. Of these infants, only 140 are discharged home from the SCN. The rest of the infants have had brief stays in SCN and are transferred back to the mother until discharge. Data analysis clearly revealed DRG relative weights to vary widely among the infants despite the same length of stay in SCN. This data stood out and represented different payor sources. A gap was identified in the documentation of care at discharge where provider discharge summaries were not incorporating the SCN stay that was impacting CMI and reimbursement.

Robust clinical documentation improvement (CDI) support was limited and the presence of two computer documentation platforms further complicated physician documentation at discharge. While some education was done around carrying diagnoses all the way to discharge, we lack automation to support this work. A system was created to tag the SCN notes and have the last note from the SCN automatically sent to the discharge folder in the consolidated electronic medical record (EMR) for the

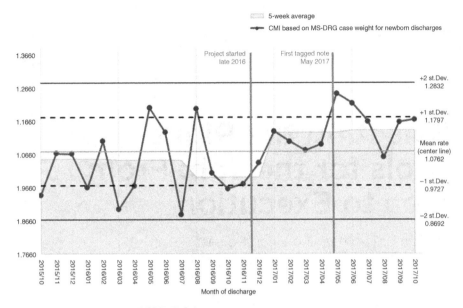

FIGURE 2.1 Newborn case mix index (CMI).

baby. CMI for newborn discharges has increased 10% since this project was implemented in late 2016 and more since our first tagged note in May 2017, illustrated in Figure 2.1.

Provider documentation in the discharge summary determines what the hospital can include for consideration when the hospital is reimbursed. This process aligns revenue to more accurately reflect the complexity and cost of the care provided throughout the stay versus the last entered notes. Without continuous documentation during hospitalization and at discharge, the potential for limited communication, safety issues, quality outcomes, and fiscal stewardship will create numerous issues that result in income loss and lost opportunities related to the CMI.

REFLECTION QUESTIONS

1. How does case mix index (CMI) impact documentation, quality, and value in health care?
2. What steps can be initiated to ensure documentation entries reflect the care provided and acuity levels for coding and billing purposes?

Selecting the Right Tools for the Job: From Idea to Execution

Patricia L. Thomas and Brian Collins

OBJECTIVES

1. Establish common models and frameworks for improvement.
2. Examine the cost-quality equation and how to build it into quality improvement.
3. Consider cost avoidance and cost benefit as strategies to guide practice and policy change.
4. Describe how to select and use quality improvement, frameworks, models, and tools.

CORE COMPETENCIES

- Understanding healthcare delivery, sources of data, reliability, and validity
- Knowledge of process and quality improvement
- Appreciation for the disciplined and systematic approach required for improvement

INTRODUCTION

This chapter focuses on different quality improvement methods and selection of tools to support interprofessional improvement work. To strengthen data-driven decisions and next steps, recommendations are provided to assist teams make data visible and actionable using tables, graphs, and improvement tools.

PRINCIPLES OF QUALITY IMPROVEMENT

The aim of quality improvement (QI) is to implement systematic activities to monitor, assess, and improve care through continuous actions that result in measurable improvement. These cyclical activities are intended to produce higher levels of performance that optimize clinical, operational, and financial outcomes.

Four principles are common in quality improvement. The principles include: (a) a focus on systems and processes, (b) a focus on patient, (c) being a member of a team, and (d) the use of data (Health Resources and Services Administration [HRSA], 2011; Institute for Healthcare Improvement [IHI], 2020a). Each of these principles are described below.

Systems and processes are pivotal to QI and focus on an organization's understanding of the delivery system. Quality improvement is most effective when it is individualized to meet the delivery system needs. Donabedian (1980) recognized that quality in healthcare was complex and offered a way to analyze care delivery noting resources (inputs) and activities (processes) which together establish the foundations for care improvement (outputs/outcomes). Activities or processes concentrate on "what is done" or the care provided and "how it is done" (by who, when, and where). While quality improvement can be achieved by examining the what or the how, it is most effective when both are addressed (HRSA, 2011; IHI, 2020a; Johnson & Sollecito, 2020; Sables-Baus & Armstrong, 2020).

While recent national attention has concentrated on the cost of care, a central principle in QI is focus on the patient and the extent to which needs and expectations are met. When considering any quality initiative, several factors should be considered by answering the following questions:

- How will this impact patient care?
- Is the care evidence-based?
- What impact will this have on safety?
- What support is present to encourage patient engagement?
- What coordination will be needed with other parts of the larger system?
- How will cultural competence and health literacy be incorporated into patient communication? (HRSA, 2011).

The landmark report from the Institute of Medicine (IOM), *Crossing the Quality Chasm: A New Health System for the 21st Century*, captured the attention of policy makers and the public that despite best efforts, healthcare delivery in the United States was not delivering the quality of care it espoused in evidence and redesign. Transformation of care delivery therefore evolved as an imperative to eliminate fragmentation and redundancy of care. To address the imperative, the IOM developed six aims (patient-centered care, patient safety, timeliness or responsive care, efficient care, effective care, and equitable care) that have guided improvement and safety work for nearly two decades (HRSA, 2011; IOM, 2001). The need to address quality and safety was also highlighted in the IOM report *To Err is Human: Building a Safer Health System* (1999) that directed national awareness to the 44,000 to 98,000 unintended hospital deaths annually from preventable errors or accidents costing $29 billion.

Unlike other aspects of care delivery, QI cannot be accomplished through the efforts of an individual and requires focus on being part of the team. A key to any successful improvement initiative resides in the clear scope of work for a defined problem or issue and the engagement of an interprofessional team. As a team sport, harnessing the collective wisdom of each team member who brings unique knowledge, skills, and abilities makes it more likely an improvement initiative will succeed. As improvement teams engage in activities, several considerations must be present to ensure effectiveness and deliverables follow. They include the following:

- The process or system is complex.
- No single person in the organization knows all the dimensions of a problem or issue.
- The work involves more than one discipline or work area.
- Creativity and innovation are needed.
- Support and commitment by team members are needed (HRSA, 2011; IHI, 2020a).

Unlike many hierarchy-driven activities in healthcare delivery, QI teams rely on leveraging insights from the person on a team who has the knowledge or experience to best address a need. Defined by the charter of an improvement team, the power of members resides in the fundamental requirement that each participant is an equal contributor. Traditional hierarchical titles are not the drivers for the role a person assumes on an improvement team. Instead, each person's perspective, relative to the improvement, establishes the weight or influence their contributions will make in the teams decision-making process (Agency for Healthcare Research and Quality [AHRQ], n.d. a; AHRQ, 2015; IHI, 2020b).

The Agency for Healthcare Research and Quality (AHRQ) and the Department of Defense (DOD) developed TeamSTEPPS®, an evidence-based teamwork model that describes the skills and behaviors necessary for team outcomes. The model includes skills for leadership, mutual support, situation monitoring, and communication necessary for quality improvement and team-based results. A focal point of this work involves communication, standardization of work, and building a shared purpose that contribute to effectiveness. Inherent in the TeamSTEPPS process are feedback cycles that focus team members on both the work and the evaluation of it to enhance outcomes (AHRQ, n.d. a, n.d. b; AHRQ, 2015; Danna, 2013; Thomas & Winter, 2019). This cycle of evaluation helps to create awareness of performance, where significant changes to outcomes are more likely the result of an intervention or have another identifiable, assignablecause.

Focus on use of the data and its analysis is the cornerstone of QI. Data are used to describe the current state, what happens when changes are made, and to document successful performance. Data provide a new appreciation and awareness of organizational practices and processes by making processes visible. Traditional beliefs and assumptions are often challenged when data are presented. The dissonance between what one thought was true and what the data represent is a significant motivator for improvement initiatives (HRSA, 2011; IHI, 2020a; IHI, 2020c).

In a digital era, there are multiple sources of data including electronic health records, practice management systems, registries, administrative data, and financial or cost data. Big data provides new sources of information including self-reported data from health risk assessments, health kiosks, patient satisfaction results, and publicly reported provider specific databases as invaluable benchmark resources. As QI commences, it is important to consider structured and unstructured data sources, as well as the need for data that may not be readily available, a critical tool to communicate results (HRSA, 2011; IHI, 2020a; IHI, 2020c).

In healthcare QI, descriptive statistics are commonly used because they are familiar to healthcare professionals. The average or mean, range, frequency, percentages, and standard deviation can be visually displayed using different QI tools. The visualization of the data becomes a platform to communicate progress in improvement work and assists team members recognize the impact of efforts.

While most improvement efforts rely on quantitative data, qualitative data are also helpful. Qualitative data derived from focus groups, patient satisfaction surveys, and staff surveys can offer information on patterns, themes, relationships between systems, and add context to support improvement (HRSA, 2011; IHI, 2020c).

THE COST-QUALITY EQUATION AND HOW TO BUILD IT INTO QUALITY IMPROVEMENT

Any discussion on improvement would be incomplete if it did not offer guidance on ways to identify cost-benefit, cost avoidance, or cost-effectiveness. Historically, the focal point of improvement work resided in improving outcomes for patients or the practice environment. Today, an additional focus on cost has entered decision-making processes with expectations for improvement activities to not only demonstrate patient-centered, evidence-based, efficient and effective interventions, but also reasonable cost.

The ability to link financial considerations to improvement are becoming the norm and often are the linchpin in decisions about policy and whether a program, project, or benefit will be continued in organizations or payer reimbursements. This requires healthcare practitioners and providers to expand knowledge and incorporate financial and cost evaluation into how they articulate the value of clinical interventions. This makes the case for improvement teams to include finance and data analyst experts in improvement activities at the onset of project so financial considerations are integrated into each phase of the work. While it is beyond the scope of this chapter to detail the methods in cost effectiveness, cost benefit, and cost avoidance, it is important to have an understanding about how a business or financial case can be made using data from QI work (Hwang & Christensen, 2008; Thomas, Harris, & Roussel, 2018).

Cost avoidance is a common metric attributed to QI initiatives because it is easily understood. It represents costs that would not be incurred in the future if an intervention or improvement is started. In terms of QI work, streamlining processes, preventing complications, or implementing clinical practice guidelines that improve clinical outcomes, often demonstrate cost avoidance. A challenge and potential pitfall in using cost avoidance is an incomplete or inaccurate calculation of the baseline expenses and the future orientation that has potential to be inaccurate. As a means to address this, many quality or process improvement projects choose cost savings as they represent tangible reductions in costs like reduced overtime or lower cost products or equipment that are visible on financial statements (Gerald R. Ford School of Public Policy, n.d.).

Cost benefit analysis places a monetary value on health outcomes and interventions to establish a net benefit by examining the cost of the intervention and the result in terms of monetary units. The net benefit is the monetized unit less the cost to implement the intervention. The cost benefit is often described as a ratio with the program cost as a ratio to benefit. It can also be expressed as the benefit to cost ratio with every dollar spent on a program the dollar benefit achieved. The advantage in using this approach is the clarity it provides to establish if the cost of a program is worthwhile (Gerald R. Ford School of Public Policy, n.d.).

Cost effectiveness analysis includes costs, but the effectiveness is measured in nonmonetary units described by a desired outcome. For example, this intervention (program) cost $X to avoid a hospital admission or an ED visit. This approach allows comparisons between interventions or programs with the same outcome and is often desired in health services were benefits cannot always be converted to dollars. In this approach, effectiveness can be described in terms of the impact on patients or those served (Gerald R. Ford School of Public Policy, n.d.).

SELECTING AND USING QUALITY IMPROVEMENT FRAMEWORKS, MODELS, AND TOOLS

Healthcare has only recently embraced QI frameworks, yet the history of improvement and distinction between approaches is important to understand. The philosophy or tenets in each framework, model, or tool helps guide the work and provides a focus for what is most important as a team engages in improvement work. Being consistent in and true to a framework or model in an improvement initiative is essential.

Alignment between the defined problem or purpose of the work, information gathered, the methods or approach to the work, and analysis of data is what offers substance and structure to improvement projects. This means clarity in the definition of the problem or purpose of the work, stating the model or framework for improvement, and ensuring consistency in how data will be collected and analyzed starts before any action by the interprofessional team. Although this sounds simple, it is not and represents the space and place that quality improvement teams often go awry. If this strategic alignment and work is not done at the onset of an improvement initiative, it will likely create delays and rework and could render the work unreliable for decision-making. Or, it will lead to little or no impact on anything important.

Organizations need to ask which activities are most core to their success within the defined problem or purpose and address those activities. Otherwise, organizational energy is wasted on peripheral, less strategic activities (Shortell et al., 1998). Beyond the scope of this chapter, but critical to improvement work, are skills in project management and what leading a project entails. Some resources for this project work are included in the Table 3.1.

What follows are the common improvement frameworks, models, and tools used in healthcare QI initiatives. This is not an exhaustive list but rather what is frequently seen in health systems.

Total Quality Management (TQM) has its roots in industry and was applied widely in healthcare in the early 1980s. Before TQM, quality in healthcare was a monitoring function that retrospectively examined work to confirm completeness. Quality departments were primarily focused on generating reports and interaction

TABLE 3.1 Project Management Resources

PROJECT MANAGEMENT RESOURCE	CONTENT	WEBSITE
Agency for Healthcare Research and Quality (AHRQ)	Quality improvement (QI) toolkit with templates, instructions, and examples	www.ahrq.gov/evidencenow/tools/qi-essentials-toolkit.html
HealthIT.gov	How to establish a continuous quality improvement process	www.healthit.gov/faq/how-do-we-establish-continuous-quality-improvement-process
Institute for Healthcare Improvement (IHI)	Resources for QI project management	www.ihi.org/resources/Pages/Tools/QI-Project-Management.aspx
Harvard T.H. Chan School of Public Health	A primer on project management for healthcare	www.hsph.harvard.edu/ecpe/a-primer-on-project-management-for-health-care
Project Management Institute	Project management for healthcare information technology	www.pmi.org/learning/library/project-management-healthcare-information-technology-6133
Health Resources and Services Administration (HRSA)	Developing and implementing a QI plan	www.hrsa.gov/sites/default/files/quality/toolbox/508pdfs/developingqiplan.pdf

with the people doing the work was very limited. Leaders and clinicians either celebrated or felt disappointment, but little information was available about the change needed to achieve a desired result. Around this same time, concerns about rising costs, efficiency, and efficiency caused healthcare leaders to look to other industries with similar concerns.

As a business solution to poor quality in manufacturing after World War II, Japan initiated quality improvement using principles from engineering and statistical process control to gain competitive advantage in the automotive industry. Although slow to adopt these principles implemented in Japan and other parts of the world, the United States brought these quality principles to the automotive industry when they were losing competitive advantage. A longstanding belief in the United States was that productivity and quality could not co-exist. This new approach to quality in productivity-dependent manufacturing processes demonstrated this belief was false (Berwick, 1989; Sollecito & Johnson, 2020).

TQM is an umbrella termed used to encompass the principles of continuous improvement, customer focus, and teamwork. TQM represented a paradigm shift in the approach to quality. TQM brought into focus that leaders alone do not have all the answers, improvement is continuous and requires learning, and not all change represents an improvement (Sollecito & Johnson, 2020). TQM has evolved into what is now recognized as continuous quality improvement that underpins accreditation, safety, and regulatory expectations. Central to these continuous improvements frameworks are data and measurement.

Fundamentals of TQM are drawn from the scientific management era of the early 20th century centered on management with facts and was influenced by the human resources era that brought attention to the abilities of people in an organization that influence results (Sollecito & Johnson, 2020). W. Edward Deming and Walter A. Shewhart are considered the major contributors to TQM and continuous improvement as we know it today in healthcare. Deming's *System of Profound Knowledge* identified appreciation of the system, understanding variation, psychology, and epistemology as the lenses necessary to understand organizations. From this, he defined 14 key principles for leaders to use to transform business effectiveness. Deming published these principles in his book *Out of the Crisis* (1986) that launched Total Quality Management however never used these terms.

In review of the 14 Principles, the focus on learning, eliminating fear and punishment, and engaging staff in improvement are cornerstones set forth by Deming as a platform for success. The constancy of purpose and focus on continually improving is a shared vision but leaders, managers, and supervisors are responsible for creating the space where this work can occur. Deming also placed emphasis on removing inspection as the method to validate quality noting cost would be driven out if attention was centered on service and production improvements. Placing attention on the role of leaders and management with placement of responsibility and accountability on each person who contributes in the work, Deming put prominence on leadership competence and learning. In this emphasis, Deming acknowledged organizational norms and leadership as important influencers. Today we see this work in designations of executive sponsors or champions and interprofessional improvement teams.

Shewhart's work is threaded throughout Deming's approach as it highlights statistical quality control. It is through understanding variation and the use of statistical process controls that changes in interventions and the results are made visible by data. With disciplined analysis and measurement, decisions can be made guided by the data results depicted in visual representation. Shewhart introduced the control chart and defined common cause and special cause variation that have become a centerpiece of quality management and continuous improvement lexicon (Berwick, 1989; Sables-Baus & Armstrong, 2020; Sollecito & Hardison, 2020).

The Lean Model focuses on identifying the root cause of a problem and understanding work processes so quality improvement would be focused on reducing waste and adding value. Value is defined by what the customer (or patient) wants, thereby supporting a basic tenet of quality improvement work (Lighter, 2011; Nelson et al., 2007; Popovich et al., 2020).

The Lean approach to quality improvement is often attributed to the automotive industry, and Toyota especially, but has historic roots in the work of Shewhart, Deming, and Fredrick Taylor's *Principles of Scientific Management* originally published in 1911 (Taylor, 2011). Fredrick described how managers could apply scientific management with a foundation that rests on laws, rules, and principles. As such, his approach centered on studying workflow processes so unnecessary or inefficient activities could be eliminated to improve productivity (Taylor, 2011). Shewhart's statistical process control (SPC) was then added to establish quality control methods where data is regularly analyzed to identify patterns of variation to establish common or chance-cause versus special or assignable-cause variation (Shewhart, 1923). This method was created with the understanding that a manufacturing process may have one standard method, however, the outcome of that process may vary nonetheless. The variation was less like flipping a coin and more like observed nature and a normal distribution of behavior or outcomes.

The Five Principles of Lean include the following:

1. Specify value from a customer perspective.
2. Identify the value stream. Establish the steps in a process and eliminate those that do not contribute to the goal
3. Establish flow without interruption. Efficiency is achieved by eliminating waste between steps.
4. Customer "pulls" services. Aallow customers to receive or request products when needed. Said differently, be timely.
5. Pursue perfection. Ccontinuously adapt and change to deliver products and services of the highest quality. (UL Knowledge Services, 2013, p. 4).

Given the elimination of waste is a central focus in Lean, identification of the most common categories of waste and how they are embedded in process is warranted. Initially the automotive industry identified seven categories of waste. Healthcare revised the labels and identified eight categories: defects, overproduction, transportation, waiting, inventory, motion, over-processing, and human potential (Graban, 2016).

Defects include the time spent doing something incorrectly or inspecting for errors. Overproduction is doing more than is needed or doing something before required. This is readily apparent in healthcare in diagnostic tests. Transportation is the movement of a product in a system and encompasses people, supplies, and materials. Waiting is the time spent anticipating the next activity or event in a workflow. Examples of this would be waiting for the next patient on a schedule or staff time not utilized when they wait for supplies. Inventory relates to the cost held in inventory storage, spoilage, movement, or waste. This might include too much inventory or expired medications. Motion describes movement of staff in an organization represented by the location or layout of a unit. Overprocessing is nonvalue added work that does not contribute to meeting patient needs or collecting too much information that is not used. Putting the date and time of every document and specimen can represent overprocessing. Human potential refers to loss or waste when employees are not engaged in work or when their ideas and suggestions for improvement are not valued or considered (Mark Graban & Constancy Inc., 2020).

Six Sigma is another measurement-based strategy for quality improvement and problem reduction. The name Six Sigma is a derivative of Shewhart's work in statistical process control where the six sigma are three standard deviations above the mean and three standard deviations below the mean that 99.73% are observations are to fall in a normal distribution. The focal point in Six Sigma is defects, distinguishing it from the Lean method focus on waste. The most common Six Sigma model is the DMAIC process that categorizes improvement activities sequentially to define, measure, analyze, improve and control processes. With attention on defects and variation, the intent is to streamline processes and ultimately reduce costs and improve care (Armstrong & Sables-Baus, 2020; Lighter, 2011; Johnson & Sollecito, 2020).

In the define phase the team ensures that the scope of the project is clear, supported by data, and is focused on patients. In the measure phase, decisions about what improvement will look like in terms of metrics and measurement of elements in the process are considered. In the analyze phase, data is collected and analyzed using quality tools. In the implementation phase, evidence-based interventions are implemented to bring about change. Last, in the control phase performance is monitored using data to sustain the improvement (Lighter, 2011; Nelson et al., 2007; Ramaswamy et al., 2020).

The IHI Improvement model relies on systematic and cyclical change to plan, do, study, and act in realtime. This model first offers three questions for the team considering improvement. The questions are: (a) What are we trying to accomplish?, (b) How will we know the change is an improvement?, (c) What changes can we make that will result in improvement.

Once the team answers each question, they engage in an interactive process by cyclically moving through phases that make rapid tests of change with evaluation that leads to another cycle that includes plan, do, study act. At the end of each cycle, the team decides what changes to make to continuously improve the process (IHI, 2020a).

In the plan phase, the team makes decisions about the test of change or observes the process and considers what data is needed and how it will be collected. At this time, the team is making predictions about what the change will bring, what will happen, and why. Decisions will be made about who will make the change, what the change will be, when it will occur, and what data needs to be collected. In moving to the do phase, the team trials the change and documents problems or unexpected observation and analyzes the data. In the study phase, all the data is analyzed and compared to the predictions offered in the planning phase. Data is summarized and the team reflects on and describes what has been learned. Moving to the act phase, decisions are made about what modifications are needed and they start to plan for the next test of change (HRSA, 2011; IHI, 2020f).

USING DATA

In quality improvement, data is the basis for decision-making because it allows us to describe how well the current process is working, what happens when change occurs, and documents performance success. Data separates beliefs about what is happening from what actually is happening. It establishes the baseline of performance and offers a means to monitor activities and results that helps team members determine if improvements have been sustained.

It is beyond the scope of this chapter to dive deeply into data analysis but it is important to gain knowledge and seek expertise to ensure valid and appropriate application of analytic methods for decision-making. Quality improvement work is best accomplished by a team, it is highly recommended that from the onset of any quality improvement initiative, an essential team member is one who has knowledge and expertise in data and data analytics. The individual for this work could hold a variety of titles including quality analyst, biostatistician, health information special-ist, data scientist, or a financial analyst to name a few. The determination about who best to invite to the team rests in the deep understanding of who could best select, organize, and analyze the data in support of the teams focus.

VARIATION

A cornerstone of quality improvement rests in the ability to establish that differences in results, or the variation in a process, warrant intervention. If unclear about what variation is and what it represents, leaders might choose to intervene unnecessar-ily and make matter worse (Bowen & Neuhauser, 2013; Stoecklein, 2015). Bowen and Neuhauser (2013) identified that common cause and special cause variation are the types of variation quality improvement is most concerned with. Common cause variation represents random variation present in a stable healthcare processes. This variation is expected and anticipated as it comes from the system or process, its com-ponents, and how they interact. In contrast, special-cause variation represents unpre-dictable deviations in a process from a cause that is not part of a process. Special cause variation can be identified through tools and methods to help determine if a quality or process improvement initiative is needed. Not all special-cause variation is negative. It may actually be used to help organizations achieve outcomes through replication when one unit or area consistently outperforms compared to their counterparts. The determination about the type of variation is critically important because it is foundational to the decision about whether a quality improvement team is needed (Bowen & Neuhauser, 2013; Stoecklin, 2015). In healthcare, process and outcome measures are often monitored using real-time data to learn from and manage variation. Comparing past, present, and desired performance, the management of variances can inform quality improvement and implementation of best practices (Bowen & Neuhauser, 2013; Stoecklein, 2015).

SELECTING INDICATORS

A common pitfall and point of frustration for improvement teams resides in selecting the indicators to best represent a change. This is a critical point in the planning process and cannot be overstated. Data and indicators are the focal point of improvements and serve as the single most important lever in determining success or failure. Given improvement activities will be evaluated based on the defined problem and whether the indicators or results demonstrate an improvement, it is imperative that appropriate indicators are chosen.

A clear line of sight between the data element or indicator and the problem or desired outcome is one piece of the equation. Many improvement team initiatives are deemed unsuccessful because the data or indicators selected do not demonstrate the change was an improvement. Another pitfall is selection of an indicator that is influenced by so many extraneous processes that the connection back to the improvement work is questioned. If conducting a project on one nursing unit intended to improve patient satisfaction survey results, be sure that survey results are reportable at the unit level and by discharge date versus when the survey was received. Otherwise, any impact will be diluted by other nursing units and the timing relative to intervention will be distorted.

While many quality improvement initiatives generate data, there are often existing datasets, registries, or reports that can be repurposed to support quality improvement. In making the case or providing background for an improvement initiative, a secondary data analysis or analysis of existing data that was collected for a different purpose, often provides the trend or performance history to justify chartering an improvement team. Common sources of secondary data are organizational data and data collected for third-party payers or by governmental agencies.

As teams consider the two or three key pieces of data that demonstrate the impact of the improvement activities, the determination about process and outcome indicators and leading and lagging indicators needs to be stipulated. Process indicators are measures of specific key processes that lead to an improvement contrasted with outcome indicators that measure the impact of one or more clinical interventions that lead to a desired result (AHRQ, 2018). An example of a process indicator would be the percentage of stable coronary artery disease patients who got lipid lowering agents prescribed. An outcome indicator example would be the risk-adjusted rate of inpatient hip fractures in acute care patients aged 65 years and over, per 1,000 discharges (AHRQ, 2018).

Recently, patient experience indicators have been established to ascertain how a patient's values and preferences were taken into consideration in the provision of care. This includes perceptions and observations about how they participated in healthcare or assessments leading to changes in health (AHRQ, 2018). Patient satisfaction surveys are common sources of this information.

Another important consideration is to determine if an indicator is a leading or lagging indicator. A leading indicator represents processes influencing a change were a lagging indicator demonstrates results. These are important distinctions for quality improvement teams as a leading indicator can reinforce that improvement interventions are having the impact that were hoped for. They anticipate or predict what will happen. Often, they are process indicators that help teams appreciate a practice change is consistently implemented. Lagging indicators demonstrate impact at the conclusion of activities and are often the measure that organizations are tracking or monitoring because they represent an outcome. A combination of leading and lagging indicators help teams appreciate the effort of the work during and after a change. To demonstrate this, a leading indicator for fall prevention would be the completion of fall risk assessments on all admitted adult patients on admission. A lagging indicator would be the fall rate with or without injury. Healthcare organizations often use leading and lagging indicators as measures on dashboards to help visualize how complex problems are being addressed in real time and how the activities bring about results or outcomes that are part of reimbursement or pay for performance indicators.

QUALITY IMPROVEMENT TOOLS AND TOOL SELECTION

There are several common tools used in quality and process improvement activities, each with a distinct purpose but all offering a mechanism to make data visible. In addition to tables, graphs, and charts, these tools serve the improvement team by structuring volumes of data so discussion, understanding, and decision-making can occur.

Selecting the ways data are displayed and offered to team members, stakeholders, and decision-makers is one of the most important decisions made in a quality improvement project. Selecting the most appropriate and relevant display tool not only aids in understanding the project, data, or processes but also builds credibility with an audience (HRSA, 2011; IHI, 2020a).

Fishbone Diagrams or Cause and Effect Diagrams

As organizations decide how and where to allocate resources for improvement, a common starting point is risk management. Often, when errors occur there is not one simple cause for the problem and no single intervention to prevent the error in the future. It is through the recognition of systems and complex processes that underlay the problem and contributed to the error that an improvement can be instituted. When this is the case, a cause and effect diagram can help organize the factors contributing to the problem to help improvement teams become clear about where to focus improvement activities.

A cause and effect diagram, also called an Ishikawa or fishbone diagram, is a graphic representation to explore possible causes of a certain effect. When developing a fishbone diagram the common categories for exploration includes materials, methods, equipment, environment, and people. These categories represent the bones on the diagram with the head of the fish as the issue. For each category, the team identifies contributing factors and documents them so the relationship of the factors in each category can be visualized. The relationship between the cause and effect can determine where to focus so that improvement work can be prioritized for team engagement. (IHI, 2020d). Figure 3.1 provides an example of a fishbone diagram created to address excess or length of stay in a hospital.

Failure Mode Effect Analysis

Failure Mode Effect Analysis (FMEA) focuses on cause and effect, but differs in how and when used. FMEA is an anticipatory approach to a concern where a team considers potential failure points where a cause and effect diagram reflects a known and defined issue or problem. FMEA is a tool to evaluate possibilities in new processes with an aim to prevent adverse events or outcomes. When conducting a FMEA review, the team analyzes the steps in the process, what could go wrong, what would happen if the process failed, and potential consequences of failure (IHI, 2020e; Lighter, 2011).

A distinction in FMEA is the assignment of risk and severity if the process fails. After generating a process map or flowchart of the process, the team explores all the possible points of failure (using a brainstorming process) and assigns a numerical

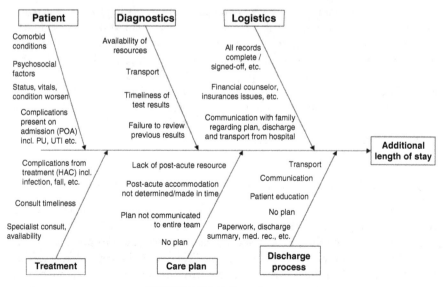

FIGURE 3.1 Fishbone diagram.

value to the severity of the risk. Each potential point of failure is reviewed for severity, likelihood of occurrence, and the effect or impact so an action plan can be generated to mitigate the risks. Prioritization of risks is completed, and improvements initiated based on the teams assessment. Each potential failure is reviewed, improvements defined, and revisions made until all the potential failure points are addressed (IHI, 2020e; Lighter, 2011).

Process Mapping/Flowcharting

Process mapping and flowcharting are common ways to generate a visual depiction of the sequence of events or steps in process that lead to an outcome. At the start of a QI project a process map or flowchart can help the interprofessional quality improvement team appreciate where work is being done, how different steps are affected by the work in other departments or areas, and where decisions influence results. Most of us have deep and detailed information about the part of a process we are responsible for but may not have an understanding of the nuances and complexity in steps others perform. This tool can be used to help interprofessional teams see the work others are doing and to establish common definitions of terms to establish a common language for work moving forward (Lighter, 2011; Nelson et al., 2007). This is an essential step in improvement projects as it establishes an understanding of the current state, which is associated with current performance.

To create a process map or flowchart each step in a process is identified. Sometimes the steps represent what occurs in a process start to finish. At other times the steps highlight where decisions are made before taking action. Irrespective of the purpose or focus, what is held in common is the need to establish activities that lead to a result or outcome. In reviewing each step, opportunities for improvement can be identified. By identifying the steps in a process and the individuals or department members involved in work, team members (and by extension the organization) are able to see the 'what is done' and 'how it is done', how they contribute to it, and offer input about what may be missed or overlooked by those not intimately engaged in the work. In addition to identifying efficiency in a process, it can aid teams in identifying care redesign opportunities. By aligning process map steps to clinical guidelines, optimal results occur (HRSA, 2011; Nelson et al., 2007).

Figure 3.2 starts and ends with oval shapes which should be clear and obvious milestones. They are followed by a series of steps or a process within the larger workflow indicated by rectangles. Each rectangle has one outbound arrow leading to the next shape. Decision points are diamond shaped and have two outbound arrows, one for "Yes" and one for "No" that lead to different shapes in the flowchart.

To get started in process mapping or flowcharting, it is helpful to observe the process yourself and interview people who have an interest in the process you aim to improve. Once the information has been collected, draft a step-by-step depiction of the process based on all of input gathered. For team discussions, it can be helpful to use "sticky notes" to display each step so the team can see each step and revise the order and come to agreement and establish the current process before deciding what step or steps need improvement. Once the team has done this work, the information can be

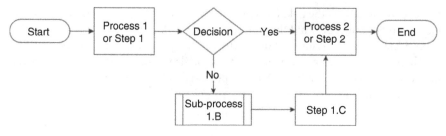

FIGURE 3.2 Process map.

transferred to an electronic document in Word, Excel, PowerPoint, or other software (Nelson et al., 2007; Sollecito & Hardison, 2020). The example provided above was created in Microsoft Visio which is designed specifically for such charts, diagramming, and vector graphics. With any of these tools, workflow diagrams should be created and used to model new ideas and processes, and continually adjusted as the team defines the ideal process.

More advanced flowcharts may also include probability factors within the decision points to indicate historical trends, where 15% or 0.15 are "Yes" or are "Admitted to Inpatient" within a process. For complex processes involving many distinct departments and professionals, some flowcharts may evolve to having "swim lanes" where two to five different roles are distinguished throughout the larger workflow. To do this, the roles (Nurse, Doctor, PT, Ops) are represented by rows (for charts flowing left to right) or columns (for charts flowing top to bottom) and their respective steps within the larger process are within their swim lane. Hand-offs, parallel processes, and other interdisciplinary discoveries may be made with this approach.

Brainstorming

At different points in the improvement cycle brainstorming can be used to engage team members. As a technique, brainstorming is a facilitated process to gather ideas and information from stakeholders. It is often used to inform process mapping and identification of innovative strategies for improvement because the ground rules in brainstorming expect the removal of judgments or criticism of ideas when generating solutions. It creates a venue for creativity and engagement while encouraging as many ideas as possible from members of the interprofessional team. Once ideas are identified, the team can combine ideas to generate a path to improvement. If the team is not able to pare down the list to prioritize a path forward, nominal group voting can be used.

Using office tools, white boards, stickie notes, or large poster-sized paper taped to walls in a conference rooms, teams will collaborate to develop cause and effect diagrams, failure points (FMEA), and flowcharts. Those closest to the process will likely have the best ideas and a PICK chart is an easy way to visualize and rate opportunities for improvement. A PICK chart rates the expected resources or effort needed to support the intervention (X-axis) versus the potential impact (Y-axis) (Figure 3.3). High impact, low effort projects identified in the upper left corner are "Implement"

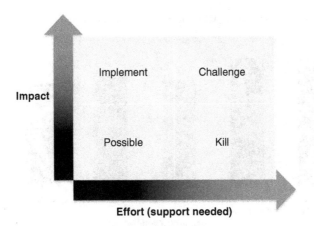

FIGURE 3.3 PICK chart.

or quick-wins. While high impact, high effort "Challenge" projects will need more thought, estimates, and planning for a better informed decision to proceed; potentially including budget requests for more staff, software, and other resources. Low-impact, high-effort project ideas are "Kill"; and low-impact, low-effort projects are "Possible." Using this framework and two scales for effort and impact, groups can focus on the handful of hundreds of possible interventions.

Bar Charts

Bar charts are a common and simple way to display data when you want to offer points of comparison, perhaps over time or across categories, such as nursing units or service type. They are very common in healthcare improvement because they are easily understood and familiar to most people. The bar length is proportional to the data value and the data is typically nominal or ordinal data (Chartblocks, 2018). In constructing a bar chart one axis represents a numerical value and the other offers a description of the categories of comparison. Figure 3.4 displays Medicare Average Length of Stay (ALOS) by Acute Care Hospital Type for the 2,731 hospitals included in the Centers for Medicare and Medicaid Services (CMS) Value-Based Purchasing (VBP) for FY2020 with publicly reported results, as well as information from the FY 2020 Final Rule and Correction Notice Inpatient Prospective Payment System (IPPS) Impact Files.

Pareto Charts

Pareto charts are similar to a bar chart that ranks related measures in decreasing order of occurrence. They are intended to analyze data about the frequency of problems in a process. Pareto charts separate the significant aspects of a problem from trivial ones. By graphically separating elements using distribution in a Pareto chart, teams can focus effort where the greatest impact is seen. The Pareto principle is based on distribution related to the significant few and the trivial many. Stated a different way,

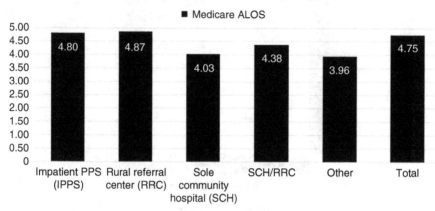

FIGURE 3.4 Bar chart example.

ALOS, average length of stay.

the significant few generally makes up 80% of the whole while the trivial many makes up the remaining 20%. The largest or longest bars will represent where improvement efforts will do the most good (IHI, 2020g).

The Pareto principle, known as the 80/20 rule, is often cited when improvement work is undertaken. The rule highlights the idea that 20% of the effort generates 80% of the results. This 80/20 rule is often used to help teams recognize that if they can identify the portion of a process that likely leads to the desired outcome, improvement in that process will likely bring success (IHI, 2020g).

Pareto charts help teams sort through situations where there are many possible causes by separating each cause into a component for analysis. Another benefit of a Pareto chart is it can provide the rationale for why a team chose to put their effort in one place when it defies the beliefs or assumptions of others (IHI, 2020g).

Pareto charts identify not only the frequency or a cause but also include a cumulative line. The steepness of the cumulative line with little arch signifies the first few problem areas make up a large percentage of the total problem and therefore represent the place to focus improvement activities. If the cumulative line is straight or flat, it signifies the elements that follow have similar contribution. This identifies that no problems stand out as being more bothersome than the rest, which limits problem solving (IHI, 2020g; Tiwari, 2018). Figure 3.5 uses the same data displayed in the Medicare ALOS chart by Hospital Type for the 2,731 Acute Care Hospitals with publicly reported CMS VBP FY2020 performance.

Histograms

Histograms are a numerical representation of a frequency distribution; essentially, they are bar charts that help teams see patterns in data, such as performance among the average. Histograms are used in continuous datasets representing things like time, weight,

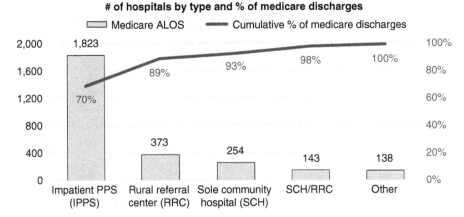

FIGURE 3.5 Pareto chart.

size, or temperature. Histograms are commonly used to see if there is a normal distribution of results and by charting standard deviations from the mean (average) to display the distribution of data (IHI, 2020h). Using the same set of data from above with the 2,731 Acute Care Hospitals included in CMS VBP FY2020 and the average payment adjustment of 0.16% (CMS VBP, 2019) as the line down the middle of the following chart, the frequency distribution is displayed by gray bars with the height corresponding to the % of total hospitals (Figure 3.6). The distribution of hospitals by standard deviation from the mean adjustment factor (+0.16%), represented by the gray bars and area, present something similar to a bell-shape, indicating a normal distribution.

Also charted is the CMS VBP Adjustment factor as a green bar and a green trend line, illustrating the 'linear exchange rate' used to re-distribute the 2% withhold from Medicare Inpatient Discharge payments. The average VBP adjustment factor 0.16% is net the -2.00%; as in, a hospital has earned back 2.16%; and a bonus payment of +0.16% is paid on top of each Inpatient Discharge in the current Fiscal Year (FY2020). This program is self-funded with penalties from hospitals with scores below 0.00% funding the bonus payments of those with adjustment factors above 0.00%. From this distribution, we can see the most common performance is below the average but within 0.5 standard deviations of the mean; as 602 hospitals are ≥ -0.5 and <0 standard deviations from the mean, representing 22% of all hospitals. While a traditional normal distribution has 38.2% falling within one standard deviation from the mean, this distribution is extremely similar with 38.8% within ≥ -0.5 and <0.5 standard deviations. Moreover, 95.4% of CMS VBP hospitals (2,606 of 2,731) fall within two standard deviations from the mean (≥ -2.0 and <2.0), which is the traditional normal distribution falling within that range.

Run Charts

Run charts are displays of data over time that can detect small changes in process stability so the effect of a change can be detected. Run charts help improvement teams determine how well a process is performing and help teams determine if the change

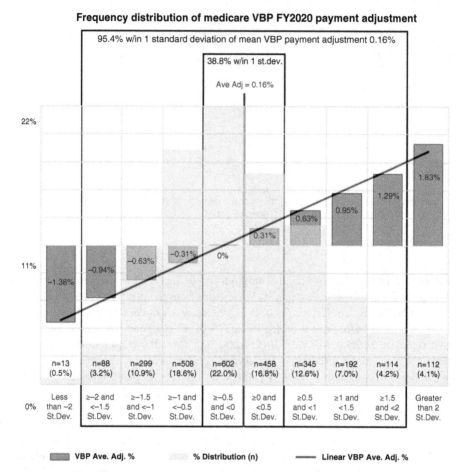

Frequency distribution of medicare VBP FY2020 payment adjustment

FIGURE 3.6 Histogram.

that was made is really an improvement. An advantage of run charts is the data can be displayed in real time so patterns can be observed. Run charts are line graphs where data is plotted over time so it helps establish effectiveness of a change. (IHI, 2020i; Sollecito & Hardison, 2020).

Figure 3.7 displays inpatient discharges per day, by month for a hospital. The chart indicates performance ranging from 31 to 38 discharges per day, with a 36-month (three-year) average of 33.7 discharges per day. The simple representation of the average within a line chart of monthly performance provides a 'run chart' where the goal is to make runs above the average, or below depending on the measure. If ALOS was being trended, a key-driver of discharges per day, or infection rates, readmissions and other adverse events; the goal would be to make a run below the average. Continuous improvement entails many small improvements intended to move the average performance over time. In addition to performance on either side of the average, a run could be consecutive time periods moving in one direction; where five to seven consecutive time periods moving up or down would indicate a level of significance.

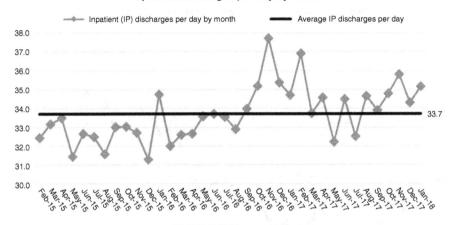

FIGURE 3.7 Run chart.

Control Charts

Control charts help organizations study how a process changes over time and build on a run chart. Similar to trended performance over days, weeks, or months with the average or mean rate drawn as a straight line to deduce 'runs', a control chart includes straight lines for standard deviations from the mean, typically at +/- 1 and 2 standard deviations, maybe +/- 3 standard deviations (6 sigma) where 99.7% of observed performance exists in a normal distribution. Control charts should be used throughout an improvement initiative and are very easy to construct in Excel or other spreadsheet applications that allow the calculation of an average and standard deviation (st. dev.). Figure 3.8 was constructed in Excel using those formulas, calculations for mean x -2, x -1, x +1, and x +2, cells that run parallel to monthly performance repeating each of those limits along with mean, and creating six rows of data to chart: Monthly performance, -2 st. dev., -1 st. dev., mean, +1 st. dev., +2 st. dev.

At the start of improvement activity, the control chart offers the baseline of performance; indicated in the control chart below by orange markers. As cycles of improvement or tests of change occur the control informs the team about the impact the change is having and what kind of variation exists. After an improvement activity, control charts help the team and the organization appreciate whether the change is sustained (Nelson et al., 2007; Sollecito & Hardison, 2020).

SUMMARY

This chapter offers information to guide selection of appropriate tools and measures to assist change leaders in rigorous use of improvement tools and highlights the value of interprofessional project teams to address the cost-quality dilemma. The complex and changing practice environment provides a venue steeped with situations

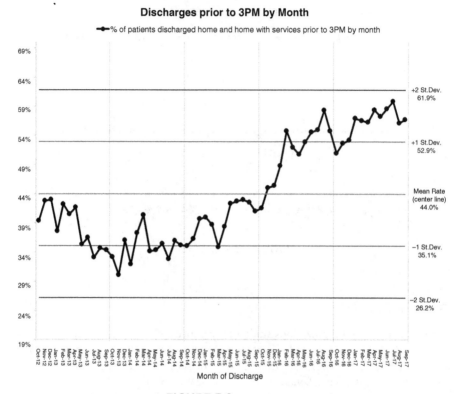

Discharges prior to 3PM by Month

—●—% of patients discharged home and home with services prior to 3PM by month

FIGURE 3.8 Control chart.

worthy of attention aimed at improvement however, staying true to a disciplined and systematic approach without stifling creativity and innovation often becomes a larger obstacle.

- Data can be used to tell the story one desires to tell. Likewise, the inappropriate use of tools can lead to misleading results. A challenge for any improvement project rests in detailed planning and judicial use of data and tools.
- Irrespective of the role on the team or professional discipline, each team member has the responsibility to approach improvement projects committed to the integrity of the work through appropriate application of models, methods, and tools.
- The ability to embrace the unique contribution, knowledge, and skills of inter-professional team members distinguishes mediocre improvement from the exceptional.
- Working to achieve sustainability of improvement projects, the definition and establishment of competencies related to leadership and participation in inter-professional quality improvement teams is an expectation.

- Thoughtful and disciplined quality improvement creates value and is the foundation for organizational learning that influences a pipeline of activity leading to safe, high quality care, and outcomes that extend to patients, populations, and communities.

REFLECTION QUESTIONS

1. You have been asked to lead a quality improvement project. What steps would you take to plan the work?
2. You are working in an ambulatory clinic and clinicians tell you that they are following all the steps of an evidence-based clinical guideline process to improve a quality metric for a large payer, but the trended reports show a decline. What would you do first to understand the disconnect between the reported outcome and the clinicians' statements?
3. A hospital department is trying to improve the efficiency in the care provided. If addressing the cost of doing business without compromising quality is the goal, what questions would you ask to gain an appreciation for the data they will need to analyze?
4. Identify what is the value of one or more of the figures provided in the chapter. Provide rationale for your answer(s).

REFERENCES

Agency for Healthcare Research and Quality. (n.d. a). *Team STEPPS National Implementation.* http://teamstepps.ahrq.gov/about-2cl_3.htm

Agency for Healthcare Research and Quality. (n.d. b). *TeamSTEPPS: Strategies and tools to enhance performance and patient safety.* http://www.ahrq.gov/professionals/education/curriculum-tools/teamstepps/index.html

Agency for Healthcare Research and Quality. (2015). *TeamSTEPPS 2.0.* https://www.ahrq .gov/teamstepps/instructor/fundamentals/index.html

Agency for Healthcare Research and Quality. (2018). *NQMC measure domain definitions: Health care delivery measure domains.* https://www.ahrq.gov/gam/summaries/domain -definitions/index.html

Armstrong, G., & Sables-Baus, S. (2020). *Leadership and systems improvement for the DNP.* Springer Publishing Company.

Berwick, D. M. (1989). Sounding board, continuous improvement as an ideal in health care. *The New England Journal of Medicine, 320*(1), 53–56. https://doi.org/10.1056/ nejm198901053200110

Bowen, M., & Neuhauser, D. (2013). Understanding and managing variation: Three different perspectives. *Implementation Science, 8,* S1. https://doi.org/10.1186/1748-5908-8-s1-s1

Centers for Medicare and Medicaid Services. (2019). CMS hospital value-based purchasing program results for fiscal year 2020. *Fact sheet, CMS Newsroom, October 29, 2019.* https://www.cms.gov/newsroom/fact-sheets/cms-hospital-value-based-purchasing -program-results-fiscal-year-2020

Chartblocks. (2018). *When to use a bar chart.* https://www.chartblocks.com/en/support/faqs/faq/when-to-use-a-bar-chart

CMS Hospital Value-Based Purchasing Program Results for Fiscal Year 2020. https://www.cms.gov/newsroom/fact-sheets/cms-hospital-value-based-purchasing-program-results-fiscal-year-2020

Danna, D. (2013). Organizational structure and analysis. In L. Roussel (Ed.), *Management and leadership for nurse administrators* (6th ed.). Jones & Bartlett Learning.

Deming, W. E. (1986). *Out of the crisis.* MIT Press.

Donabedian, A. (1980). *The definition of quality and approaches to its assessment.* Health Administration Press.

Gerald R. Ford School of Public Policy. (n.d.). *Comparison of approaches to measuring cost impact: Cost benefit, cost-effectiveness, and cost utility analyses.* http://www.mihealthfund.org/wp-content/uploads/2018/05/Resource-Sheet_ComparisonsCostMethods.pdf

Graban, M. (2016). *Lean hospitals: Improving quality, patient safety, and employee engagement* (3rd ed.). CRC Press.

Mark Graban & Constancy Inc. (2020). *Mark Graban's lean blog: Types of waste in healthcare.* https://www.leanblog.org/eight-types-of-waste-in-healthcare

Health Resources and Services Administration. (2011). *Quality improvement.* https://www.hrsa.gov/sites/default/files/quality/toolbox/508pdfs/qualityimprovement.pdf

Hwang, J. & Christensen, C. (2008). Disruptive innovation in health care delivery: A framework for business-model innovation. *Health Affairs, 27*(5), 1329–1335. https://www.healthaffairs.org/doi/full/10.1377/hlthaff.27.5.1329

Institute for Healthcare Improvement. (2020a). *Quality improvement essentials toolkit.* http://www.ihi.org/resources/Pages/Tools/Quality-Improvement-Essentials-Toolkit.aspx

Institute for Healthcare Improvement. (2020b). *Science of improvement: Forming the team.* http://www.ihi.org/resources/Pages/HowtoImprove/ScienceofImprovementFormingtheTeam.aspx

Institute for Healthcare Improvement. (2020c). *Science of improvement: Establishing measures.* http://www.ihi.org/resources/Pages/HowtoImprove/ScienceofImprovementEstablishingMeasures.aspx

Institute for Healthcare Improvement. (2020d). *Cause and effect diagram.* http://www.ihi.org/resources/Pages/Tools/CauseandEffectDiagram.aspx

Institute for Healthcare Improvement. (2020e). *Failure mode effect analysis.* http://www.ihi.org/resources/Pages/Tools/FailureModesandEffectsAnalysisTool.aspx

Institute for Healthcare Improvement. (2020f). *Science of improvement: Testing changes.* http://www.ihi.org/resources/Pages/HowtoImprove/ScienceofImprovementTestingChanges.aspx

Institute for Healthcare Improvement. (2020g). *Pareto diagram.* http://www.ihi.org/resources/Pages/Tools/ParetoDiagram.aspx

Institute for Healthcare Improvement. (2020h). *Histograms.* http://www.ihi.org/resources/Pages/Tools/Histogram.aspx

Institute for Healthcare Improvement. (2020i). *Run charts.* http://www.ihi.org/resources/Pages/Tools/RunChart.aspx

Institute of Medicine. (1999). *To err is human: Building a safer health system.* National Academies Press.

Institute of Medicine. (2001). *Crossing the quality chasm: A new health system for the 21st century.* National Academy Press.

Johnson, J. K., & Sollecito, W. A. (2020). *McLaughlin and Kaluzny's continuous quality improvement in health care* (5th ed.). Jones & Bartlett Learning.

Lighter, D. (2011). *Advanced performance improvement in health care: Principles and methods.* Jones & Bartlett Publishers.

Nelson, E., Batalden, P., & Godfrey, M. (2007). *Quality by design: A clinical microsystems approach.* Jossey-Bass.

Popovich, E., Wiggin, H., & Barach, P. (2020). Lean and six sigma management: Building a foundation for optimal patient care using patient flow statistics. In *McLaughlin & Kaluzny's continuous quality improvement in healthcare* (5th ed.). Jones & Bartlett Learning.

Ramaswamy, R., Johnson, J., & Hirschhorn, L. (2020). Integrating implementation science approaches into continuous quality improvement. In *McLaughlin & Kaluzny's continuous quality improvement in healthcare* (5th ed.). Jones & Bartlett Learning.

Sables-Baus, S., & Armstrong, G. (2020). Quality improvement: The essentials. In G. Armstrong & S. Sables-Baus (Eds.), *Leadership and systems improvement for the DNP.* Springer Publishing Company.

Shewhart, W. A. (1923). *Economic control of quality of manufactured product.* D. Van Nostrand Company, Inc.

Shortell, S. M., Bennett, C. L., & Byck, G. R. (1998). Assessing the impact of continuous quality improvement on clinical practice: What it will take to accelerate progress. *The Milbank Quarterly, 76*(4), 593–624. https://doi.org/10.1111/1468-0009.00107

Sollecito, W., & Hardison, D. (2020). Understanding variation, tool, and data sources for CQI in health care. In *McLaughlin & Kaluzny's Continuous quality improvement in healthcare* (5th ed.). Jones & Bartlett Learning.

Sollecito, W., & Johnson, J. (2020). The global evolution of continuous quality improvement: From Japanese manufacturing to global health services. In *McLaughlin & Kaluzny's continuous quality improvement in healthcare* (5th ed.). Jones & Bartlett Learning.

Stoecklein, M. (2015). *Understanding and Misunderstanding Variation in Healthcare: Case Study.* ThedaCare Center for Healthcare Value. https://createvalue.org/wp-content/uploads/Understanding-and-Misunderstanding-Variation-in-Healthcare.pdf

Taylor, F. (2011). *The principles of scientific management.* Prism Key Press.

Thomas, P. L., Harris, J. L., & Roussel, L. A. (2018). Creative and meaningful clinical immersions. In J. L. Harris, L. Roussel, & P. L. Thomas (Eds.), *Initiating and Sustaining the Clinical Nurse Leader Role: A practical Guide* (3rd Ed., pp. 109–122). Jones & Bartlett Learning.

Thomas, P., & Winter, J. (2019). Synergistic interprofessional teams: Essential drivers of person-centered care. In J. L. Harris, L. Roussel, C. Dearman, & P. L. Thomas (Eds.), *Project planning and management: A guide for nurses and interprofessional teams* (3rd ed.). Jones & Bartlett Learning.

Tiwari, A. (2018). *Pareto chart and its uses.* https://anexas.net/Blog/pareto-chart-and-its-uses

UL Knowledge Services. (2013). *Applying lean principles to improve healthcare quality and safety.* https://legacy-uploads.ul.com/wp-content/uploads/sites/40/2015/02/UL_WP_Final_Applying-Lean-Principles-to-Improve-Healthcare-Quality-and-Safety_v11_HR.pdf

CASE EXEMPLARS FOR APPLICATION

An Actionable Immunization Plan That Collects and Presents Improvement Outcomes

John Deckro

In order to immunize and protect hospitalized patients from influenzas, the importance of an actionable and responsive data collection and dissemination is paramount to spreading influenza. This exemplar describes the collaboration by an interprofessional team to create a daily summary of the patients, their flu immunization status, and outcomes.

Vaccination of hospitalized patients needing a seasonal influenza (flu) shot is an important health-promotional activity. While efficacy varies with each flu season, vaccination is considered one of the most cost-effective ways to decrease associated morbidity and mortality. The Centers for Disease Control and Prevention (CDC) states: "To avoid missed opportunities for vaccination, providers should offer vaccination during . . . hospitalizations" (Grohskopf et al., 2019). Inpatient flu shots are also a Joint Commission quality marker. While obtaining the needed data was a critical underpinning of this plan, developing 'buy-in' among stakeholders from administration, nursing, pharmacy, medical support services, physicians, informatics, case managers, and respiratory therapy was the key to success.

A small community medical center, part of a national organization, had low inpatient flu vaccination rates. Respiratory therapists, social workers, and pharmacists also participated in discharge rounds and were among some of the influential advocates for the timely ordering of vaccines. Overall, and with the medical center, nursing, and pharmacy leadership's endorsement, a position that 'flu shots were everybody's responsibility' was introduced. The *Daily Flu Shot List* was also distributed to the unit clerks, nurse managers and unit champions to provide another avenue to address vaccination before patient discharge.

As with many improvement plans, inherent barriers exist. Such barriers specific to this plan included: 1) vaccinations were considered an outpatient responsibility; 2) vaccines were not routinely stocked on the units; 3) medical center policies specified that all medications/vaccinations administered to inpatients require a provider's order in the electronic medical record, and 4) nurses assigned to the clinical units often found it challenging to secure the required order from the busy prescribers in a timely manner.

Building upon the work of Cohen et al. (2015), several Plan-Do-Study-Act (PDSA) cycles were executed and a successful paradigm evolved. Pertinent and timely data was sought-out, analyzed, and distributed to a variety of stakeholders. A staff member with expertise in programing developed and assisted in the testing and refinement of a programming routine known as Structured Query Knowledge (SQL). The SQL routine queried the Corporate Data Warehouse for admitted patients, their flu vaccination status, and possible contraindications and/or a history of vaccine refusals during the current flu season. This routine was run each morning. In conjunction with medical center quality management personnel, a document template was prepared that listed: 1) inpatients, stratified by unit, needing a flu shot or documentation of a refusal during the current admission; 2) the prescribing clinicians for the patient; and 3) known contraindications to vaccination. The *Daily Flu Shot List* was made available for morning discharge rounds for review with prescribing clinicians. Respiratory therapists, social workers, and pharmacists also participated in discharge rounds and were among some of the most influential advocates for the timely ordering of vaccines. Overall, and with the medical center, nursing, and pharmacy leadership's endorsement, a position that 'flu shots were everybody's responsibility' was introduced. The *Daily Flu Shot List* was also distributed to the unit clerks, nurse managers and unit champions to provide another avenue to address vaccination before patient discharge.

While obtaining the needed data was a critical underpinning of this effort, developing 'buy-in' to the effort among stakeholders from administration, nursing, pharmacy, medical support services, physicians, informatics, case managers, and respiratory therapy was the key to success. The medical center was able to raise the percentage of inpatient acceptance of flu vaccination or documentation of a refusal for each admission from below the organization's national average to ~7% above the national average.

REFLECTION QUESTIONS

1. As a healthcare professional or administrator, what initial steps are required when developing an improvement process that includes data collection and analysis?
2. What role does each member of an improvement team play in any improvement team and why? What ways can improvement outcomes be disseminated?

High Reliability Organizations Through Collaborative Communication, Education, Innovation, and Data Sharing

Coy L. Smith and Erika DeMartinis

A nursing leadership team developed and implemented an innovation framework that relies on interprofessional communication, education, innovation, and collaborative data sharing commensurate with national and international agency models. The positive impact of the interprofessional collaboration and communication was foundational to quality and safety outcomes, primarily decreased fall rates and restraint use, toward a high reliability healthcare system. Using multidirectional and concurrent data, patient outcomes were improved.

Using a 'Unit Tracking Board', safety huddles occurred where nursing, during each shift, communicated key safety concerns based on available data and daily when interprofessional teams were present. This communication forum provided the platform to bridge continuous communication between disciplines and reduce patient safety issues. Key quality and safety metrics were focal points for huddle discussions that had been identified and entered on the Unit Tracking Board. This process provided a method for continuous tracking of improvements.

Incorporating safety huddles, using a Unit Tracking Board, is an innovative approach to a cultural change that fosters innovation, interprofessional communication, and change directed at quality and safety outcomes. This supports data present in the literature that focuses on how interprofessional teams are pivotal to continuous quality improvement and are essential for innovation to occur. With spread of this innovation throughout healthcare organizations, quality and patient safety will become a culture dedicated to improvement, supported by all staff.

REFLECTION QUESTIONS

1. Consider that you have been tasked as a unit champion to assist with a system wide improvement initiative. What considerations and steps will you take to ensure staff are active participants in the initiative and how will you communicate results?
2. What are the key drivers associated with a high reliability organization and how may this be accomplished by all staff?

REFERENCES

Cohen, E. S., Ogrinc, G., Taylor, T., Brown, C., & Geiling, J. (2015). Influenza vaccination rates for hospitalised patients: A multiyear quality improvement effort. *BMJ Quality Safety*, *24*(3), 221–227. https://doi.org/10.1136/bmjqs-2014-003556

Grohskopf, L. A., Alyanak, E., Broder, K. R., Walter, E. B., Fry, A. M., & Jernigan, D. B. (2019). Prevention and control of seasonal influenza with vaccines: Recommendations of the advisory committee on immunization practices – United States, 2019-20 influenza season. *MMWR. Recommendations and Reports, 68*(3), 1–21. https://doi.org/10.15585/mmwr.rr6803a1

Using Data to Calculate Quality and Opportunity Cost

Teresa Pazdral

Sustainability for a community hospital could mean data mining for an existing opportunity and calculating the value of quality. Our disproportionate share hospital on the Massachusetts/New Hampshire border serves a population which is 80% public pay. The hospital is a medium-sized facility with 186 licensed beds and an outsized emergency room (ER) with 68,000 annual visits. The ER's rate of patients that 'Left without being seen' (LWBS), a publicly reported measure, creates an inability to move people from the ER into the hospital. Providers cannot see patients without the precious commodity of a bed. Or can they?

Fifteen years ago the facility started segmenting the care of the population by creating a rapid assessment zone (replace 'room' with rapid assessment zone) staffed 14 hours a day by an Advanced Practice Provider (APP) for the 15% of patients triaged as low acuity. Recent improvement projects across the country have tried to further segment the population into those who need a moderate amount of diagnostic evaluation and treatment but still, to the clinical eye of the triaging personnel, look like that evaluation and likely discharge could take place in 2 to 3 hours. In order to determine the value of such a space in the facility, an analysis of data on admissions and discharges from the previous year has been completed.

The two work projects followed the data analysis. The first was to establish the financial value of the streamlined care of the segmented population using a predictable admission rate of 12% with a rate of 3.7% for LWBS. By predicting a decrease in the LWBS rate and calculating the expected income from the admissions lost, a range of increased revenue was identified.

The data were also used to further model information about the time of day of arrivals, the mode of arrival, the triage severity of the patient and the ultimate disposition of the patient, replicating the unit flow unit based on the number of beds required. The peak volume day and hour are modeled in Figure 3.9, with 15 patients arriving (the far left of this graphic) and 2.6 patients being admitted to an inpatient unit (in the lower left corner of the graphic), 4.3 patients leaving from an ER exam room (in the lower right corner of the graphic), and 8.1 patients leaving directly from

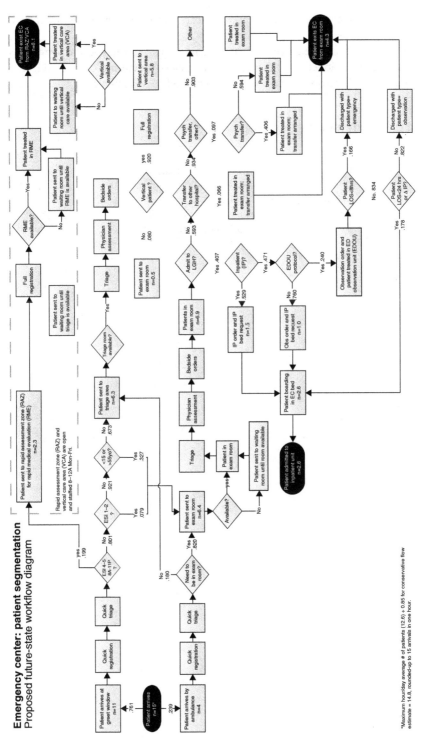

FIGURE 3.9 Emergency center segmentation.

the rapid assessment zone or a new proposed care area (in the upper right corner of the graphic).

The combination of the need for the redesigned space, with specific operational plans based on our modelling and a tangible financial opportunity, convinced leadership to prioritize investment in a project-constrained environment.

REFLECTION QUESTIONS

1. Consider all the data you routinely collect as you provide patient care. What clinical issues can you identify that have both cost and quality implications that might benefit from an analysis of data?
2. As you consider the design and workflow of your practice, what changes in space configuration and workflow would improve cost, quality, and efficiency?

4

Data as the Centerpiece of Administrative and Clinical Decisions

James L. Harris and Patricia L. Thomas

OBJECTIVES

1. Identify the value of data to inform administrative and clinical decisions.
2. List key attributes of performance, strategic thinking, and operational thinking necessary to achieve peak efficiency in healthcare organizations.
3. Determine the importance of analyzing data in order to create sustainable change in organizations and clinical practice.
4. Explain how tools and techniques are essential to successful problem identification and achievement of defined outcomes.

CORE COMPETENCIES

- Adaptability to change, challenge assumptions, and remain data oriented and patient-centric
- Develop quality and value-based care models for sustainability
- Knowledgeable of information technology and future developments in healthcare
- Knowledgeable of reliability and utility of data for decisions
- Ability to formulate new perception of education, employment, and entrepreneurship in response to the fourth industrial revolution

INTRODUCTION

Managers who operate in vision versus circumstances offer clarity when healthcare infrastructures require change. None of the changes are more discerning than understanding the value of how reliable and evidence-based data can inform administrative and clinical decisions (Marjanovic et al., 2017). Data has become the new currency of power underpinning decisions in the current healthcare landscape.

While governance and culture are significant in any organization, data are pivotal for successful leadership decisions. Meaningful data are a key ingredient for quality, safety, and sustainable outcomes. All data, including the historical processes of collection, analysis, and subsequent actions must be considered in any organization when changes are required. Processes that are not linked to outcomes lose value and sustainability over time. If outcomes do not inform and discipline the process, loss occurs and decisions may become a distractor (Porter-O'Grady & Malloch, 2015). To avoid this scenario, data must be a primary driver for administrative and clinical decisions. Otherwise, the absence of meaningful data that guides strategy, operational thinking and clinical decisions has limited value to an organization (Marzorati & Pravettoni, 2017).

Throughout this chapter, the concept of value, as it relates to data, will be discussed as well as its influence on administrative and clinical decision-making. Attributes of performance, strategic initiatives, and operational thinking will also discussed in order to achieve peak performance. Data analysis and evidence-based tools are identified and the value they have when identifying problems, solutions, and achievement of defined outcomes.

VALUE

Regardless of the size and services provided by a healthcare organization, value has become a distinguishing theme that guides administrative and clinical decisions. In the recent decade, incentives have shifted from volume to value (Fulford, 2011; Wieten, 2015). As a result, the value of data cannot be underestimated. Data informs healthcare decisions and operations daily. Without meaningful data and managers who connect the right people together, decisions are unsystematic and deleterious outcomes arise. Hence, correlation can be mistaken for causation (McAfee & Brynjolfsson, 2012). Without data that has value and cross-function cooperation among users, decisions are made that could jeopardize the viability of any healthcare organization and patient outcomes.

Today, consumers are demanding more value for healthcare services provided. To guide operational thinking and clinical decisions, healthcare organizations collect data constantly from patients that focus on experiences, perceived quality, communication, access, and shared decision-making (Mohammed et al., 2015). Leaders and clinicians alike must consider a new lens to organize, analyze, and evaluate the data that are collected. Likewise, administrators and clinicians must also remain mindful that patient centeredness is essential in the current environment. Patient experiences must remain meaningful along the care trajectory in order to remain competitive.

Leaders and clinicians must challenge current assumptions of care delivery and create new models of care based on patient value (Porter & Lee, 2013; Porter & Teisberg, 2006). According to Porter in 2009 and 2010, a value-based care model must be guided by three key principles: (a) value provided to the patient according to the health outcomes per dollar spent, (b) care and treatment provided should be based on medical conditions, and (c) outcomes must be quantifiable and documented to include the patient's preferences within a team perspective. Minot (2009) supports the third principle and challenges leaders and clinicians to develop processes that measure and account for what is valued and managed.

Healthcare organizations and providers need and use data. Capturing the value of data requires much coordination and collaboration among users. This ensures effective use and alignment of data and its ongoing value to administrators and clinicians as decisions are made. While there is no single strategy that captures all the opportunities of how data can generate value for administrators and clinicians, value-chain thinking and value-chain mapping are useful in understanding the processes and activities associated with value (Marjanovic et al., 2017).

For over three decades, value chain has been associated with activities in an organization performed to deliver a valuable product to consumers. By definition, value chain represents activities that an organization performs to deliver a valuable product to a specific market (Porter, 1985; Simatupang et al., 2017). While its origin dates to application in operations management and process engineering for various industries, it has relevance today for healthcare in terms of providing value of care delivered in order to retain consumers (Ilyas et al., 2006; Porter, 1985; Womack et al., 1990). Value chain thinking and healthcare relevance can be best operationalized for healthcare when one considers four steps that include: (a) "value discovery (what intended value is going to be created?), (b) value design (how is value created?), (c) value delivery (how is value realized?), and (d) value capture (how is value captured?" (Simatupang et al., 2017, p. 11).

Value chain mapping on the other hand is another process useful for understanding healthcare value as its utility is recognized through identifying activities central to improvement opportunities aligned with a specific service offered or product line. Value chain mapping offers improvement teams a starting point for discussions, identifies gaps in services, service volume, and the identification of new metrics for monitoring outcomes and ultimate service sustainability (Mooney, 2014). As discussed, both value chain thinking and mapping are valuable in the turbulent and emerging healthcare market.

ATTRIBUTES OF PERFORMANCE, STRATEGIC THINKING, AND OPERATIONAL THINKING

Performance, strategic thinking, and operational thinking are intrinsically linked by attributes that revolve around efficient use of data in a constantly changing healthcare landscape. By definition, an attribute is a quality, charter, or characteristic ascribed to something or someone (Merriam-Webster, 2001). The foundational importance of performance, strategic thinking, and operational thinking attributes remains relevant as administrators and clinicians use data to reduce costs, improve flexibility and care delivery, and ensure the centrality of individuals are representative of the distinctiveness of an organization (Crema & Verbano, 2013). For purposes of this chapter, each attribute will be considered separately.

Using data to optimize performance require a shared culture across an organization and attention to what is being attributed as high performance. A detailed vision must be inclusive of multiple individuals and departments depending on the intended process and outcomes. While processes are more sensitive to differences, outcomes reflect all aspects of an issue. Processes cannot have value if not linked to an outcome (Mant, 2001).

Whatever is tolerated, one endorses. If one does not attribute data to achieving peak performance, what may one ascribe to the quality of an organization and its leaders? Several attributes and benefits of performance are integral to a successful journey in healthcare as cited in the literature (Greene & Green, 2017; McMurchy, 2009). Performance attributes and benefits for purposes of this chapter are listed in Table 4.1.

TABLE 4.1 Performance Attributes and Benefits

ATTRIBUTES	BENEFITS
Continuous Quality Improvement	Improved continuity and quality of care Improved operational efficiency and flow of information Data driven Reduced costs Improved satisfaction of employees and patients Stakeholder involvement/participation Effective planning
Patient-Centeredness	Improved access, flow, and seamless/coordinated care Clinical quality becomes a priority Patient and family involvement is encouraged and supported Equitable distribution of health resources
Information Oriented	Data are translated into transparent and actionable information Information and reporting requirements are prioritized Data are leveraged to gain market share Population health incentives are architected The effects of interventions and patterns of care delivery are recognized and encouraged Care access and comprehensiveness of care improved Care needs and service provision-based on market trends and user patterns are longitudinally predicted

(continued)

TABLE 4.1 Performance Attributes and Benefits (continued)	
ATTRIBUTES	**BENEFITS**
Adaptability	Strategy is pursued in order to find value Project goals are synergistic Goals are prioritized that align with strategy Evidence is used and new models of care created commensurate with identified needs and trends in healthcare
Fiscally Disciplined	Capital improvements balance fiscal capacities Fiscal goals and strategies are defined and communicated to accomplish each Inputs and outcomes are measured and adjustments made accordingly
Accountability	Individuals and teams assume responsibilities for successes and failures Effective transitions and corrective actions are based on data and evidence Pathways are created for bi-directional input Individual and group contributions are valued Opportunities are extended to create new and ongoing partnerships
Creativity	Individuals and teams are inspired to achieve excellence and generate new ideas Enthusiasm spreads throughout the organization Results-oriented activities are commonplace that engenders focused actions by others
Collaborative	Opportunities are created for life-long learning and team collaboration Strong and lasting partnerships are created An organizational culture of discovery and innovation are encouraged and rewarded

As presented in Table 4.1, performance attributes benefit the organization, patients, and employees. As a result, multiple strategies and objectives are developed that foster ongoing development, a culture of inclusiveness, and environments that value data-based performance.

Strategic thinking is a way of life in healthcare and includes several attributing characteristics. It requires fluidity and adaptability when internal and external forces require transformative actions and reconfiguration of goals and objectives. Linear thinking is shifted to collateral thinking that is multidirectional and supportive of the information age (Porter-O'Grady & Malloch, 2015; Schwab, 2017). Strategic thinking is developed with the big picture in mind and guides organizational direction.

Strategic thinkers as leaders value imagination, experimentation, and varying inputs as teams identify what works and what does not. Once leaders and teams identify this information, a new strategy is identified to improve outcomes across the organization (Githens, 2019; McCulloch, 2019).

Operational thinking on the other hand is purposeful and productivity oriented. Productivity dominates thoughts and actions. Operational thinking is attributed to data generation and methods that are sequential and concrete. The methods are beneficial to the organization in reducing risk and uncertainty, development of clinical guidelines, and validation of effective strategy. An additional benefit of operational thinking is predictability. Predictability linked to productivity is valued today as limited resources must be maximized with the shift from revenue management to cost management (Githens, 2019; McCulloch, 2019).

The attributes of performance, strategic thinking, and operational thinking are integral to organizational success. Balancing each offers organizational leaders and clinicians multiple opportunities to move from idea to action and envision the future.

CREATING SUSTAINABLE CHANGE THROUGH DATA ANALYSIS

The interacting and intersecting roadmap of data continues to change how administrative and clinical decisions are made. Understanding and using data offer opportunities for organizations to respond to individuals, the environment, and competing forces when change is imminent. Being adaptive and responsive to data in an organization are normative requisites for any decision-making infrastructure. Data provide signals and guideposts for actionable change as volume has shifted to value at the point-of-care. Failure to identify what is quality data and its importance, challenges data integrity and its analysis, and data variances will limit successful change in the long term. Just because data provides evidence of statistical significance, clinical significance may be absent. Conversely, clinical significance may be evident that would impact clinical outcomes with no evidence of statistical significance (Miller, 2019).

There is no question that data quality influence successful change in an era of unparalleled advancements in technology. While there are numerous data sources available for any healthcare organization that guides decisions and structural improvement, not all data are specific, dependable, and value-added. Understanding the different types of healthcare data and how it is presented offer much value when change is required. Healthcare data continues to inform treatment, cure, health promotion and prevention, global public health initiatives, volume indicators, and predictive models to forecast patient needs based on demographics (Marjanovic et al., 2017).

Regardless of the type of data available to any healthcare organization, the perplexing question remains, what is quality data? Universally, authors have sought to answer this question. Dating to the 1950s, investigators sought to examine the quality of products, definitions, product use, and conformance requirements. Inquiry in future decades will be focused on data quality (Crosby, 1988; General Administration of Quality Supervision, 2008; Wang & Strong, 1996; Zhu, 2015). In 2015, a hierarchical data quality assessment framework including quality dimensions, quality elements, and indicators were proposed. Subsequently, a two-layer data quality standard for assessing data quality followed to include availability, usability, reliability, relevance, and presentation quality (Cai & Zhu, 2015). The relevance of both offers the importance for assessing data quality.

There is little agreement on how data in healthcare should be measured, analyzed, and used. Differences continue to vary regarding the quality of care between organizations and how data are analyzed to formulate a conclusion. The differences require organizations to consider the selection of patients, randomization, and any inconsistency in data collection and analysis. This calls for organizations to use data from national databases that demonstrate utility and that is presented in user-friendly terms (Utzon et al., 2009). Likewise, administrators and clinicians must constantly identify what forces are in play when a change in operations or clinical practice is required. This requires a review of objective and measureable data, challenging other's thinking, questioning data accountability of teams, and the ability to infuse new sources of evidence in an organization. In other words, individuals and teams must study the process of data collection and analysis and stakeholders involved. This does not occur in a vacuum nor without considering what internal and external forces may be operating within the setting. Such forces may include resistance to change, poor quality data and analysis, and any reimbursement or accreditation requirements. Otherwise, sustainable change is jeopardized.

Good data quality and analysis have several beneficial advantages. Moreno (2017) offered insight into the advantages. Confidence in the data by users is pivotal to mitigating risk, compliance, efficiency, market advantage, and engendering a culture of data integrity. Without data quality and integrity, missed opportunities prevail, reputation deteriorates, and costs soar. To ensure the advantages and any changes are sustained in organizations, sustainable plans that promote data quality and analysis, required accountability of analysts, and a governance system is standardized when decisions regarding data corrections are necessary (SAS Insights, 2019).

TOOLS AND TECHNIQUES TO GUIDE PROBLEM IDENTIFICATION AND ACHIEVEMENT OF OUTCOMES

Advances in technology guide how we live, identify opportunities, and arrive at decisions. Technology offers individuals and groups the power to transform infrastructures that are critical to achieving quality, value, efficiency, and high-value care. Technology also provides various tools and techniques for users in order to achieve optimal outcomes. The use of tools and techniques are contingent on having reliable data infrastructures that eliminate artificial variability and provide data to reengineer processes for how problems are identified and meaningful outcomes are achieved.

There is no argument that problems that occur in healthcare and administrative decisions affect clinical decisions and vice versa. How healthcare organizations identify administrative or clinical problems vary. Many tools, techniques, and metrics only capture information that is specific to a select element. This information is used to inform the totality of the organization that may not specifically address the root cause of a problem or ways to correct an issue. No single tool, technique, or metric should stand alone when a decision is required (Porter-O'Grady & Malloch, 2017). Transparency in what tools, techniques, and metrics that are being used to identify problems and reach decisions creates a culture of value and inclusiveness of others. As a result, individuals and teams become fiscal and patient-centered stewards that ultimately benefit the organization, employees, and consumers of care.

Although it is unrealistic to anticipate all problems and consistently achieve sustainable outcomes from decisions made, there are tools and techniques that are useful in reducing risk and enhancing the well-being of individuals. Industrial tools and techniques for identifying problems and guiding decisions are central to continuously improving healthcare quality, safety, and value. Many of the tools and techniques were adopted over previous decades with their utility validated by organizational sustainability and value-added outcomes (Crema & Verbano, 2013; Deming, 1993; Feng & Manuel; 2008; Radnor et al., 2012; Varkey et al., 2006). Examples include, but are not limited to, use of a PDSA (Plan, Do, Study, Act) cycle, an analysis of the five Ps of a microsystem, root cause analysis, continuous quality management, process re-engineering, Lean, Six Sigma, SWOT analysis, evidence-based practice, value-based medicine, and evidence-based medicine. More recently, mind mapping, the Geographical Interface System (GIS) model, and scenario planning have been adopted to gain insight into valuation (Porter-O'Grady & Malloch, 2017). For purposes of this chapter, a selection of the right tools for the job from idea to execution of a project was presented in Chapter 3.

Regardless of the size of a healthcare organization, tremendous challenges are present and change is inevitable. The importance of using reliable data, tools, and techniques to inform administrative and clinical decisions cannot be underestimated. New models, tools, and techniques will be necessary as the fourth industrial revolution evolves. New technologies will affect all disciplines, organizations, and economies. They will inspire and innovate individuals toward progressive thought and inquiry necessary to succeed and navigate during turbulent times (Schwab, 2017).

Gwata (2019) identified a prerequisite necessary for organizational success in the fourth industrial revolution: to formulate new perceptions of education, employment, and entrepreneurship. Education must be organized where students have specialized knowledge in a field with complimentary information outside their specialization. As knowledge is broadened and new skill sets are acquired, individual opportunities for employment expand. Technology will continue to intensify and employees must embody an entrepreneurial spirit of innovation and continuous improvement. As new perceptions are formed of education, employment, and entrepreneurship and accompanied by cogent actions, objectives are achievable and technology will guide business processes and ultimately success.

SUMMARY

- Vision offers managers clarity to when and how to manage change.
- Data are the new currency of power.
- Processes not linked to outcomes lose value.

- Outcomes inform and discipline processes necessary for sound administrative and clinical decisions.
- Incentives in healthcare have shifted from volume to value.
- Data and cross-functional cooperation among users enhance value in healthcare.
- Patient experiences and their value must remain meaningful.
- Value-based care models are guided by health outcomes per dollar spent, conditions, and care outcomes.
- No single strategy, tool, or technique captures opportunities for value and sustainability.
- Value-chain technology and mapping assist administrators and clinical leaders to understand value.
- Adaptability and data responsiveness are normative requisites for a decision-making infrastructure.
- Data quality assessment and standards offer exemplars to assess data quality.
- No agreement exists on the best strategy to measure, analyze, and use data to guide healthcare decisions.
- Technology offers the power to transform infrastructures to achieve quality, value.
- Artificial variables must be eliminated in order to achieve optimal outcomes.
- No single tool, technique, or metric captures the totality of a problem.
- Data transparency creates an overarching culture of value and inclusiveness.
- Multiple tools and techniques exist to guide data collection, analysis, and decision processes.
- New metrics, tools, and techniques will evolve in the fourth industrial revolution.
- New perceptions of education, employment, and entrepreneurship must be reconfigured in the future.

REFLECTION QUESTIONS

1. From your previous and current experiences, what steps would you take to ensure data are collected, analyzed, and used to guide administrative and clinical decisions?
2. Discuss and describe how would you assess the current organizational culture in order to reconfigure perceptions of education, employment, and entrepreneurship based on the fourth industrial revolution.
3. Assess recent patient satisfaction data. What strategies would you use to ensure data are reliable and what steps would you take to change negative outcomes?

REFERENCES

Cai, L., & Zhu, Y. (2015). The challenges of data quality and data quality assessment in the Big Data Era. *Data Science Journal, 14*, 2. http://doi.org/10.5334/dsj-2015-002

Crema, M., & Verbano, C. (2013). Future developments in health care performance management. *Journal of Multidisciplinary Health, 6,* 415–421. https://doi.org/10.2147/JMDH.S54561

Crosby, P. B. (1988). *Quality is free: The art of making quality certain.* McGraw-Hill.

Deming, W. E. (1993). *The new economics.* MIT Press.

Feng, Q., & Manuel, C. M. (2008). Under the knife: A survey of six sigma programs in US healthcare organizations. *International Journal of Health Care and Quality Assurance, 21,* 535–547. https://doi.org/10.1108/09526860810900691

Fulford, K. W. (2011). The value of evidence and evidence of values: Bringing together value-based and evidence-based practice in policy and service development in mental health. *Journal of Evaluation in Clinical Practice, 17*(5), 976–987. https://doi.org/10.1111/j.1365-2753.2011.01732.x

General Administration of Quality Supervision Inspection and Quarantine of the People's Republic of China. (2008). *Quality management systems-fundamentals and vocabulary* (GB/T19000-2008/ISO9000:2005).

Githens, G. (2019). *How to think strategically. Sharpen your mind. Develop your competency. Contribute to success.* Maven House Press.

Greene, D., & Green, R. (2017). *10 characteristics of high-performing healthcare organizations.* https://uscan.gehealthcarepartners.com/insight-detail/top-10-characteristics-of-high-performing-healthca

Gwata, M. (2019). *To flourish in the fourth industrial revolution, we need to rethink these 3 things.* https://www.weforum.org/agenda/2019/08/fourth-industrial-revolution-education/

Ilyas, R. M., Banwet, D. K., Shankar, R. (2006). Value chain relationship-A strategy matrix. *Supply Chain Forum: An International Journal, 7*(2), 56–72. https://doi.org/10.1080/16258312.2007.11517176

Mant, J. (2001). Process versus outcome indicators in the assessment of quality of health care. *International Journal for Quality in Health Care, 13*(6), 475–480. https://doi.org/10.1093/intqhc/13.6.475

Marjanovic, S., Ghiga, I., Yang, M., & Knack, A. (2017). *Understanding value in health data ecosystems.* Rand Corporation.

Marzorati, C., & Pravettoni, G. (2017). Value as the key concept in the health care system: How it has influenced medical practice and clinical decision-making processes. *Journal of Multidisciplinary Health, 10,* 101–106. https://doi.org/10.2147/JMDH.S122383

McAfee, A., & Brynjolfsson, E. (2012). Big data: The management revolution. *Harvard Business Review, 90*(10), 60–66.

McCullouch, B. (2019). *Strategic vs. operational thinking: What's the difference?* https://www.bobmcculloch.com/articles?blogid=22668&&modex=blogid&modexval=22668

McMurchy, D. (2009). *What are the critical attributes and benefits of a high-quality primary healthcare system?* https://www.researchgate.net/publication/237374751_WHAT_ARE_THE_CRITICAL_ATTRIBUTES_AND_BENEFITS_OF_A_HIGH-QUALITY_PRIMARY_HEALTHCARE_SYSTEM

Merriam-Webster. (2001). Attribute. In *Merriam-Webster's new collegiate dictionary.* Random House.

Miller, R. J. (2019). Evaluating statistical approaches in nursing. In C. R. King, S. O. Gerard, & C. G. Rapp (Eds.), *Essential knowledge for CNL and APRN nurse leaders* (pp. 283–295). Springer Publishing Company.

Minot, J. (2009). *Geographic variation and health care cost growth: Research to inform a complex diagnosis.* http://www.rwjf.org/en/library/research/2009/10/geographic-variation-and-health-care-cost-growth.html

Mohammed, K., Nolan. M. B., Rajjo, T., Shah, N. D., Prokop, L. J., Varkey. P., & Murad. M. H. (2016). Creating a patient-centered health care delivery system a systematic review of health care quality from the patient perspective. *American Journal of Medical Quality, 31*(1), 12–21. https://doi.org/10.1177/1062860614545124

Mooney, C. L. (2014). *5 reasons CR professionals need a value chain map.* www.greenbiz.com/blog/2014/01/09/5-reasons-cr-professionals-need-value-chain-map

Moreno, H. (2017). The importance of data quality—Good, bad, or ugly. *Forbes.* https://www.forbes.com/sites/forbesinsights/2017/06/05/the-importance-of-data-quality-good-bad-or-ugly/#292180cf10c4

Porter, M. E. (1985). *Competitive advantage-Creating a sustaining superior performance.* The Free Press.

Porter, M. E. (2009). A strategy for health care reform-toward a value-based system. *New England Journal of Medicine, 361*(2), 109–112. https://doi.org/10.1056/NEJMp0904131

Porter, M. E. (2010). What is value in health care? *New England Journal of Medicine, 363*(26), 2477–2481. https://doi.org/10.1056/NEJMp1011024

Porter, M. E., & Lee, T. H. (2013). The strategy that will fix health care. *Harvard Business Review, 91*(12), 24.

Porter, M. E., & Teisberg, E. O. (2006). *Redefining health care: Creating value-based competition on results.* Harvard Business Press.

Porter-O'Grady, T., & Malloch, K. (2015). *Quantum leadership: Building better partnerships for better health.* Jones & Bartlett Learning.

Porter-O'Grady, T., & Malloch, K. (2017). *Quantum leadership: Creating sustainable value in health care.* Jones & Bartlett Learning.

Radnor, Z. J., Holweg, M., & Waring, J. (2012). Lean in healthcare: the unfilled promise? *Social Science Medicine, 74,* 364–371. https://doi.org/10.1016/j.socscimed.2011.02.011

SAS Insights. (2019). *The importance of data quality: A sustainable approach.* https://www.sas.com/en_us/insights/articles/data-management/importance-of-data-quality-a-sustainable-approach.html

Schwab, K. (2017). *The fourth industrial revolution.* Penguin Random House.

Simatupang, T. M., Piboonrungroj, P., & Williams, S. (2017). The emergence of value chain thinking. *International Journal of Value Chain Management, 8*(1), 1–19. https://doi.org/10.1504/IJVCM.2017.082685

Utzon, J., Petri, A. L., & Christophersen, S. (2009). Analysis of quality data based on national clinical databases. *Ugeskr Laeger, 171*(38), 2723–2727.

Varkey, P. K., Reller, M., & Resar, R. K. (2006). Basics of quality improvement in health care. *Mayo Clinic Proceedings, 82,* 735–739. https://doi.org/10.1016/S0025-6196(11)61194-4

Wang, R. Y., & Strong, D. M. (1996). Beyond accuracy: What data quality means to data consumers. *Journal of Management Information Systems, 12*(4), 5–33. https://doi.org/10.1080/07421222.1996.11518099

Wieten, S. (2015). *What the patient wants: An investigation of the methods of ascertaining patient values in evidence-based medicine and values-based practice.* https://doi.org/10.1111/jep.12471

Womack, J. P., Jones, D., Roos, D. (1990). *The machine that changed the world.* Macmillan Publishing.

Zhu, Y. Y., & Wu, F. (2009). *Datalogy and Data Science.* Fudan University Press.

CASE EXEMPLARS FOR APPLICATION

Knowing More About Heart Failure Readmissions

Sean Collins

Clinicians in acute care hospitals have a working knowledge of heart failure readmissions. Seeing the same individuals return repeatedly seemingly unable to stay stable at home for very long. It is reaffirming to know that this working knowledge is well supported by national level data as it is useful for clinicians to consider what can be learned for their practice.

In a review of published models based on national readmission data, Collins and Dias (2015) provide some clear facts and suggestions for how to consider experiences and data to learn from these models in practice. Simply stated, patients that have been readmitted are more likely to be readmitted again. Once patients have been readmitted, future readmissions occur at shorter intervals. More precisely, the time between hospitalizations decreased by 40% with each repeat admission and each admission was associated with a 28-day (95% CI, 22–35) reduction in time out of the hospital (Bakal et al., 2014).

With this understanding a stepwise approach to interventions by clinicians could consider the model predicted time before the next admission and provide individualized interventions to include timing. Success starts by simply extending readmission beyond the prediction. What we need to understand - fundamentally - what is happening with recurrent readmissions during a time that there are likely no pathophysiological changes to cardiac function.

Based on the data and published models Collins and Dias (2015) provide a framework and possible approaches to consider. First, we must include a more thorough assessment of the unmet need in activities in daily living (ADLs). Second, we should adopt a more holistic perspective on the implications of heart failure to include the International Classification of Function (ICF), disability and health to consider reduced activity tolerance, ability to perform ADLs, and quality of life as integrated, inherent, and integral components of the readmission problem.

Clinicians need to understand the data that is driving models that are leading to policies so that they can communicate with data analysts about clinically relevant information to include in models. The relationships between physiology, activity, behavior, and daily needs are tightly connected in reality and need to be more tightly connected in data-driven decisionmaking.

Whether approaching the problem of HF readmissions as a clinician with one patient at a time or as a data analyst with a sample or population patient data, each one makes inferences to possible causes for readmission with hopes that manipulation of possible causes will favorably alter outcomes (Collins, 2018). Therefore, our search for data-driven decision-making must heed the advice of Bradford Hill and our dialogue must consider alternative and interacting explanations (Fedak et al., 2015).

REFLECTION QUESTIONS

1. Consider a long-standing problem faced in your practice or organization. What questions could you ask to bring new or different data to the improvement process?
2. If you were going to make the business case to initiate an improvement team for the problem you identified in question 1, what data would you ask a data analyst to pull?

REFERENCES

Bakal, J., McAlister, F., Liu, W., & Ezekowitz, J. A. (2014). Heart failure re-admission: Measuring the ever shortening gap between repeat heart failure hospitalizations. *PLoS One, 9*(9), e106494. https://doi.org/10.1371/journal.pone.0106494

Collins, S. (2018). Synthesis: Causal models, causal knowledge. *Cardiopulmonary Physical Therapy Journal 29*(4), 134–143. https://doi.org/10.1097/CPT.0000000000000101

Collins, S., & Dias, K. (2015). Heart failure: Stability, decompensation, and readmission. *Cardiopulmonary Physical Therapy Journal, 26*(3), 58–72. https://doi.org/10.1097/CPT.0000000000000011

Fedak, K. M., Bernal, A., Capshaw, Z. A., & Gross, S. (2015). Applying the Bradford Hill Criteria in the 21st Century: How data integration has changed causal inference in molecular epidemiology. *Emergency Themes Epidemiology, 12*(1), 14. https://doi.org/10.1186/s12982-015-0037-4

Using Data From a Different Lens to Guide Change and Advance Human Capital

Karen L. Spada

The role of a healthcare consultant can be stimulating and at times stressful. This is especially true when one assumes an interim role as a Chief Nursing Officer for a system that is completing the selection and vetting process for a vacant position. This requires the interim consultant to possess acumen of cultural sensitivity, collegiality, strong interpersonal skills, and strategy. Strategy must be grounded in proven methods and data driven approaches that use available internal resources and evidence to produce sustainable change and enhance human capital.

The strategy is fundamentally linked to a commonality among all healthcare systems; data collection, analysis of findings, and actions to ensure that quality, safety, and measurable value is sustained. While there are numerous individuals involved in this process, nurse managers play a pivotal role. Nurse managers are at the point-of-care in all systems and may lack the expertise to use data to benefit sustainable change, clinical successes, and have not been provided opportunities to strengthen intellectual capital that will be useful when assuming different positions.

As an interim consultant, I work with nurse managers to understand data collection as a method to understand "where we are" and "where we need to go." Without data and understanding its value, one is clueless as to progress or deficits until later when receiving feedback or reviewing quarterly productivity reports. Evidence and instilling accountability guide each interaction with managers. An environment where it is okay to make a left or right turn or reverse a course of action when needed is encouraged and accepted. Using daily reports of common metrics and outcomes such as falls, readmission rates, hospital-acquired pressure ulcers, and others, managers assume ownership of improvement and can value data. What follows are interventions such as hourly rounds, improved documentation that captures outcomes, improvement accountability among staff, and confidence levels that foster ongoing change, improvement, and intellectual capital.

Central to all success is celebrating and recognizing positive outcomes. There are multiple ways this is accomplished. Celebration and recognition paradoxically engender change, interest, and ownership in using data to guide continuous healthcare improvement and operational efficiency. As I depart each interim assignment, I reflect on what worked, the successes, and what could be changed or improved with the strategy as an individual process for improvement.

REFLECTION QUESTIONS

1. Consider that you are a healthcare consultant that works with organizations on a time-limited basis to increase performance outcomes. How would you approach the task? What evidence supports your approach?
2. What are the key factors that drive organizational improvement in healthcare organizations? Support your answer with evidence.

Using Administrative Data to Establish Improvement in Billing and Accounts Receivable

Brianne Burke and Tamara VanKampen

The importance of a continuous stream of revenue in any organization cannot be overstated. A standalone nurse-managed primary care clinic in an urban setting struggled for years with its billing and revenue processes. Billing services were provided by a contracted service provider that resulted in issues that went both unnoticed and unaddressed. When the billing processes were scrutinized, several issues were brought to light. An interprofessional team comprised of the practice manager, patient services manager, billing consultant, accounts receivable (A/R) specialist, provider, and consultant engaged in a gap analysis to identify gaps, barriers, and opportunities in the current process. Several areas of focus for improvement were identified in billing processes, collections, communication, and patient and staff satisfaction.

The time of service collection rate was appalling for a multiple reasons. Office staff were not trained to collect money from patients. Patient questions about billing, co-pays, and charges went unanswered as there was no one in the clinic who could help them because the biller worked in another location. When messages were left for the biller by office staff there was a delay in response or no response at all. This generated dissatisfaction for patients.

Another issue was lack of communication between the biller and providers at the practice. In addition to not understanding the billing and coding practices, there was no feedback mechanism to communicate with the providers on documentation required for specific codes that often resulted in reimbursement changes. While monthly reports summarized revenue generation and reimbursement, providers were not able to adjust their documentation to address gaps in real time that led to frustration and repeated errors. The overall billing process was unnecessarily long and drawn out. One reason for this was the time between services provided and a claim being created. Backlogs of claims to be submitted adversely affected revenue flow.

After mapping the current billing process, the team recognized there were gaps and delays that could be addressed by bringing the billing process internal to the practice. The patient services manager worked with a billing consultant to learn best practices. Providers were engaged in the work and offered education about ways the electronic health record (EHR) supported documentation of required billing fields. Work processes at the front office were modified to enable office staff to complete billing processes each day and automated reports were identified for providers and the patient services manager to expedite documentation and submission of claims. After the training was completed for the office staff, the decision to bring billing in-house occurred. The results of this decision have been impressive.

Diligent management of accounts receivable (A/R) accelerated potential cash flows by $16,800 in a three-year span (2016–2019). Daily charges increased by 216% and days in A/R have decreased by 44% over that same time span. Claims needing additional work have decreased by 17% in the past year (Figure 4.1). There is now a constant flow of charges and payments. Billing, claims submission, and claim denials are done on a daily basis as opposed to only once or twice a month. This has eliminated the overwhelming backlog that existed prior to implementing the new process.

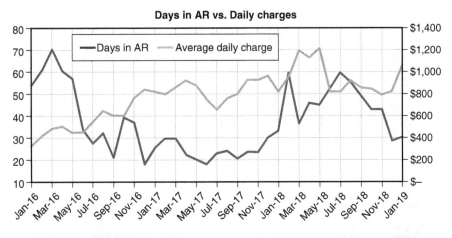

Days in AR				Average Daily Charge		
Jan-16	**Jan-19**	**Δ**		**Jan-16**	**Jan-19**	**Δ**
54.4	30.2	−44.46%		$334	$1.0K	215.80%

Diligent management of AR has accelerated potential cashflows by **$16.8K**

FIGURE 4.1 Charges and cashflows. We want to focus on the beginning and the end of the data; the information between tells a story of what happened. We always want to see the average daily charge increasing and the days in accounts receivable (AR) decreasing. Have there been any changes?

AR, accounts receivable.

TABLE 4.2 Live Benchmarks

LIVE BENCHMARKS

	7-DAY AVERAGE	FIRST PLACE	SECOND PLACE	THIRD PLACE	COUNT	CHARGE ENTRY LAG (DAYS)		HOLD LAG (DAYS)		MGRHOLD LAG (DAYS)		% OF SELF PAY > 90 DAYS	
						MEDIAN	YOUR RANK	MEDIAN	YOUR RANK	MEDIAN	YOUR RANK	MEDIAN	YOUR RANK
Your Practice						2.3	N/A	1.4	N/A	14.0	N/A	42.1%	N/A
Primary Care Practices in Michigan					48	4.9	12	3.4	20	11.9	22	33.7%	30
Primary Care Practices in the Midwest					250	3.4	71	3.4	75	11.9	102	35.1%	154
All Primary Care Practices					1561	3.2	451	3.7	431	13.8	571	34.8%	913
All Michigan Practices					209	3.8	54	3.0	74	10.8	99	33.5%	127
All Midwest Practices					1215	3.4	336	3.6	349	12.6	463	37.4%	683
Medium Practices					1378	4.0	334	4.3	323	13.6	626	36.6%	763
National					7587	3.2	1,885	3.9	1,951	13.3	2,932	37.0%	4,194

(continued)

91-DAY AVERAGE

	COUNT	CHARGE ENTRY LAG (DAYS)		HOLD LAG (DAYS)		MGRHOLD LAG (DAYS)		% OF SELF PAY > 90 DAYS	
		MEDIAN	YOUR RANK	MEDIAN	YOUR RANK	MEDIAN	YOUR RANK	MEDIAN	YOUR RANK
Your Practice		2.9	N/A	5.5	N/A	14.3	N/A	32.5%	N/A
Primary Care Practices in Michigan	49	6.0	12	5.7	21	36.3	11	38.9%	20
Primary Care Practices in the Midwest	253	5.0	77	7.3	100	38.3	56	35.9%	107
All Primary Care Practices	1577	5.1	469	8.1	589	42.0	364	38.8%	635
All Michigan Practices	212	6.8	49	5.7	101	24.7	69	34.7%	90
All Midwest Practices	1223	5.2	361	7.0	496	33.7	309	39.6%	460
Medium Practices	1387	5.2	339	6.5	604	27.8	431	38.8%	543
National	7637	4.9	2,308	7.6	3,004	33.8	2,014	39.2%	2,897

Live Benchmark analyze your practice's performance across four "best practice" metrics, and compare your practice with other Athena practices in your state, region, specialty, and group size (provided there are at least 5 practices to be compared. You are shown your overall rank in each category over a 7-day average for a real-time view and a 91-day average for a quarterly view.

As a result of this work, the practice meets or is above both state and national benchmarks based on the EHR trended data reports (Table 4.2). Having an onsite biller has improved communication and satisfaction as questions can be addressed immediately. The staff have been working together to improve the entire billing process and have seen an improved revenue flow that has created staff enthusiasm and a more positive work experience. Overall, the practice now has fewer billing errors, a better trained front desk staff that understand how to collect payments and read explanation of benefits (EOBs), and most importantly, the cash flow and revenue continues to improve.

REFLECTION QUESTIONS

1. What billing processes will improve cash flow and cost avoidance?
2. What outcomes can be realized through improved communication between billers and providers?
3. Consider that you are opening a freestanding clinic as an advanced practitioner in a rural setting. What steps would you take to ensure sustainability for the future?

5

Application of Data Science in Healthcare

Patricia L. Thomas and James L. Harris

OBJECTIVES

1. Define data science.
2. Trace the origin of data science.
3. Discuss how data science emerged in response to big data.
4. Explore how data science is applicable to contemporary healthcare.

CORE COMPETENCIES

- Knowledge of healthcare delivery, big data, and the value of data science
- Decision-making strategies and frameworks to guide innovative approaches to healthcare change
- Evaluation methods
- Relationship and network builder

INTRODUCTION

The catalyst for healthcare success requires practitioners and leaders to understand data and the emerging field of data science. If innovative discovery, improved decision-making, and a data-driven environment advance, individuals must engage in action-oriented approaches directed at using data for continuous improvement and future scientific discovery. This chapter defines data science, provides an overview of its origin, how it emerged in response to big data, and the applicability to contemporary healthcare demands and efficient operations.

DATA SCIENCE

Data science is a multidisciplinary field that uses scientific methods, processes, algorithms, and systems to extract knowledge and insights from structured and unstructured data. Data science recognizes that in isolation, data accrual is insufficient to guide innovation and foster change. It is not about creating models or frameworks. Rather, data science is the use of data to create a visualization that generates meaning as it is produced and used regardless of the healthcare settings (Masica & Escarce, 2019).

Ahalt et al. (2014) define data science in healthcare as, "the systematic study of the organization and use of digital data in order to accelerate discovery, improve critical decision-making processes, and enable a data driven economy" (p. 3). Data science encompasses the principled acquisition, curation, exploration, manipulation, and interpretation of big datasets (Brennan & Bakken, 2015).

Data science offers a means to take thousands of data points and organize them using mathematic equations and process engineering to discover associations, patterns, and trends to make recommendations, solve issues, or manage complex problems. This requires collective actions by teams of clinicians and individuals with expertise in big data analytics, bioinformatics, technology, engineering, healthcare administration, business and entrepreneurship, and healthcare policy to ensure data are managed and used for an implicit purpose (Bhavnani et al., 2016; Topol, 2015).

The Origin of Data Science

The history of data science offers the backdrop for the evolution of the field and provides insights for the future. In the early to mid-1990s as electronic interfaces in healthcare organizations were becoming more common, data mining and database information was initiated. In 1996, Fayyad, Piatetsky-Shapiro, and Smyth wrote *From Data Mining to Knowledge Discovery in Databases* that framed how data mining had the potential to transform data and identify patterns that could be analyzed and used to generate knowledge. The premise of this article established the foundation from which data science evolved. Notably, the article highlighted that machine thinking and artificial intelligence (AI) could and would require investment and development to reach their full potential for discovery and knowledge generation into the future.

In 2001, William Cleveland merged computer science and data mining to create a source of innovation and knowledge generation. As a result, Cleveland coined the term data science to represent a new discipline through an ambitious plan to link data analytics to statistics. Through these actions, the groundwork for theory development, application, and evaluation emerged creating a foundation upon which learning from data was conceptualized (Cleveland, 2001). During the same time period, social media and shared experiences through YouTube came into the lexicon and offered new opportunities for data analysis. From the origin until today, data science continues to emerge and offer opportunities for managing change and creating new knowledge applicable to multiple situations.

Data Science Emergence in Response to Big Data

Data science in healthcare has emerged in response to big data and encompasses the analysis and understanding of many sources of data. Combining statistics, mathematics, computer science, and information science, it supports moving data from disparate and disconnected points to information that is actionable as new knowledge (O'Connor, 2018). In addition to modeling and computer programming, data science incorporates computer engineering strategies for visualization, data warehousing, and high-performance computing (Brennan & Bakken, 2015). Methodologies for developing and analyzing complex and large healthcare datasets are emerging with great promise surrounding improved outcomes, efficacy, and fiscal stewardship (Masica & Escarce, 2019; Raghupathi & Raghupathi, 2014).

Data science has similarities to work in census collection, public health data sets, or patient registries where data are structured and aggregated for population trends to support care paths and clinical guidelines. New citizen science incorporating crowdsourcing to leverage public and patient participation to collect health data through open and online data repositories is needed to advance the science (Bhavnani et al., 2016; Topol, 2015). Volumes of data are available as individuals use smart phones, applications (apps), the Internet, mobile devices, and technology. This data can be used to streamline wait times, gather information, and improve operational efficiency throughout healthcare organizations.

Recent interest in healthcare data science centers on the ability to use data to improve practice or outcomes (both clinical and financial) in complex situations. Data aggregated from medical records, social media, genomics databases, and wireless and wearable mobile health devices are being analyzed using techniques like machine learning and AI for structured and unstructured data (Bhavnani et al., 2016). Established big data sources like electronic medical records, health insurance claims databases, and digitalized radiography images are used in a variety of analytic methodologies like decision trees, computer-assisted diagnostics, and ridge regression to produce learning models for disease classification and prediction (Bhavnani et al., 2016). New initiatives to provide open access infrastructures to search, download, and analyze biomedical research and post publication clinical trial data sets are available through OpenImmport (www.immport.org) and the Yale Open Data Access (www.yoda.yale.edu).

In terms of data analytics, the healthcare industry is using analytical methods including machine learning, AI, and cloud-based analytics that were once only found outside healthcare settings. The translation to healthcare has generated clinical decision support, predictive modeling, and personalized treatment planning. Although attractive, some caution is warranted given the unknowns, particularly related to issues that could arise from diagnostic, risk, and therapeutic decisions based on these new analytics (Bhavnani et al., 2016).

There are few clinicians trained to understand and assimilate big data analytics. In addition to learning about clinical informatics and the electronic health record, understanding data heterogeneity (for accuracy and formatting), data fragmentation (when data comes from several sources), data availability and handling (management, access, querying, and sharing), data privacy and integrity (prevention of corruption and hacking), and data conceptualization (ontologies) are necessary. Several online and open curriculum-based training and certification courses are available at IBM's Big Data University (www.bigdatauniversity.com) and Cloudera University (www.cloudera.com) to help clinicians learn best practices in data analytics for translation to research or patient care (Bhavnani et al., 2016).

Data science has expanded into the healthcare industry with the extensive adoption of electronic medical records and Internet and app-based health interfaces. This digital era has brought science, technology, and healthcare together and with it, the need for new skills in how data are used to make decisions and predictions about interventions and desired outcomes. Big data and predictive analytics are new ways to use data to improve personalization of care, improve care design and delivery, and automate reporting through both structured and unstructured datasets (Bhavnani et al., 2016).

To make actionable the possibilities that reside in leveraging big data and predictive analytics, a significant paradigm shift is needed. No longer bound by structured datasets, open-source and unstructured data can now be utilized to inform individualized care for patient populations. The convergence of demographic, epidemiologic, and economic trends have created the imperative to accelerate change. Likewise, economic data has influenced how we utilize data to innovate care delivery systems and models. While the challenge before us is both daunting and audacious, other industries have used big data to transform services and the healthcare industry is now poised to revolutionize how treatment and management decisions are made in response to patients, providers, and consumer demands (Bhavnani et al., 2016; Masica & Escarce, 2019).

Current and Future Application of Data Science in Contemporary Healthcare

The boundaries associated with application of data science are endless. Data science promotes analysis that culminates in identification of impacts of data, strategy, and problem-solving abilities. As in the past and the immediate future, strategic and problem-solving abilities are pivotal markers for future healthcare innovation.

With the maturation of data science and adoption in healthcare settings, new opportunities to utilize machine learning and machine-driven data decisions are possible and offers intensive and substantial learning. As AI becomes more acceptable and utilized in healthcare settings, additional experimentation, utilization of research methods, and developmental opportunities for a future generation of data scientist is possible.

Practitioners and managers often voice opposition concerning the vast amounts of data and data points required for collection, the administrative burden, and the relative low return on the time and effort as measured in patient care impact and outcomes. Data science and data scientists are offering new ways to turn data points into relevant insights, trends, and foundational elements to support predictive analytics.

Predictive analytics are sets of analytical procedures that use existing data to forecast probabilities. The annotated data are used to derive models that support health decisions. While more common today in business or operational decision-making centered on customers, products, and competitors, data at the population or individual level is now being used to influence care delivery and decision-making. Drawing from diverse data sources including epidemiology, disease burden, and socioeconomics, predictive analytics will continue to offer advantages in healthcare settings.

Defined as healthcare based on data, algorithms, and molecular tools, precision medicine is another application. Precision medicine combines knowledge of disease prevention, treatment, and care with sophisticated data analytics for decision-making about interventions that will add value by improving cost structures and clinical outcomes. Precision medicine teams merge discipline knowledge and tools from physical and natural scientists and engineers as they engage with clinicians, social and behavioral scientists, and population investigators to produce and share a computational "learning system." This knowledge network aggregates, integrates, accesses, and analyzes information from large patient cohorts, health populations, and experimental systems to reveal testable hypotheses to classify diseases by mechanisms for precise individualized prevention, diagnosis, and treatment options (Dzau et. al., 2016).

Breakthroughs in precision medicine have led to the launch of the U.S. Precision Medicine Initiative to understand how a person's genetics, environment, and lifestyle can help determine the best approach to prevent or treat disease. Initially focusing on knowledge in genetics and biology to establish more effective cancer treatments, the long-term goal focuses on applying tools in big data analytics for precision medicine to guide decision-making in healthcare broadly. The NIH, *All of Us Research Program,* engaged one million volunteers who will provide genetic data, biological samples, and other health information to encourage open data sharing. Participants can access personal health information and data from information used for research. Researchers can use the data to predict disease risk, study disease, understand how diseases occur, and develop improvements in diagnosis and treatment (National Institutes of Health [NIH], 2020).

The implications of precision medicine are far-reaching. In addition to the potential revealed in diagnosis and treatment of disease, research initiatives to develop the knowledge for a robust evidence base, innovation in pharmaceutical interventions, health policy development, establishment of population based clinical standards, and revisions to reimbursement structures are possible. The data sharing and infrastructure needs will be significant, and the incorporation of structured and unstructured data will be essential when engaging a variety of stakeholders. Attention to data access, privacy, and security will remain constant and new challenges in common datasets, interfaces, oversight, and administration will emerge (Dzau et.al., 2016).

Consumer demand and requirements for patient engagement have changed interaction with the healthcare system and are also linked to data science. A new subspecialty in clinical informatics, consumer health informatics, (CHI) focuses on how patients or consumers interact with Health Information Technology (HIT). CHI incorporates the patient perspective in healthcare decision-making and is a critical component associated with population health strategies (American Medical Informatics Association [AIMA], 2017; Austin & LaFlamme, 2021). Examples of consumer data sources include telehealth, mobile health technology apps, patient monitors and sensors, and fitness tracking devices. Ongoing efforts are a top priority to remove barriers that prevent patients from accessing personal health records.

With the growth of Internet connectivity, wireless technology, and sensor devises, the way patients, families, and communities connect with health services will continue to expand and benefit data science application. As an example and according to the American Telemedicine Association (ATA), the benefits of tele-medicine are improved access, cost effectiveness, improved quality of care and patient demand for clinical diagnosis and monitoring. Telehealth, a more common term, refers to using technology for clinical diagnostics, care management, patient education, and routine follow-up visits for rural health accesses (Center for Connected Health, 2020).

In addition to new sources of data in mobile devices and mobile apps, wearable devices, and data kiosks, healthcare organizations are taking nontraditional approaches to the uses of big data and adopting ways to advance data science. As one considers disruption in the health industry, companies once focused on consumers in other sectors are now entering the healthcare space. Unique and industry disrupting partnership arrangements have been formed that many will embrace and propel data science to new levels. For example, the opportunity to use existing strengths from other industry sectors to address dissatisfaction with healthcare has catapulted outsiders into the healthcare landscape. With expertise in supply chain, big data, data management and storage, technology, and customer service, companies once focused on services outside the healthcare arena are now ready to revolutionize it. With acknowledgment that the healthcare industry is slow to address longstanding challenges, these industry leaders are prepared to use strategies they have refined outside healthcare as a lever for innovation and improvement.

The next decade promises disruption in healthcare industry on a magnitude not previously experienced. When one considers the transformation of telecommunication, transportation, and interconnectivity, healthcare is well positioned to embrace change beneficial to society. Opportunities to advance data science and its application will remain constant as the healthcare industry responds to evolving technology, yet to be introduced into the global market.

SUMMARY

- The healthcare industry is poised to revolutionize how decisions and interventions are made and deployed.

- Big data and data science introduce new stakeholders and interdisciplinary team members supporting innovation and care delivery.
- Data science is a systematic study of an organization and uses digital data to accelerate discovery, improve clinical decisions, and enable a data driven economy.
- Clinicians and administrators will require knowledge and skills in big data and data analytics to further advance decision-making processes.
- Data science has immeasurable potential and will drive clinical care standards, policy, how technology supports change, and methods to evaluate measurable outcomes.
- Data science has application in healthcare as evidenced by the potential generated by machine learning, AI, predictive analysis, precision medicine, and consumer demands.
- Disruptions in healthcare settings will remain constant and intensify in the future requiring action, team collaboration, and evaluation of outcomes.

REFLECTION QUESTIONS

1. You are in a meeting where evaluation of a program is undertaken. As you listen to the conversation you recognize the evaluation methods are simplistic and the engagement of a data scientist would benefit the team. How would you describe the value of bringing a data scientist to the group?
2. You are approached by a colleague who is overwhelmed with the amount of time spent on computers rather than in direct interactions with patients. While you appreciate the lack of interoperability between systems, what benefits would you highlight about collecting points of data as it relates to what you now know about knowledge discovery?
3. A friends' child is in high school considering future health related study and is uncertain about what major to declare. What questions would you ask them to help elucidate whether the role of a data scientist might be a good career choice?
4. As you consider disruptors in the health field and look to the next five years, what do you think the next disruption to improve healthcare delivery will be? What influenced your thoughts?

REFERENCES

Ahalt, S., Bizon, C., Evans, J., Elrich, Y., Ginsberg, G., Krishmanmurthy, A., Lange, L., Maltbie, D., Masys, D., Schmitt, C., & Wilhemsen, K. (2014). *Data to discovery: Genomes to health. A whitepaper from the National Consortium of Data Science.* RENCI, University of North Carolina. https://datascienceconsortium.org/wp-content/uploads/2016/02/NCDS-white-paper-FORPUBLICATION.pdf

American Medical Informatics Association. (2017). *Nursing informatics.* www.amia.org/programs/working-groups/nursing-informatics

Austin, R., & LaFlamme, A. (2021). Information systems/technology and patient care technology for the improvement and transformation of healthcare. In M. Zaccagnini & J. Pechacek (Eds.), (4th ed.). *The doctor of nursing practice essentials: A new model for advanced practice nursing.* Jones & Bartlett Learning.

Bhavnani, S., Munoz, D., & Bagai, A. (2016). Data science in healthcare: Implications for early career investigators. *Circulation: Cardiovascular Quality Outcomes, 9,* 683–687. https://doi.org/10.1161/circoutcomes.116.003081

Brennan, P. F., & Bakken, S. (2015). Nursing needs big data and big data needs nursing. *Journal of Nursing Scholarship, 47*(5), 477–484. https://doi.org/10.1111/jnu.12159

Center for Connected Health Policy. (2020). Center for Connected Health Policy. https://www.cchpca.org/

Cleveland, W. (2001). Data science: An action plan for expanding the technical areas of the field of statistics. *International Statistical Review / Revue Internationale De Statistique, 69*(1), 21–26. https://doi.org/10.2307/1403527

Dzau, V., Ginsburg, G., Chopra, A., Goldman, D., Green, E., McClellan, M., Plump, A., Terry, S., & Yamamoto, K. (2016). *Realizing the full potential of precision medicine in health and healthcare: A vital direction for health and health care.* https://nam.edu/realizing-the-full-potential-of-precision-medicine-in-health-and-health-care-a-vital-direction-for-health-and-health-care

Fayyad, U., Piatetsky-Shapiro, G., & Smyth, P. (1996). *From data mining to knowledge discovery: Advances in knowledge discovery and data mining,* 1–34. AAAI Press/The MIT Press.

Masica, A., & Escarce, J. (2019). Innovative data science to transform health care: All the pieces matter. *Generating Evidence & Methods to Improve Patient Outcomes (eGEMS), 7*(1), 47. https://egems.academyhealth.org/articles/10.5334/egems.314

National Institutes of Health. (2020). *What is the Precision Medicine Initiative?* https://medlineplus.gov/genetics/understanding/precisionmedicine/initiative/

O'Connor, S. (2018). Big data and data science in healthcare: What nurses and midwives need to know. *Journal of Clinical Nursing, 27,* 2921–2922. https://doi.org/10.1111/jocn.14164

Raghupathi, W., & Raghupathi, V., (2014). Big data analytics in healthcare: Promise and potential health. *Information Science and Systems, 2,* 3. https://doi.org/10.1186/2047-2501-2-3

Topol, E. (2015). *The patient will see you now: The future of medicine is in your hands.* Basic Books.

CASE EXEMPLARS FOR APPLICATION

Interprofessional Care Coordination Conferences and Improved Transitions of Care for Medically Fragile Pediatric Patients

Tamara VanKampen

Medically complex and fragile pediatric patients are high utilizers of healthcare resources. Although they represent less than 1% of the general population, the group accounts for more than 30% of pediatric healthcare costs (Murphy & Clark, 2016). This group of patients tends to have longer lengths of stay in the hospital, higher readmission rates, and frequent emergency department visits (Berry et al., 2014). Medically complex and fragile pediatric patients often require multiple healthcare providers, leading to an increased risk of miscommunication between providers or providers and families.

For purposes of this exemplar, the pediatric healthcare organization where the author completed the project utilizes hospitalists to care for admitted patients. A literature review revealed while having hospitalists and specialists is often beneficial, communication between multiple providers can be challenging, potentially leading to suboptimal outcomes for patients (Auger et al., 2016). Approximately 60% of sentinel events with this group are rooted in lack of communication (Solan et al., 2016). Coordinated care can lead to cost reductions related to healthcare utilization, improved health outcomes, and increased key stakeholder satisfaction.

One strategy to improve communication is through the use of care coordination conferences (CCC), where providers, key stakeholders, and family members meet to discuss inpatient and outpatient care. The interprofessional team members that participated in this work included physicians, residents, nurses, nurse practitioners, and discharge planners/care management staff. Without conferences, coordinated care opportunities were lost, higher readmission rates occurred, poorer patient outcomes were evident, and lower satisfaction with care by both providers and families were documented. These concerns were the impetus for the project that was two-fold: (a) evaluate streamlined care conference processes and (b) improve transitions of care communication between hospitalists or medical residents and PCPs for medically complex patients.

Streamlining the CCC process was a priority for this organization, as there was no standard format, conferences took too long, provided little value, and key stakeholders were often not in attendance. Another issue was lack of a standard process for communicating with PCPs who desired more communication both when medically complex pediatric patients were admitted and throughout the course of hospitalization.

Respondents to a survey sent by this author to local PCPs provided useful feedback and gave direction for this project. The PCPs admitted an average of fewer than three patients each month, and of those, approximately 43% were medically complex. Sixty-seven percent of respondents were unfamiliar with the CCCs at the organization, with 80% stating they would like more involvement with the conferences. Of those who were familiar, 62.5% were either not at all satisfied or somewhat satisfied with the conferences. As for communication upon admission of a medically complex patient, 80% of respondents were either not at all satisfied or somewhat satisfied, with 20% stating they were very satisfied. Drawing on thematic information from the surveys, it was determined better communication between inpatient and primary care providers was needed. After meetings with a pediatrician, a hospitalist, a resident, and the pediatric resident chiefs, it was determined the best way to notify PCPs of an admission was to have the physician residents send a secure text to the PCP upon patient admission. A brief script for the text was created and a list of PCP phone numbers was posted for medical residents and hospitalists on each floor of the organization.

For the CCCs, standard work was written by a care coordination committee. A baseline average for three months was chosen to be used as a comparison to the same three months the following year. Goals of the streamlined process included reduced in-patient length of stay, decreased 30-day readmissions, and more inclusion of all key stakeholders. New care conferences followed analysis of the data with key players participating.

Post implementation surveys related to patient admission communication showed a 50% improvement. The most common means of contact was a secure text (66.67%) or a phone call (33.33%). However, due to the low number of respondents to the second survey, the results did not have statistical significance. Time constraints of the project were a factor in obtaining follow-up data from the organization related to streamlined CCC processes. Although overall length of stay did not show a decrease, overall 30-day readmission rates did decrease more than 10% in the three months following implementation.

Improved communication for transitions of care and care coordination is a necessity for improving patient outcomes and decreasing healthcare utilization.

Tracking quality indicators and continuous quality improvement is standard at this organization. This commitment ultimately highlighted areas in need of improvement and allowed for needed changes to occur. It is important for this organization to continue to improve care coordination for their medically complex patients while admitted and when transitioning to and from the PCP. Improving the care coordination conferences through streamlining and standardization, as well as regular inclusion of PCPs, should result in a more valuable process for all. By ensuring all key stakeholders are involved in care processes for medically complex patients, improved care, reduced utilization costs, and improved patient outcomes and satisfaction is possible as concluded by this project.

REFLECTION QUESTIONS

1. What are ways that teams can improve communication and increase quality outcomes?
2. What ways can a root cause analysis provide opportunities to collect and use data for improvement? Explain your response.

REFERENCES

Auger, K. A., Mueller, E. L., Weinberg, S. H., Forster, C. S., Shah, A., Wolski, C., & Davis, M. M. (2016). A validated method for identifying unplanned pediatric readmissions. *The Journal of Pediatrics, 170*, 105–112. https://doi.org/10.1016/j.jpeds.2015.11.051

Berry, J. G., Hall, M., Neff, J., Goodman, D., Cohen, E., Agrawal, R., & Feudtner, C. (2014). Children with medical complexity and Medicaid: Spending and cost savings. *Health Affairs, 33*(12), 2199–2206. https://doi.org/10.1377/hlthaff.2014.0828

Murphy, N. A., & Clark, E. B. (2016). Children with complex medical conditions: An underrecognized driver of the pediatric cost crisis. *Current Treatment Options in Pediatrics, 2*(4), 289–295. https://doi.org/10.1007/s40746-016-0071-7

Solan, L. G., Sherman, S. N., DeBlasio, D., & Simmons, J. M. (2016). Communication challenges: A qualitative look at the relationship between pediatric hospitalists and primary care providers. *Academic Pediatrics, 16*(5), 453–459. https://doi.org/10.1016/j.acap.2016.03.003

A Team Approach to Building Precise Outcome Measures

John Nelson

Over the last 19 years, I have learned outcomes measures that inform the most were developed by a team. Most important within the team are the front-line staff and the mathematician. Once a mathematic model of the care elements of interest are developed, it is the information technology experts who are critical to move the data collection process from a full or partial manual method to be fully automated for real time and proactive management of outcomes. This short perspective exemplar highlights one analyst's experience in the deployment of a method of analysis that has saved millions of dollars for organizations each time it has been used.

Model specification is a bit of an academic term but it is important if outcomes are to be improved using measures with precision. A specified model displays all the variables that relate to the outcome of interest. This can be, for example, all the reasons patients fall in an organization. This could also be patient related: i.e., medication side effects, delirium, and weakness when ambulating. The reasons could also be staff related: i.e., staff not educating patient regarding identified falls risks, inattentiveness, and so on. Finally, it can be environment related: i.e., a wet floor. Whatever the actual or suspected reason, it should be in the model. This first phase of model development is referred to as a structural model. It is front-line staff who are best equipped to identify the reasons based on their intimate knowledge of patient care and closest proximity to patients. Quality staff may also provide reasons based on case studies or root cause analysis within the organization but nothing can replace the knowledge derived from staff who live the patient care experience every day.

Once the structural model is developed, the more difficult phase of measurement modeling is required that encompasses how to measure the patient, employee, and environmental variables that were identified as risks for the outcome of interest. In continuing with the example of falls, one can identify many variables like medications and fall history variables that are easily measured. The challenge rests in latent variables like attitudes and beliefs of the staff that are very important but often not measured. If one does not measure the variables staff report as important to outcomes, the models will be wrong. In leaving out these latent variables measurement remains on the peripheral variables and because pieces are missing, there is model misspecification and the outcome of interest remains unsolved.

Measurement model error can be solved by including a psychometrician on the improvement team who is trained in developing measures of invisible variables like attitude, caring, and incivility. The psychometrician is a key team member because they bring a wide lens to measurement and a focus to whether a variable is demonstrated consistently on all units, within all within all disciplines, and on all shifts. Description of measurement testing is beyond this brief exemplar, but the absence of a psychometrician on any quality team is a major flaw in healthcare quality improvement work nationally and globally. An example to demonstrate this from my own work rests in the 106 unique instruments used to measure job satisfaction. None were found to rigorously test the measure's accuracy across groups and contexts. Most of the research in nurse job satisfaction use measures developed by the staff or an instrument that has limited testing in the sample using the measure.

The final team member that is critical, and yet to be discovered, is the expert who works with the staff members, quality staff, analyst, and psychometrician to automate the measurement model so the structural model can be studied in relationship to the outcome. If an interface expert (for lack of a specific title) were to assist the team and assimilate the data from the measurement model, and interface to inform what is relating to the outcome in real time, the historical data used to study a retrospective act could be used to study trends and predict risk for proactive management of outcomes. The possibility would be staff units based on identified risk and skills and abilities of each staff member.

Currently, there is a reliance on machine learning and artificial intelligence to solve these issues. It is almost as if we have this "new guy" who is going to solve the issues using big data. However, from a science perspective, nothing can replace theory as the foundation for good structural models and associated measurement models. It begins with the staff sharing their story, where the "hunch" begins, and giving birth to belief, which is theory. It is this nuanced story that is then measured and tested for operational refinement.

In sharing my perspective, I have an interesting story of discovery experienced by staff who worked with me to transform their story to a structural and measurement model. They used their model to study the same variables in both patients who fell and patients who did not fall. They had been studying only the falls patients, and were intrigued to learn by studying fall patients and non-fall patients they could compare why one group fell and one did not. Using the comparative data to understand falls, they reduced falls from 4 per 1,000 days to 0.6 falls per 1,000 days which saved the organization $1.6 million.

Several reasons for falls occurring were identified and actions were taken to resolve them. One of most interesting findings was related to having the bed closest to the bathroom occupied by a high-risk fall patient compared to having the low-risk fall risk patient furthest from the bathroom. It was unit policy to put at the high-risk fall patients close to the bathroom. What was discovered within the data was that the bed closest to the bathroom led patients to believe it was a short distance they could make without falling, regardless of their risk. Patients were "teased" into believing they could make that short distance! If staff did not respond quickly to the call-bell of the patient needing to get to the bathroom, the patient felt they could take a few short steps alone. The patient's perception was that the risk they were taking was reasonable only to fall after a few steps. Policy changed to put the high-risk fall patients in the bed farthest from the bathroom which contributed to fewer falls. The resulting conversation between staff and patients regarding rationale for the bed placement took place and enhanced patient education related to their personal fall risk factors.

Using data science and analytics I have proven many times over that outcomes can be improved by using staff built structural models and quality staff help with good measurement models. What has yet to be discovered is an interface expert who can help outcome management move from retrospective or rearview mirror management to forward looking proactive risk management.

REFLECTION QUESTIONS

1. Consider the falls data presented in this exemplar. What did you identify that could be used in your current practice and why?
2. What value does theory play in developing precise outcome measures and why?
3. Do you have models of outcomes that are validated by staff? What variables do they suggest are missing in the model?
4. What variables do you find impact an outcome that are not found in literature?
5. What ways can a root cause analysis provide opportunities to collect and use data for improvement? Explain your response.

6

Big Data: Understanding Its Value

Brian Collins

CHAPTER OBJECTIVES

1. Define information systems and the relation to data, information, and knowledge.
2. Discuss big data as a concept and the potential volume, data types and sources, and velocity as it is created.
3. Explain the importance of veracity; including data integrity, accuracy, and relevance of information.
4. Determine the value of big data and future priorities for its management.

CORE COMPETENCIES

- Management of information systems and big data
- Big data analysis, synthesis, and statistical process control
- Understand value and its relation to data
- Apply business principles using reverse engineering principles, information systems, and data

---

INTRODUCTION

To understand big data and its value in healthcare, reverse engineering of information and knowledge from information systems (IS) is necessary. This requires tracing the footprint of data from the initial human computer interaction and the larger information system to integration of data, decision support processes, and workflow as discrete electronic inputs are produced. Such inputs yield data that are available for clinical and administrative teams as strategic planning and evidence-based decisions are made.

This chapter presents an overview of the footprint of data origin. The five Vs of big data, (volume, velocity, variety, veracity, and value), are defined and discussed. Understanding each of the five Vs is critical to outcomes measurement and continuous improvement. Quality improvement requires understanding and revising the production of processes on the basis of data (Berwick, 1989). One of the most impactful advantages of electronic transaction processing and clinical documentation is the ability to enter data once and use it multiple times and in multiple ways (Sensmeier, 2015). This includes the abstraction and ability to extract, transform, and load (ETL) that data into analytical and communication platforms. As the invaluable bi-product of federal reporting regulations, publicly available data sets with benchmarks, thresholds, examples, and targets are created.

TRACING THE FOOTPRINT OF DATA

One of the historical sources credited with tracing the footprint of data is the Data-Information-Knowledge-Wisdom (DIKW) hierarchy introduced by organizational theorist Russell Ackoff and presented is in Figure 6.1 (Rowley, 2007).

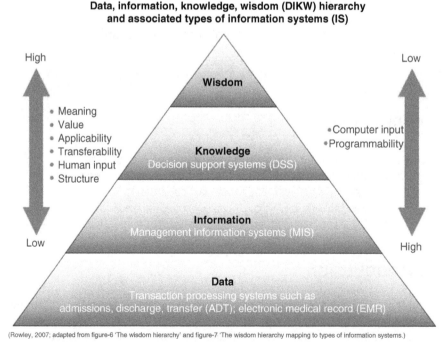

(Rowley, 2007; adapted from figure-6 'The wisdom hierarchy' and figure-7 'The wisdom hierarchy mapping to types of information systems.')

FIGURE 6.1 Data-Information-Knowledge-Wisdom Hierarchy.

The model provides context for understanding data and its value in the current healthcare landscape. Ackoff (1999) suggested that understanding the model is to consider that when less time is devoted to transmission of knowledge and ways of its attainment, with little or no time spent to transmit understanding or ways of obtaining distinction between data, information, and wisdom, its application is lost.

Compared to Maslow's Hierarchy of Needs (Ermine, 2018), DIKW is pivotal to any organization achieving value and sustainable performance with data; otherwise, data remains at the lowest, most basic level and its "Purpose" is to "Know-nothing" (Zeleny, 2006). Providing a functional view of the DIKW hierarchy, Table 6.1 illustrates the level, effect, purpose, and manifest of each level in the hierarchy as posed by Zeleny (2006).

Data are symbols, transactional records essential for operations and archived for retrieval or use; in an electronic environment, data exists and we know nothing from having it alone. Information is processed data, where meaning is added and it becomes useful; it is descriptive (what, who, where, when) and allows us to do things right (efficiency). Knowledge is familiarity gained through experience or association. It is the range of understanding from being aware to circumstance of apprehending through reasoning and condition of having information. Knowledge is the sum of what is known; the acquired body of truth, information, and principles used to guide decisions that create quality outcomes (Carper, 1978). Knowledge and information are a circulatory system; interconnected in an integrated, mutually enhancing system of autopoietic self-production cycle (Zeleny, 2006). This "autopoiesis," or the production of itself, is parallel to the Theory of Continuous Improvement and revising the production of processes on the basis of data about the processes themselves (Berwick, 1989). Zeleny describes four essential transformations in this circulatory system:

- **Articulation: knowledge → information**
  - Describes, records, and preserves the acquired, tested, proven, and effective knowledge and experience. Symbolic description, records, manuals,

TABLE 6.1 Functional View of the Data-Information-Knowledge-Wisdom Hierarchy

LEVEL	EFFECT	PURPOSE	MANIFEST
Data	Exist	Know-Nothing	Symbols; transactional and archived records
Information	Efficiency	Know-What	Data that are processed to be useful; provides answers to who, what, where and when
Knowledge	Effectiveness	Know-How	Application of data and information; answers how question
Wisdom	Explicability	Know-Why	Appreciation of why; evaluated understanding

databases, graphs, diagrams, expert systems, "cookbooks," and procedures help to create a symbolic memory of the enterprise. This creates the information necessary for subsequent forms suitable for new and effective action.

- **Combination: information → information**
  - Transforms one symbolic description into another, more suitable (actionable) symbolic description; this is the content of traditional information and technology (IT). Involving data and information processing, data mining, data warehousing, documentation, databases, and other combinations; the purpose is to make information actionable and useful in the coordination process.
- **Internalization: information → knowledge**
  - Uses information for effective action and constructive knowledge. Information has to be actively internalized in human abilities, coordination, activities, operations, and decisions. Only through action does information attain value.
- **Socialization: knowledge → knowledge**
  - Shares and propagates the learning and transfer of knowledge among organizations. Without such sharing through the community of action, knowledge loses its social dimension and becomes ineffective. Learning organization can emerge and become effective only through socialization of knowledge.

As this occurs, organizations are able to appreciate the value of data through transformative processes where new information, knowledge, and future inquiry emerge. But for this to occur, the assumption that data can be used to create information is germane to knowledge and wisdom.

Wisdom originates from intelligence and effectiveness that is linked to data, information, and knowledge. The boundless nature of wisdom is integrated across disciplines as an integrated whole, greater than the sum of the parts. This wholeness creates a dependency on value and judgment when making decisions for organizational effectiveness. Leaders need wisdom when considering which of the 100+ publically reported measures of any hospital's performance to focus actions necessary to achieve the largest impact. Otherwise, attempting to respond to the myriad of outcomes and associated variables simultaneously is not effective for deployment of resources in today's healthcare industry (Zeleny, 2006).

Fortunately, decision support systems (DSS), dashboards, balanced scorecards and other tools are available to easily produce, present data, information, and introduce new knowledge. But wisdom is knowing the answer before anyone can ask how, why, or what? Knowing an answer or explanation regarding data provides the rationale, impetus for action, and is more important than who, what, when, and how many. The why engages teams, provokes thought, and drives creativity for improvement team innovation and continuous quality.

Keys to Making Big Data a Massive Business: The Five Vs

As discussed in previous chapters, the purpose of data is to produce value and function as a primary driver for administrative and clinical decisions. In order for this to occur, data must be transformed where value shapes business principles and frames healthcare decisions and ultimately measurable and sustainable outcomes. The expanding understanding of big data and its use in health care is evolving as demonstrated most succinctly when one considers the definition and five Vs of big data (Brennan & Bakken, 2015; Broome, 2016; Laney, 2001).

Understanding big data can be elusive. Reducing the intangibility, an indefinable definition, and facilitating big data use in health care requires consideration of its definition and conceptualize it as a pyramid with volume as the foundation. For purposes of this chapter, big data represents the collection of datasets that are massive posing difficulty when using legacy and traditional processing applications (Press, 2014).

As the definition of big data continuously advances, becomes commonplace in healthcare, and driving business success, the five Vs of big data will require reflection and understanding if maximum benefit is attained. Beginning with the foundation, the original three dimensions or "3D Data Management: Controlling Data Volume, Velocity, and Variety" (Laney, 2001) was intended for industry where data was the actual commodity and these were the major dimensions of the product. Still applicable, but instead of the market value of data, we intend to harness the strategic and operational value for improvement activities. As data is information about the process by which is was created and we intend to use it, to create a body of knowledge, and act wisely for the improvement of the process and outcomes.

Volume is the size of data that is beyond typical handling without the appropriate tools. Figuratively, this means enormous potential to be distracted by unimportant data and consumed with inconsequential data management. Literally, for example, this means the current version of Microsoft Excel (2019) cannot open files with more than 1,048,576 rows or 16,384 columns and you need to start your analysis in a database management system (DBMS) like Microsoft Access, Oracle, SQL Server Enterprise Manager, or Hadoop or another tool supported by your organization. Knowing "why" you are looking at the data is far more important than the specific data tools and skills that will have to be learned per your organizations information infrastructure. Rest-assured, if left to your own devices and looking for information in a database, you would likely "SELECT Patient ID, Admission date/time, Discharge date/time FROM the Encounter table WHERE Unit = Telemetry" if you wanted to create a table of patient data to calculate length of stay on a specific unit. And just that easy, you are speaking Structured Query Language (SQL). Or using Crystal Reports, COGNOS, Power BI, Tableau or countless alternatives with little learning curve assuming your understanding of the data and information being analyzed.

Velocity is descriptive of data rates being generated and often is considered more important than volume. Originally described as point-of-interaction (POI) speed, or point-of-care (POC) in healthcare, system performance and the ability to act on this data is a competitive differentiator. Having back-up databases, Operational Data Stores (ODS), Data Warehouses, Online Analytical Processing (OLAP), and other tools will allow analysts access to data without compromising core system performance. You do not want to run a large report in your EMR and hear multiple co-workers ask, "Is the system locking-up for anyone else?" Ideally, there is a reporting environment to run large analyses that is separate from the production database where data is constantly being written and retrieved.

Variety concentrates on the multiple sources and types of data. Even within a single source such as CMS Hospital Compare, the variety of data types is as numerous as the measures themselves. From patient satisfaction survey results often measuring "% Always" responses and higher is better, to Hospital-Acquired Conditions (HACs) measures per 1,000 days and lower is better. Understanding and managing the variety of information is essential in harnessing the value of big data.

Veracity focuses on the reality that data integrity is questionable to inform decisions. A very important factor, this "refers to the level of uncertainty associated with data elements and their source, and alert the user to the inherent uncertainties in data that may have been collected under unanticipated or untraceable conditions." (Brennan & Bakken, 2015). Someone serving in a role functionally described as a "Data Hygienist" by Health Information and Management Systems Society (HIMSS) would "unify and normalize data while ensuring accuracy" (Kwiatkowski, 2018). Errors may not be immediately visually obvious, such as letters appearing in a numeric data field; versus an anomaly to expected performance.

Value is at the apex of the pyramid offering opportunities for healthcare organizations to transform the tsunami of data into a cost-benefit analysis (Brennan & Bakken, 2015; Broome, 2016; Laney, 2001). Value is what you make of the data, from the negative perceived cost of compiling and submitting data to CMS per regulatory requirements, to the opportunity of being on the positive side of a linear exchange where your achievement bonus is being funded by those performing below average. Value will be further explored in Chapter 9 with the business case for change.

Big data builds on the fact that a substantial amount of public data, at the provider level with aggregate performance for thousands of measures, is readily available. This includes numerators, denominators, rates, risk adjusted factors, and qualifying information as the bi-product of regulations. The majority of this data is linked to reimbursement and performance. The calculations, such as the linear exchange rate, are fully transparent as is the data for each provider setting the performance thresholds. This includes up- and downhill calculations on the linear exchange. It is assumed that the downhill calculations optimizing the value of data will be shift to an uphill position and the current average will become below average. Similarly, top performing provider organizations will respond to increasing penalties where opportunity exists, turning a $500k penalty into a $500k payment becomes a million dollar proposition.

Including and beyond top performing provider organizations, optimizing the value of data can improve substantially, without addressing actual performance versus data capture measure by measure. The following examples illustrate this improvement idea.

- Is the operating room really that bad with regards to accidental punctures or lacerations, or is a surgeon performing a procedure with strikingly similar vernacular to those diagnoses codes?
  - Successfully removing a tumor could leave a hole in the remaining tissue.
- Is a primary care practice really that bad managing annual diabetic office visits, or do you actively manage patient status, such as inactive or deceased?

- ◎ The latter, especially does not visit for regular office visits, anywhere.
- • Is a hospital truly that bad managing C.Diff., or is a medication and test ordered too close in sequence or over ordered?
  - ◎ Including timing of order, result and diagnosis; this and other measures can go from "Present on Admission" (POA) indicators that boost risk adjustment and payment to Hospital-Acquired Condition (HAC) penalties overnight, literally.

These obvious, but potentially huge, opportunities are exploited across measures and organizations actively seeking to understand and gain value from big data. Eventually, these examples and various practices conform to standard with optimal performance with little deviance and minimal emphasis. Measures peak, becoming statistically inconsequential and potentially excluded from aggregate ratings, and maybe not reported. Or consider the scientific process yielded the null hypothesis and the measure is no longer of consequence. Regardless, big data exist because information and knowledge were used to synthesize topics, measures, standards, and the results reported publically.

The aggregate circumstance of competing in hundreds of measure outcomes across thousands of provider organizations is exponentially challenging and is contingent on the business and value of big data. Maintaining suboptimal performance in a measure, outside of the top 25% for instance, could eventually lead to below-average results and bottom 25% over a few reporting cycles. With significant performance difference in evidence-based practice, all measures potentially will continue to be significant in the business of health care.

Regulations, evidence-based medicine (EBM), predictive analytics, and artificial intelligence (AI) are grounded by information and knowledge generating policies, mandates, measures, and mechanisms requiring production of data. The burden to produce this data is also a bi-product, but only if used, value is obtainable. Poor performance in publicly reported measures echoes a quote in Chapter 4 of this book, "Whatever is tolerated, one endorses."

Defining and harnessing the most value from big data is a continuous process as healthcare organizations use reverse engineering, information, and knowledge generated from information systems and big data. Big data will continue to drive business principles and the healthcare economy in the future as mandates and regulations ensue.

INFORMATION SYSTEMS AND DATA

Similar to the cyclical process of information and knowledge is information systems and data. While most will offer data on a distribution of information, one must assume that it is a manufactured product. This assumption is founded and defined using the definition of big data. For purposes of this discussion and chapter, data must be linked and generated from IS that include, but are not limited in healthcare organizations to the electronic medical record (EMR); admission, discharge, and transfer (ADT); patient registry; billing; and other data convergence in healthcare systems. Data exist and flow between each of those systems within a provider organization and results in an extract, transform, and load (ETL) process for measures for reporting by regulatory mandates.

Information Systems for Healthcare Management identifies categories of information systems. The categories include the following: Clinical (i.e. Electronic Medical Record, EHR); Management (i.e. Admission, Discharge, Transfer systems, ADT); Strategic Decision Support Systems (DSS); Electronic Networking: and, e-Health applications (Glandon, Smaltz, & Slovensky, 2013; Wager et al., 2009). Each system or product interfaces and shares data across categories to create an effective and efficient process available to inform teams and organizations about the current data. Vendors often purport, the ideal software solution for each endeavor, will meet multiple needs. This is an epic assertion. Either sole-source or off the shelf applications are often designed to produce transactions from patient encounter documentation via template to codifying an International Classification of Disease (ICD) code. These are used for submission as a Uniform Billing (UB) form for payment.

Let there be no intimidation or apprehension when approaching big data. It is intended to provide information, knowledge, and wisdom that healthcare organizations and any business may use to produce value. If you know why you are looking at the data and what you are trying to accomplish, the rest is more readily learnable.

SUMMARY

- The footprint of data and cyclical process of information systems provide an understanding of the value of data in today's healthcare market.
- Big data and its inherent value in healthcare cannot be understated.
- When data integrity is questioned, the five Vs of big data are foundational to processes necessary to resolve what is in question and apply modifications for sound decisions.
- Reverse engineering is a technique where the value of data is captured.
- Information and knowledge are pivotal for organizational stability.

REFLECTION QUESTIONS

1. How can teams use reverse engineering in healthcare organizations to an advantage?
2. Consider the myriad of performance indicators available to any healthcare organization. Identify three indicators and how are they used to measure efficiency and maintain peak performance.
3. How can the five Vs of big data be used for large dataset analyses?

REFERENCES

Ackoff, R. L. (1999). *Ackoff's best*. John Wiley & Sons.

Berwick, D. M. (1989). Sounding board, continuous improvement as an ideal in health care. *The New England Journal of Medicine, 320*(1), 53–56. https://doi.org/10.1056/NEJM198901053200110

Brennan, P. F., & Bakken, S. (2015). Nursing needs big data and big data needs nursing. *Journal of Nursing Scholarship, 47*(5), 477–484. https://doi.org/10.1111/jnu.12159

Broome, M. E. (2016). Big data, data science, and big contributions. *Nursing Outlook, 64*(2), 113–114. https://doi.org/10.1016/j.outlook.2016.02.001

Carper, B. A. (1978). Fundamental ways of knowing in nursing. *Advances in Nursing Science, 1*(1), 13–24. https://doi.org/10.1097/00012272-197810000-00004

Ermine, J. (2018). *Knowledge management: The creative loop*, Vol. 5. Wiley.

Glandon, G. L., Smaltz, D. H., and Slovensky, D. J. (Eds.). (2014). *Information systems for healthcare management* (8th ed.). Health Administration Press.

Kwiatkowski, M. (2018, July 30). Making big data accessible to your business: How to staff & support distributed analytics teams. *Healthcare Information and Management Systems Society Clinical & Business Intelligence Community*. https://www.himss.org/resources/making-big-data-accessible-your-business-how-staff-support-distributed-analytics-teams

Laney, D. (2001). *3D data management: Controlling data volume, velocity, and variety*. https://blogs.gartner.com/doug-laney/files/2012/01/ad949-3D-Data-Management-Controlling-Data-Volume-Velocity-and-Variety.pdf

Press, G. (2014). 12 big data definitions: What's yours? *Forbes*. https://www.forbes.com/sites/gilpress/2014/09/03/12-big-data-definitions-whats-yours/#1c1d64ec13ae

Rowley, J. (2007). The wisdom hierarchy: Representations of the DIKW hierarchy. *Journal of Information Science, 33*(2), 163–180. https://doi.org/10.1177/0165551506070706

Sensmeier, J. (2015). Big data and the future of nursing knowledge. *Nursing Management, 46*(4), 22–27. https://doi.org/10.1097/01.NUMA.0000462365.53035.7d

Wager, K., Lee, F. W., & Glaser, J. P. (2009). *Healthcare information systems: A practical approach for health care management* (2nd ed.). Jossey-Bass. A Wiley Imprint.

Zeleny, M. (2006). Knowledge-information autopoietic cycle: Towards the wisdom systems. *International Journal of Management and Decision Making, 7*(1), 3–18. https://doi.org/10.1504/IJMDM.2006.008168

CASE EXEMPLAR FOR APPLICATION

Big Data and Its Utility in Health Care

Brian Collins

Big data are immeasurably generated and consistently shared globally. Big data has multiple advantages across various industries, research enterprises, and academic settings. Specifically, big data offers the healthcare industry great potential for decision-making and new insights into innovative efficiency and operational processes. As big data are generated and analyzed, new tools for predictive analysis will be required. Efficient algorithms will also be required to avoid data pitfalls such as inaccurate correlation (Gandomi & Haider, 2015; Sivarajah et al., 2017).

For purposes of this exemplar, consider information displayed in Exhibit 6.1 below and how the Centers for Medicare and Medicaid Services (CMS, 2019a; 2020a) has captured and used big data to illustrate overall performance by acute care hospital type. While this is only one example of how healthcare can use big data for analysis and comparison purposes, this information informs opportunities for current and future opportunities related to quality, safety, and efficiency.

REFLECTION QUESTIONS

1. What value does big data have for health care, research enterprises, and academia? Elaborate on each area and provide examples relevant to practice.
2. How will big data of the future guide innovation and new healthcare technology? Identify a potential role you will play in this future area.

EXHIBIT 6.1 Centers for Medicare and Medicaid Services Value-Based Purchasing FY2020 Overall Performance and by Hospital Type

MEAN (AVERAGE)	RCC	IPPS PROPRIETARY/ PHYSICIAN	IPPS GOVERNMENT	IPPS NON-PROFIT PRIVATE	IPPS NON-PROFIT CHURCH/ OTHER	SCH/RRC	SCH	MDH/ OTHER
				RESULTS BY ACUTE CARE HOSPITAL TYPE				
Count (n)	2,731	373	388	230	864	341	143	254	138
Average # of Beds	218	300	196	249	247	239	166	86	67
Average Daily Census	130	190	110	161	153	143	84	36	24
Est. Medicare Discharges	3,208	4,680	2,588	2,996	3,714	3,494	3,057	1,352	1,015
Est. MCR $ per Disch. (CMI x $6k)	10,748	10,973	10,580	11,136	10,824	10,978	10,142	9,507	8,496
Actual FY2020 VBP Adj. Factor	1.001636	0.999637	0.999729	1.000128	1.001695	1.002087	1.002478	1.005438	1.005564
Est. FY2020 VBP bonus or (penalty)	56,402	(18,657)	(7,414)	4,270	68,130	80,032	76,827	69,914	47,998

Hospital Statistics

(continued)

EXHIBIT 6.1 Centers for Medicare and Medicaid Services Value-Based Purchasing FY2020 Overall Performance and by Hospital Type (continued)

	MEAN (AVERAGE)	RESULTS BY ACUTE CARE HOSPITAL TYPE							
		RCC	IPPS PROPRIETARY/ PHYSICIAN	IPPS GOVERNMENT	IPPS NON-PROFIT PRIVATE	IPPS NON-PROFIT CHURCH/ OTHER	SCH/RRC	SCH	MDH/ OTHER
KPIs									
Average Occupancy %	59.9%	63.2%	56.2%	64.4%	62.1%	60.1%	50.6%	42.1%	35.9%
Medicare ALOS	4.75	4.87	4.78	5.01	4.77	4.77	4.38	4.03	3.96
Medicare Case Mix Index (CMI)	1.7914	1.8288	1.7633	1.8559	1.8040	1.8297	1.6903	1.5845	1.4160
Quality (VBP Payment Adj. %)	0.1636%	−0.0363%	−0.0271%	0.0128%	0.1695%	0.2087%	0.2478%	0.5438%	0.5564%
VBP Domains									
Clinical Care	58.4	59.7	59.2	57.3	57.9	59.0	58.6	58.1	56.8
Community Engagement	32.0	31.5	31.4	29.5	32.7	31.9	34.4	32.7	30.8
Safety	44.3	42.6	44.1	46.6	44.6	44.8	44.4	43.9	43.7
Efficiency and Cost Reduction	19.8	17.9	20.7	20.4	20.6	18.5	20.0	18.9	21.1

MORT-30-AMI	0.8722	0.8734	0.8737	0.8722	0.8716	0.8726	0.8723	0.8701	0.8720
MORT-30-HF	0.8833	0.8847	0.8837	0.8830	0.8828	0.8837	0.8825	0.8828	0.8828
MORT-30-PN	0.8977	0.8984	0.8969	0.8968	0.8980	0.8980	0.8981	0.8968	0.8978
**COMP-HIP-KNEE	0.0256	0.0260	0.0258	0.0258	0.0255	0.0260	0.0251	0.0251	0.0252
Communication with Nurses	78.7	78.8	78.6	78.2	78.7	78.7	79.3	78.7	78.7
Communication with Doctors	79.4	79.4	79.4	78.8	79.4	79.5	79.6	79.7	79.4
Responsiveness of Hospital Staff	65.8	65.7	66.1	65.0	65.9	65.5	66.6	66.0	65.3
Communication about Medicines	63.4	63.5	63.3	62.9	63.6	63.4	63.8	63.5	63.4
Cleanliness and Quietness Env.	65.2	65.1	64.9	64.1	65.4	65.1	65.4	65.6	65.1
Discharge Information	86.6	86.6	86.5	86.3	86.8	86.7	86.4	86.3	86.4
Overall Rating of Hospital	70.5	70.8	70.2	69.1	70.6	70.6	70.9	70.8	70.9

Clinical Care: MORT-30-AMI, MORT-30-HF, MORT-30-PN, **COMP-HIP-KNEE

Community Engagement: Communication with Nurses, Communication with Doctors, Responsiveness of Hospital Staff, Communication about Medicines, Cleanliness and Quietness Env., Discharge Information, Overall Rating of Hospital

(continued)

EXHIBIT 6.1 Centers for Medicare and Medicaid Services Value-Based Purchasing FY2020 Overall Performance and by Hospital Type (continued)

	MEAN (AVERAGE)	RESULTS BY ACUTE CARE HOSPITAL TYPE							
		RCC	IPPS PROPRIETARY/ PHYSICIAN	IPPS GOVERNMENT	IPPS NON-PROFIT PRIVATE	IPPS NON-PROFIT CHURCH/ OTHER	SCH/RRC	SCH	MDH/ OTHER
Safety** CLASBI (HAI-1)	0.722	0.745	0.713	0.661	0.751	0.668	0.699	0.779	0.658
CAUTI (HAI-2)	0.812	0.824	0.865	0.794	0.806	0.832	0.783	0.790	0.715
SSI CS (HAI-3)	0.829	0.861	0.905	0.870	0.824	0.782	0.912	0.712	0.751
SSI AH (HAI-4)	0.863	0.896	0.845	0.883	0.906	0.756	0.752	0.948	0.784
MRSA (HAI-5)	0.836	0.832	0.830	0.863	0.828	0.782	0.891	0.852	0.934
CDI (HAI-6)	0.684	0.706	0.700	0.681	0.665	0.670	0.652	0.700	0.737
Elec. Del. <39wks (PC-01)	0.015	0.016	0.014	0.015	0.015	0.012	0.017	0.019	0.021

| ** | Efficiency and Cost Reduction MSPB | 0.98890 | 0.99270 | 0.98427 | 0.99138 | 0.98796 | 0.98941 | 0.98951 | 0.99353 | 0.98295 |

**1Lower values indicated better performance for these measures. Z-scores are multiplied by -1.

Sources: From Centers for Medicare and Medicaid Services. (2020a). *FY 2020 final rule and correction notice impact file.* https://www.cms.gov/Medicare/Medicare-Fee-for-Service-Payment/AcuteInpatientPPS/FY2020-IPPS-Final-Rule-Home-Page-Items/FY2020-IPPS-Final-Rule-Data-Files; Centers for Medicare and Medicaid Services. (2020b). *FY 2020 final rule and correction notice tables, hospital valuebased purchasing (VBP) program* . https://www.cms.gov/Medicare/Medicare-Fee-for-Service-Payment/AcuteInpatientPPS/FY2020-IPPS-Final-Rule-Home-Page-Items/FY2020-IPPS-Final-Rule-Tables; Centers for Medicater and Medicaid Servicest. (2019). *How to read your fiscal year* (FY) 2020 hospital value-based purchasing (VBP) program percentage payment summary report (PPSR). www.medicare.gov/hospitalcompare/Data

REFERENCES

Centers for Medicare and Medicaid Services. (2019a). CMS hospital value-based purchasing program results for fiscal year 2020. *Fact sheet, CMS Newsroom, October 29, 2019.* https://www.cms.gov/newsroom/fact-sheets/cms-hospital-value-based-purchasing-program-results-fiscal-year-2020

Centers for Medicare and Medicaid Services. (2019b). How to read your fiscal year (FY) 2020 hospital value-based purchasing (VBP) program percentage payment summary report (PPSR). https:www.medicare.gov/hospitalcompare/Data

Centers for Medicare and Medicaid Services. (2020a). *FY 2020 Final Rule and Correction Notice Impact File.* https://www.cms.gov/Medicare/Medicare-Fee-for-Service-Payment/AcuteInpatientPPS/FY2020-IPPS-Final-Rule-Home-Page-Items/FY2020-IPPS-Final-Rule-Data-Files

Centers for Medicare and Medicaid Services. (2020b). *FY 2020 final rule and correction notice tables, hospital valuebased purchasing (VBP) program.* https://www.cms.gov/Medicare/Medicare-Fee-for-Service-Payment/AcuteInpatientPPS/FY2020-IPPS-Final-Rule-Home-Page-Items/FY2020-IPPS-Final-Rule-Tables

Gandomi, A., & Haider, M. (2015). Beyond the hype: Big data concepts, methods, and analytics. *International Journal of Information Management, 35*(2), 137–144.

Sivarajah, U., Kamal, M. M., Irani, Z., & Weerakkody, V. (2017). *Journal of Business Research, 70,* 263–286. doi.org/10.1016/j.busres.2016.08.001

7

Data as an Influencer of Policy and Regulation

Michael R. Bleich and Patricia L. Thomas

OBJECTIVES

1. Analyze how data influences policy and regulation development and implementation.
2. Relate examples of the influence of policy and regulation on healthcare quality, safety, and value.
3. Identify sources and barriers germane to national and global data use when developing policy and regulations.
4. Cite exemplars of how globalization is impacting health policy and practices through information exchange.
5. Utilize reports, documents, and tools to formulate organizational and social policy and/or regulations that standardize and stabilize clinical practice and resource utilization.
6. Identify the ramifications of strategic policy and regulation development on individual practice.

CORE COMPETENCIES

- Understand how data influences policy and regulation development and implementation in a data rich environment
- Adapt strategies to managing a global healthcare environment influenced by existing evidence
- Possess knowledge and skills about legislative processes to become politically active in policy and regulation development

- Exhibit an ability to use reports, documents, and tools to improve healthcare quality, safety, and value

INTRODUCTION

Healthcare is an industry known to be data rich and information poor. This saying reflects an imbalance in the return on investment related to the human and technological cost of entering clinical, financial, and organizational data into various databases. These databases are crucial to decision-making, particularly when data are accessible, valid, reliable, and timely. Over time, the overabundance of data entry has fallen on the backs of clinicians to fulfill unfettered expectations from multiple data-demanding stakeholders. Despite this burden, data can be culled and refined into information. Information is a data set or a subset useable in practice. From data, information results when it can be retrieved, modeled, and applied with computer technology. Information provides direction and insight into health policy and regulatory standards development, all with direct care management and service reimbursement implications. For these reasons and more, data and information are influencers in policy and regulation.

Reflect on the volumes of health data generated daily and how that data is used. Skilled clinicians use data and transform it into information to guide practice at the point-of-care. Others collect data and aggregate it to reveal patterns that would be invisible in its raw form; this data guides quality and safety improvement initiatives aimed at one or more patient populations. Other analysts use information to identify fragmentation in care delivery or to improve operational efficiency.

Historically, data management was limited to its manual collection and analysis. Today, computerization permits data entry, storage, and manipulation that is limitless and nonstop, an unprecedented reality. The amount of healthcare data collected and used in formulating health policy is so massive it goes by a special name: Big Data. Data scientists have developed software used by clinicians, administrators, and researchers to store masses of data in data warehouses. Big data accounts for massive volumes of clinical and organizational data, retrieves data from a variety of sources, and has velocity in transforming it into information. Known as the three Vs, big data accommodates volume, variety, and velocity (Warren, 2017).

The advent of big data for policy- and regulatory-setters has unequaled value. So much is data and information a critical aspect of healthcare service delivery that several landmark reports and publications are credited with standardizing data usage by requiring multiple data sources, assuring data validity and reliability for its intended use, and for influencing comparative improvement initiatives so consumers have a choice in where and from whom they receive care.

In this chapter, policy and regulation is defined; landmark reports, documents, initiatives, and organizations that influence data management requirements are discussed; technology enhancements as influencers in global data sharing are proffered; the function of data in advancing global strategic policy and regulation is posited; and barriers, constraints, and ethics to open source data use in the context of regulatory environments is posted.

POLICY AND REGULATION DEFINED

As a foundation for the chapter, policy and regulation are defined. The definitions align with their linkage to healthcare delivery, operational management, policy, and mandated statutes.

In general usage, policy is defined as a directive statement developed and monitored by an authority which advances a purposeful course of action and sets direction in response to a problem or situation (Milstead & Short, 2019). Milstead and Short (2019) references policy as the standing decisions of an organization. Health policy is aimed at ways to improve the longevity and overall well-being of populations, mandates defining consumer expectations that enrich the patient experience, and directives about the human and material resources needed to effectively and efficiently fulfill these aims (Feldstein, 1999). As presented in this chapter, policy examples will begin at the individual and organizational level and evolve to reflect global examples.

To healthcare providers, one example of a health policy is a regulatory mandate specifying actions aimed at human and material waste reduction in the health system. In writing good policy, policymakers examine how a directive impacts upstream and downstream consequences to ensure that the mandate does not unduly conflict with other policies or negatively influence practices. This careful deliberation ensures equilibrium and growth toward an optimal system of care (Bodenheimer & Grumbach, 2005). During the ideal policymaking process, data informs the process. This data is drawn from clinical research, epidemiologic, financial, population-based, demographic, and other data bases. Data modeling, the computer-aided process of organizing and standardizing assorted data sets into a format that illustrates how these data interrelate to one another such that predictive analytics further informs decision-making needed for policy setting.

Policies have their authoritative genesis from state and federal law, regulatory standards, professional practice acts, association standards, or consumer groups. Any organization has multiple policies in place, and some are discordant with others. An effective set of policies results when discordance is minimized through boundary scanning sources of best practices, keeping abreast of laws and regulations, and using internal monitoring to ensure relative congruence between and among policy directives. For example, a policy developed by the risk management department may restrict clinical practices that may be allowed in a state practice act.

As noted above, policies are generated from multiple sources, including regulations. Regulation has a more prescribed policy function. One difference is that regulations result from federal, state, or local statute, making noncompliance illegal. In some cases, statutes may authorize the monitoring and compliance function of the law to private agencies. For example, an accrediting agency such as the Joint Commission is authorized by federal statute to monitor healthcare agencies to federal standards. The Centers for Medicare and Medicaid Services translate statutes into regulations, such as the Health Insurance Portability and Accountability Act (HIPAA) that protects patient privacy (U.S. Department of Health and Human Services, 2013). Simply, a regulation is defined as standard or rule with mandated oversight (Miller-Keane Encyclopedia and Dictionary of Medicine, Nursing, and Allied Health, 2003). A second difference is that noncompliance with mandatory regulations can result in fines, compulsory compliance training and intensive monitoring, and even organizational closure in extreme violations. It should be appreciated that policy and regulations are strengthened with the use of available evidence but there is no requirement that data and information be used in the development of these practices. Regardless, the use of data is a desirable contribution when health professionals are engaged in policy development.

LANDMARK REPORTS, DOCUMENTS, AND INITIATIVES INFORMING POLICY, REGULATION, AND INITIATIVES IN HEALTHCARE

The benefit of most landmark reports, such as those from the National Academy of Medicine (formerly the Institute of Medicine), are that by law they must use evidence-based sources in their policy recommendations. Users of reports that are evidence-driven are assured of objective blind reviews, use of best available evidence, and the elimination of biases, adding to the social value of report recommendations. That said, the agencies issuing reports or white papers lack the authority to mandate and monitor policy implementation and evaluation. Other authoritative resources that interpret, write, implement, and evaluate policy are left with that duty, so to the extent that the recommendations suggested by objective reports are followed, it assures that data and information are incorporated into policies and regulations.

A variety of landmark reports, documents, and initiatives have guided healthcare improvement activities, daily operations, and informed policy and regulation on local, state, national, and global levels. Each report referenced below used valid and reliable data sources in their analysis and communication strategies to achieve the maximum benefit of their intent.

When the report entitled *Best Care at Lower Cost: The Path to Continuously Learning Health Care in America* was issued, it highlighted how the better use of data would improve healthcare delivery and outcomes. The report underscored the value of bringing state-of-the-art knowledge to the field of medicine and illustrated emerging data management tools that would enrich decision science. With better use of data, the report noted its influence to better guide continuous improvement initiatives and inform leaders on methods to eliminate healthcare economic instability and threats to global competitiveness. Left unchanged, the report projected that without improved data collection, mining, and use, the healthcare industry would continue to underperform, cause unnecessary patient harm, and threaten global market stability given the relationship between health and well-being of society and overall industrial capacity. This report revealed that value of conjoining healthcare organizations, legislators, and consumers to mitigate deleterious outcomes, a required transformative partnership to improve clinical care (Institute of Medicine [IOM], 2012).

Crossing the Quality Chasm: A New Health System for the 21st Century is another Institute of Medicine seminal report that intensified a holistic approach to quality improvement. This roadmap enabled leaders to account for metrics that would comprehensively show that care delivery was safe (no harm done), effective (treatment achieved the intended purpose), patient-centered (accounting for individual differences and preferences), timely (avoiding time-sensitive treatment delays), efficient (to reduce the cost of waste) and equitable (ensuring that all people had access to care and services) (IOM, 2001).

With metrics and data collection plans reflecting a holistic perspective, decision-makers could track these metrics on dashboards, a tool to visualize the impact of attempted change initiatives on the other system components. For instance, improving the efficiency of care delivery, if taken too far, might have a negative impact on safety. Stratifying data by population characteristics in the patient-centered domain might reveal that care is inequitable.

Regardless of the healthcare system or improvement initiative, purposeful metrics and the resultant data collected are the cornerstone to provide evidence that the intent of six industry services characteristics is met internally and externally, and in compliance with regulatory and accrediting agency mandates. Institutional policies and procedures are informed with the enriched data set.

The Centers for Medicare and Medicaid Services (CMS) is replete with documents and publications reflecting directives and mandatory requirements for organizational and provider reporting and surveillance. Two examples of data collection requirements that are used for quality and outcomes assessments are the Hospital Consumer Assessment of Healthcare Providers and Systems (HCAHPS) and Hospital Compare databases (Centers for Medicare and Medicaid Services [CMS, 2019]; CMS, n.d.).

In use since 2006, HCAHPS is a standardized patient survey developed under the rigor of the Agency for Healthcare Research and Quality (AHRQ) to capture hospital care experiences. The data from this survey are designed to produce comparable data on important consumer topics. Second, this data provides incentives to hospitals to achieve high clinical standards. Third, the data is published nationally to increase public accountability and increase transparency between and among hospitals (HCAHPS Survey, 2020). Patients at least 18 years of age that are discharged with nonpsychiatric medical-surgical or maternity-based diagnoses are randomly selected to participate in the survey, conducted within 48 hours to six weeks post-hospital discharge. The survey measure nurse communication, physician communication, responsiveness of hospital staff, pain management, communication about medications, and discharge information provided, in addition to the cleanliness and noise levels of the hospital environment.

Using HCAHPS scores and other metrics determined by hospital and public sector stakeholders, Hospital Compare is a consumer service website that rates hospital performance in the topics noted above. While hospitals find the scoring system controversial, the HCAHPS scores and other measures are converted into a summary star rating system. Beyond patient satisfaction, the star rating system accounts for surgical complications and death rates, unplanned hospital visits, complications such as infection, timely and effective care administered to patients with sepsis, heart attack, and other diagnoses, and claims data captured from Medicare payments (CMS, n.d.). Each has indirect and direct impact on continuous improvement initiatives, reimbursement, and organizational sustainability. These and other examples of CMS data sets are retrievable from CMS (CMS, 2019). With widespread application and noted relevance from payors, regulators, and consumers, hospital compare has been extended into homecare (www.medicare.gov/homehealthcompare/search.html) and nursing homes (www.medicare.gov/nursinghomecompare/search.html) to compare skilled nursing facilities.

Two organizations that have ignited data collection, analysis, and management are the Institute for Healthcare Improvement (IHI) and the World Health Organization (WHO). The IHI launched in 1991 as a collaborative movement to redesign a health system that was suffering from error, waste, delays, and unsustainable costs. As it grew, IHI expanded its emphasis to include advancing innovation and become a voice in the geopolitical direction of health; it has become an influential force in the United States and multiple other nations (IHI, 2020).

Today the IHI provides multiple data collection tools and techniques for data analysis through its annual conference, its online Open School which offers courses for the novice to the expert on subjects encompassing building a culture to support quality; defining and advancing quality improvement and patient safety competencies; promoting leadership development; and guiding project management to drive improvement (IHI, 2020).

Globally, IHI has leveraged its expansive network to address its triple aim: to simultaneously improve the individual patient experience, examine patterns and trends associated with population health, and address the cost of care (Whittington et al., 2015). Recently, a fourth aim emerged as a result of clinician burnout and work dissatisfaction. The fourth aim ensures that the healthcare cultures addresses the care of the provider, the linchpin between policies, regulation, processes, and the patient (Bodenheimer & Sinksy, 2014). IHI has addressed global health and assists global entities in addressing healthcare needs that align regional initiatives and utilize a combination of foci drawn from the quadruple aim (IHI, 2015). In addition to supporting improvement initiatives in the United States, the IHI has partnered with Europe, Africa, the Middle East, Central America, and the Caribbean to address health needs of vulnerable populations across the globe to build capacity to create sustainable solutions (IHI International, n.d.).

Established through the auspices of the United Nations, The World Health Organization (WHO) was launched in 1948 and today covers 194 member states across six regions of the world. The WHO has led global standards development in public health functions such as ensuring air and water quality standards, vaccinations, and preventing and addressing problems from asthma to Zika. Through WHO, important strategies develop that address universal health coverage by focusing on primary care and health workforce training, addressing health emergencies, and addressing the social determinants of health across the globe.

Important to this chapter is the WHO's Global Health Observatory, an interactive repository of health statistics of specific health topics (WHO, 2020). With health-related statistics derived from more than 1,000 indicators, these data align with the United Nations Sustainable Development Goals (SDGs) (United Nations Sustainable Development Goals, n.d.). There are 17 goals that universal governments, businesses, medial, institutions of higher education, and local nongovernmental organizations have established to improve the lives of people globally. To meet these various goals, which range from eliminating poverty, erasing hunger, promoting health and well-being, and improving clean water and sanitation, among others, they require baseline data, data to measure the impact of initiatives, and outcomes measures (United Nations Sustainable Development Goals, n.d.).

The global health observatory data is considered a metadata repository. This means it is an open-source collection for use by clinicians, legislators, policymakers, researchers, and others and it can be searched by theme, category, indicator, or country for download in various file formats. Metadata stores hundreds of separate pieces of information, each of which has its own structured format. As a metadata repository, the user gains the benefit of easily capturing a range of data at their fingertips global data that may be been captured in multiple computer formats. WHO's work encompasses a series of regulatory and legislative actions that are consistently linked to the health goals of society. Data are systematically collected and used to advance care using available evidence in underserved and underrepresented regions (WHO, 2015).

GLOBALIZATION OF HEALTHCARE AND THE INFLUENCE OF EXISTING DATA

What is globalization and how does it impact healthcare? Globalization is the growing interdependence of the world's economies, cultures, and populations brought about by many factors such as technology, information flow, and service provision with regard for society as a whole, rather than siloed perspectives of each nation (Peterson Institute for International Economics [PIIE], 2019). Globalization is complex and has political ramifications through trade agreements, and economic factors. In healthcare globalization includes but is not limited to research partnerships crossing borders, sharing scientific advances, solving clinical problems and implementing interventions across populations and socioeconomic groups, medical tourism, and workforce credentialing.

As noted in the last section, metadata bases through WHO and coalitions between and among international nursing organizations such as the International Council of Nurses, Sigma Theta Tau, university partnerships, and others are introducing new concepts and ideas for ways to deliver care, enrich cultural awareness, share human and material resources, and influence social determinants of health that may deter from societal health and well-being. While each country adheres to cultural and legal norms, there is increased data influence contributing to actions tied to global warming, disease eradication, the effects of poverty, illiteracy, food production

and availability and factors noted in the SDGs. The availability of a healthy and productive workforce is the basis for industries to thrive and increasingly, these work-
forces may leave one country and travel to another to fill needs. Relocated people
give credence to the statement that sometimes global is local – the cross-exchange of
people with varying cultural backgrounds and perspectives and with varying views of
quality of care and health practices are integrated across the globe. Data is informing
new global perspectives and sharpened the awareness of those experiencing health
disparities, now trackable with longitudinal (Labonté et al., 2015).

In finance and business circles, globalization ostensibly relates to the economic
benefits derived from increased international trade, investment, and product integration, and associated reductions in the prevalence of poverty (Dollar, 2001). Negative
health aspects associated with globalization are cited in the literature and include
threats to public health and government's regulatory policy space from multilateral
and bilateral trade agreements, structural adjustment policies, growing income, and
wealth inequalities (Deaton, 2004). These reflect, in turn, the increasing importance
of what a *Lancet* Commission described as "transnational activities that involve
actors with different interests and degrees of power" (Marmot, 2005; Ottersen et al.,
2014, p. 630). Changing the future will require global leaders to reflect on a common
good where healthcare is accessible, affordable, and of high quality (Bodenheimer &
Grumbach, 2005).

Other studies have focused on the links between globalization and social
determinants of health (SDH), defined broadly as the working and living conditions that determine people's abilities to lead healthy lives (Labonté & Schrecker,
2007a; 2007b; 2007c; Lee, 2007). One of the arching insights documented in the
SDH literature is the health effect of globalization on lack of uniform care distribution among populations and disparities producing significant variances in SDH
(Labonté et al., 2009).

As presented, globalization in healthcare presents both a panacea of opportunity
and an increased awareness of the factors that impede health and well-being. Leaders
are urged to use data to enhance their understanding of the SDH, the multilevel economic and cultural impact from the local organizational level to a global and societal
level, and how the impact of disease and disability impacts all people, as reflected in
the transmission of SARS, Ebola, and Corona virus. At the heart of leadership is how
data informs the need for policy as a standing direction, as noted earlier in this chapter, and what level of focus sufficiently impacts population health – organizational to
federal to global. What data is collected, how it is accessed, how it is used, and how it
is secured are all influenced by leaders.

DETERMINANTS OF STRATEGIC POLICY AND REGULATION DEVELOPMENT AND HOW DATA INFORMS OUTCOMES

The rapid acceleration of data and speed with which healthcare decisions must be
made, and predominate attention focusing on improving quality, safety, and value

of healthcare can result in a cognitive dissonance as noted previously – not all policies and regulation align and there is nonlinearity in bringing each aspect of data management into play, creating what can feel like an imminent threat to survival in a turbulent healthcare situation. The paradox of how data will inform process and product is often absent because information is drawn from and not linked across sectors, further limiting the ability to determine the current state of an organization financially and operationally. This paradox justifies the important of metadata bases. Analyzing a topic of interest enables healthcare leaders and policy makers to discern patterns or relationships among discrete events and comprehend, rather than approach the situation with apprehension. Little good is produced when one pontificates with little or no understanding of the phenomenon or circumstances. Opportunity will be missed. When opportunity is missed or goes unrecognized, the ability to strategically frame a policy or regulation well, trade-offs or compromises are jeopardized and absent to the relevance of a stated objective. This requires policy and regulation development that has clarity, meets the intended objective, involves leaders and consumers, and links data to evidence as organizations validate desired outcomes and meet required indicators of performance (Hallworth et al., 2014).

BARRIERS AND GAPS USING DATA TO ACHIEVE THE INTENT OF POLICY AND REGULATIONS

Despite the progress made in data management as presented in this chapter, barriers and gaps remain to its full use. First, leaders must be trained in big data, beyond the traditional tools or applications limited to a single data set. An important part of this training combines clinical documentation reported in electronic health records, to outcomes that are publicly reported, and business intelligence reports. A second issue is that many organizations struggle with systems interoperability. Simply stated, at the organizational level clinical, human resource, financial, and operational data bases do not interact. Add to these other forms of public use data that are inoperable to internally based computer capacity and the problem of interoperability becomes even a greater barrier to effective data management. A third gap is that healthcare has been limited by nonstandardized data names, definitions, and conceptual unity. Think of all of the terms that are used in managing pain: discomfort, ache, soreness, strain, cramps, paroxysm, and throbbing. Retrieving data for pain management outcomes is challenged if the computer programs are unable to detect these variants in nomenclature. Sadly, nursing documentation is often not archived for analysis in many electronic health records. In the United States and other countries without a national health system, data retrieval is far less accessible than in those countries with a designed system (Englebright & Jackson, 2017).

To summarize, Heitmueller et al. (2014) identified three broad categories of barriers: (a) normative barriers, (b) market failures, and (c) technocratic barriers. Normative barriers include cultural and ethical norms surrounding data usage. These affect individual trust that data confidentiality will be protected with mandated regulations. This concern remains today with significant human and fiscal resources invested to ensure data security and confidentiality (Giest, 2017; Zook et al., 2017).

Market failures focus on conflicts that are inherent with how data will benefit society globally with those who control the data. While data may be spread for the improvement of health and care delivery, adverse behavioral consequences may develop and require different policy responses. What is posed as an opportunity in industry to improve health and treatment options may conversely prove to outweigh the wider benefits when individual and group privacy is at risk (Giest, 2017; Vellido, 2019).

Technocratic barriers refer to issues that include technology, government rules and procedures, and are concerned with technology, industry data standards, data system inoperability, and legislation. This requires government intervention on a global scale to ensure privacy and a balance between the collective interest of individuals, organizations, and government in respect to data use and sharing. While these concerns were identified nearly two decades ago, the ethical questions and concerns continue to influence decision making today (Giest, 2017).

NATIONAL AND INTERNATIONAL USE OF DATA TO GUIDE POLICY AND PRACTICE

Whether on a national or international level, using data to guide policy and practice is contingent on making a robust case for change. Making the case to use and interpret data for the implicit purpose of policy development requires transparency and ethical considerations for how information will be used, shared, and whether there is an incentive for individuals to gain benefit from its use. This becomes an even more important consideration when global data is used from countries or societies where values are less scrupulous or data sources less monitored.

Making the case for national and international data use and sharing requires solid evidence that is based on an identified need and explicit benefits for care delivery, spread of evidence, and generation of new knowledge. Creating a demand for data applications, incentivizing innovation, and partnerships are recognized enablers to sharing data. This will require individuals to question if existing policy and practices are achieving the balance between identified benefits and potential risks (Heitmueller et al., 2014). If deficits are found, actions by leaders, legislators, and consumers are required in order to amend policies and practices that meet the contemporary needs in healthcare noting confidentiality and data ownership warrant a deliberate and thorough assessment and evaluation prior to its use (Giest, 2017; Zook et. al., 2017).

Understanding the value of how data guide policy and practice requires legislative and practice savvy. If nations are to combat illness and promote the health and well-being of individuals in a global society, partnerships that support data sharing is justified and imperative. Otherwise, individual and potential organizational or international innovations become missed opportunities that cannot be recaptured (Biot et al., 2019; Kalkman et al., 2019; Zenooz & Fox, 2019).

SUMMARY

- Leaders have increased responsibility to make evidence-based or evidence-informed decisions in their leadership practice. This includes but is not limited to data that drives policy and regulation.
- Leaders are authors of policy, interpreters of policy, and evaluators of policy from authoritative sources including laws and regulations.
- Policy has been defined and introduced as relevant at the individual, organizational, and societal level.
- Far-reaching exemplars of policy drivers have been presented from the sources including that National Academy of Medicine, Center for Medicare and Medicaid Services, World Health Organization, Institute for Healthcare Improvement, and others.
- Expansive data bases that collect data and provide computerized tools to accommodate the volume of data from a variety of sources, with the velocity to use it in real time are presented, known as the three Vs. This data drives quality improvement and population-based best practices.
- The concept of how data has influenced globalization and the ability to address boundaryless social problems linked to health and well-being has been presented.
- While healthcare has always been a data-rich environment, it is no longer information poor.
- Information, the outcome of useable data to solve real-world problems and establish policy that gives direction to improve health status is now plausible in policymaking.

REFLECTION QUESTIONS

1. How does data drive current clinical practices? What is your obligation in data entry? What capacity do you have to identify patterns of clinical care from the electronic health record or other databases? Is there an adequate return on the investment you make at this time?
2. What is the role of research in adding data to the development of health policy?
3. Where would you secure demographic, epidemiologic, and economic data to build the case for policy setting?
4. How does the saying, "global is local" apply to your locale? What are the healthcare considerations that must be given to immigrant populations settling from their countries of origin to a different nation?
5. Globalization is usually tied to economics. Is this a fair representation of globalization? Why does economics enter into the arena of healthcare policymaking?
6. What policy would you like to introduce to improve the health and well-being of those in your care? How would you build the case for this policy using data? What would the policy directive you would like to see in place be expressed?

REFERENCES

Biot, C., Johnson, P., Massart, S., & Pecuchet, N. (2019). *Data sharing is key to innovation in health care*. MIT Technology Review. https://www.technologyreview.com/2019/09/27/132847/data-sharing-is-key-to-innovation-in-health-care/

Bodenheimer, T., & Grumbach, K. (2005). *Understanding health policy: A clinical approach* (4th ed.). Lange Medical Books/McGraw-Hill.

Bodenheimer, T., & Sinsky, C. (2014). From triple to quadruple aim: Care of the patient requires care of the provider. *Annals of Family Medicine, 12*(6), 573–576. http://www.annfammed.org/content/12/6/573.full

Centers for Medicare and Medicaid Services. (n.d.) *About hospital compare*. https://www.medicare.gov/hospitalcompare/Data/Data-Sources.html

Centers for Medicare and Medicaid Services. (2019). *HCAHPS: Patients' perspectives of care survey*. https://www.cms.gov/Medicare/Quality-Initiatives-Patient-Assessment-Instruments/HospitalQualityInits/HospitalHCAHPS

Deaton, A. (2004). *Health in an age of globalization*. National Bureau of National Research.

Dollar, D. (2001). Is globalization good for your health? *Bulletin of World Health Organization, 79*, 827–833.

Englebright, J., & Jackson, E. (2017). Wrestling with big data: How nurse leaders can engage. In C. W. Delaney, C. A. Weaver, J. J. Warren, T. R. Clancy, & R. L. Simpson (Eds.), *Big data-enabled nursing: Education, research, and practice*. Springer International Publishing.

Feldstein, P. J. (1999). *Health policy issues: An economic perspective on health reform*. Health Administration Press.

Giest, S. (2017). Big data for policymaking: Fad or fasttrack? *Policy Science, 50*, 367–382. https://link-springer-com.proxy.lib.wayne.edu/content/pdf/10.1007/s11077-017-9293-1.pdf

Hallworth, M., Parker, S., & Rutter, J. (2014). *Policy making in the real world: Evidence and analysis*. Institute for Government.

The HCAHPS Survey – Frequently asked questions. (2020). https://www.cms.gov/Medicare/Quality-Initiatives-Patient-Assessment-Instruments/HospitalQualityInits/Downloads/HospitalHCAHPSFactSheet201007.pdf

Heitmueller, A., Henderson, S., Warburton, W., Elmajarid, A., Pentland, A., & Darzi, A. (2014). Developing public policy to advance the use of big data in health care. *Health Affairs, 33*(9), 1523–1530. https://doi.org/10.1377/hlthaff.2014.0771

Institute for Healthcare Improvement. (2015). *How to improve*. http://www.ihi.org/resources/Pages/HowtoImprove/ScienceofImprovementEstablishingMeasures.aspx

Institute for Healthcare Improvement. (2020). *History*. http://www.ihi.org/about/pages/history.aspx

Institute for Health Improvement International. (n.d.). *About*. http://ihiinternational.org

Institute of Medicine. (2001). *Crossing the quality chasm: A new health system for the 21st century*. National Academy Press.

Institute of Medicine. (2012). *Best care at lower cost: The path to continuously learning health care in America*. National Academy Press.

Kalkman, S., Mostert, M., Gerlinger, C, van Delden, J. J. M., & van Thiel, G. J. M. W. (2019). Responsible data sharing in international health research: A systematic review of principles and norms. *BMC Medical Ethics, 20*(1), Article 21. https://bmcmedethics.biomedcentral.com/articles/10.1186/s12910-019-0359-9

Labonté, R., Cobbett, E., Orsini, M., Spitzer, D., Schrecker, T., & Ruckert, A. (2015). Globalization and the health of Canadians: Having a job is the most important thing. *Global Health, 11*, 19. https://doi.org/10.1186/s12992-015-0104-1

Labonté, R., & Schrecker, T. (2007a). Globalization and social determinants of health: Introduction and methodological background (part 1 of 3). *Globalization Health, 3*(1), 5. https://doi.org/10.1186/1744-8603-3-5

Labonté, R., & Schrecker, T. (2007b). Globalization and social determinants of health: Promoting health equality in global governance (part 3 of 3). *Globalization Health, 3*(1), 7. https://doi.org/10.1186/1744-8603-3-7

Labonté, R., & Schrecker, T. (2007c). Globalization and social determinants of health: The role of the global marketplace (part 2 of 3). *Globalization Health, 3*(1), 6. https://doi.org/10.1186/1744-8603-3-6

Labonté, R., & Schrecker, T., Packer, C., & Runnels, V. (2009). *Globalization and health: Pathways, evidence and policy.* Routledge.

Lee, K., World Health Organization, & Commission on Social Determinants of Health. (2007). *Globalization, global governance and the social determinants of health: A review of linkages and agenda for action.* World Health Organization.

Marmot, M. (2005). Social determinants of health inequalities. *The Lancet, 365*(9464), 1099–1104. https://doi.org/10.1016/S0140-6736(05)71146-6

Miller-Keane Encyclopedia and Dictionary of Medicine, Nursing, and Allied Health (7th ed.). (2003). Regulation. W. B. Saunders.

Milstead, J. A., & Short, N. A. (2019). *Health policy and politics: A nurse's guide* (6th ed.). Jones & Bartlett Learning.

Ottersen, O. P., Dasgupta, J., Blouin, C., Buss, P., Chongsuvivatwong, V., Frenk, J., Fukuda-Parr, S., Gawanas, B. P., Giacaman, R., Gyapong, J., Leaning, J., Marmot, M., . . . Scheel, I. B. (2014). The political origins of health inequality: Prospects for change. *Lancet, 383*(9917), 639–667. https://doi.org/10.1016/S0140-6736(13)62407-1

Peterson Institute for International Economics. (2019). What is globalization? And how has the global economy shaped the United States? https://www.piie.com/microsites/globalization/what-is-globalization

United Nations Sustainable Development Goals. (n.d.). 17 goals to transform our world. https://www.un.org/sustainabledevelopment/

U.S. Department of Health and Human Services. (2013). *Health information privacy: Summary of the HIPAA security rule.* https://www.hhs.gov/hipaa/for-professionals/security/laws-regulations/index.html

Vellido, A. (2019). Societal issues concerning the application of artificial intelligence in medicine. *Kidney Diseases (Basel, Switzerland), 5*(1), 11–17. https://doi.org/10.1159/000492428

Warren, J. J. (2017). A big data primer. In C. W. Delaney, C. A. Weaver, J. J. Warren, T. R. Clancy, & R. L. Simpson (Eds.), *Big data-enabled nursing: Education, research, and practice.* Springer International Publishing.

Whittington, J. W., Nolan, K., Lewis, N., & Torres, T. (2015). Pursuing the triple aim: The first 7 years. *Milbank Quarterly, 93*(2), 263–300. https://doi.org/10.1111/1468-0009.12122

World Health Organization. (2015). *Health policy.* https://www.who.int/rhem/policy/en/

World Health Organization. (2020). *Global health observatory (GHO) data.* About the GHO. https://www.who.int/gho/about/en

Zenooz, A., & Fox, J. (2019). *How new health care platforms will improve patient care.* Harvard Business Review. https://hbr.org/2019/10/how-new-health-care-platforms-will-improve-patient-care

Zook, M., Barocas, S., Boyd, D., Crawford, K., Keller, E., Gangadharan, S., Goodman, A., Hollander, R., Koenig, B. A., Metcalf, J., Narayanan, A., Nelson, A., & Pasquale, F. (2017). Ten simple rules for responsible big data research. *PLoS Computational Biology, 13*(3), e1005399. https://doi.org/10.1371/journal.pcbi.1005399

CASE EXEMPLARS FOR APPLICATION

Using Measurement to Create a Global Conversation About Outcomes

John Nelson

A study initiated in 2019 that includes 11 countries and 20 hospitals revealed how nurses view the work environment. The span of this work is impressive, drawing data from 20 hospitals that when examined in the aggregate house over 12,000 inpatient care beds and employ 15,000 nurses and 2,000 nursing assistants. The 30% of staff who responded to the work environment survey revealed an understanding of the concepts of caring for self, caring of the manger, and role clarity, all impacting their job satisfaction. Specifically, the relationships and systems are key influencers that enable them to do their work and enjoy it. This large sample and rigorous study would not have been possible without a committed group of nurses, academicians, and leaders in hospital operations. This short paper will review how this group came together over time, to create and sustain a conversation about the work environment that was based in evidence. The overall aim was to show how the work experience of the nurse impacts outcomes for patients.

The formation of this group went through many iterations as a result of several groups with specific interest in outcomes, job satisfaction, caring science, and models of patient care. The group members came from both academe and clinical operations. The commonality among the groups and individuals was the belief that action and relationships are what matters to outcomes. The challenge was developing measures to measure the behaviors that are understood within the context of culture and practice but illusive to measure. Those engaged in the dialogue believed the interface between the patient and nurse is the critical element driving outcomes and patient safety and measurement related to this relationship was missing from data used in most quality improvement projects.

The coming together of this group started with an understanding I had as a staff nurse. I recognized that the relationship between the patient and nurse would only happen in a system that facilitated this relationship. Having been a staff nurse in a hospital for 11 years that had a primary care nurse delivery model, I was able to maximize the application of my clinical and relational skills to care for patients. With the primary nurse care model I had continuity of care with the patient and family from admission to discharge which helped me develop an interdisciplinary care plan that the patient, family, and care team work from.

When I was informed we were going to change our model of care delivery from primary nursing to a team-based care approach, I was concerned that assignment of patient care by task and role would fragment care. I went to the literature and found there was no evidence or study of primary nursing and outcomes. There was no evidence on primary nursing because there was no measure to study the model. Primary nursing had been in practice since the 1960's (Nelson, 2000) and took hold with the work of Marie Manthey and others (Manthey, 1980; Manthey et al., 1970) at the University of Minnesota. Marie Manthey carried her work on to a company called Creative Health Care Management (CHCM) to integrate into a model of care called Relationship Based Care (Koloroutis, 2004; Koloroutis & Abelson, 2017). When I recognized there was no measure to study primary nursing, I entered a master's degree program to pursue a deeper understanding of statistics to develop a measure on how to study primary nursing related to nurse job satisfaction (Nelson, 2000).

When I graduated, I presented my findings to Marie Manthey revealing primary nursing was a central component of nurse job satisfaction. I showed her how it related to important other variables like relationships with coworkers, autonomy, workload, and intent to stay in an organization. She was delighted to see the significance of primary nursing within research and called the executive team at CHCM to present these research findings and explore how we could incorporate them into the work of the RBC model of care. This was the beginning of the international collaborative to study the work environment more deeply. Jayne Felgen, the Chief Executive of CHCM, and I started studying the concept of primary nursing within the framework of their clients who were using RBC (Persky et al., 2008; Persky et al., 2011a; Persky et al., 2011b). It was our desire to measure "everything" but beginning with the most important aspects of care delivery within the framework of RBC.

Concurrent to this work in RBC, my work in job satisfaction expanded. I was at Inova Health working with Karen Drenkard and was asked to study how Watson's 10 processes of caring connected to nurse job satisfaction (Drenkard, 2008). This was the beginning of building models to connect concepts important to the employee and patient experience. We worked with Dr. Jean Watson to develop the Caring Factor Survey (CFS) which measured the concepts of caring (DiNapoli et al., 2010). Once this work was published, I received emails from all over the world seeking to use the CFS and the six derivation measures to study caring relationships. There were approximately 75 studies using the CFS measures within the first two years of my work in Caring Science.

I called Dr. Watson and said since we could not possibly help write all 75 studies, I suggested we send out an email to all researchers and invite them to put the studies into a book with Dr. Watson and myself as the editors. This resulted in the publication of 45 studies conducted by 81 researchers from seven countries in *Measuring Caring* (Nelson & Watson, 2011) published by Springer Publishing Company.

During the work of editing this book, the work became almost untenable as it was all volunteer work for me and my company did not have the resources to help everyone. I was helping about 250 active researchers who were conducting research on job satisfaction, RBC, and caring science in 23 countries. Some of the work resided in my company, Healthcare Environment, but most did not. While sharing this with a colleague on a lobster dinner cruise in Maine during a Plexus conference, I shared that I was considering letting this significant effort go. Dr. Dan Pesut overheard me and suggested I call Sigma Theta Tau International (STTI) to see if they would be interested in "adopting" this international effort. Dr. Pesut had served as the President for STTI from 2003-2005 and thus made this connection for me.

Jayne Felgen and I flew out to Indianapolis and had a five-hour meeting with the executive team at STTI to discuss the possibility of them adopting the work. They embraced the work and its possibility and the work was "adopted" by STTI under the name the Caring International Research Collaborative. With STTI's support and endorsement, Jayne Felgen, myself, and Geraldine Murray, a colleague from Ireland oversaw this group.

Within STTI, the people who signed up to study various concepts grew to 1,600. The work was organized in "sharing groups" comprised of individuals studying a specific construct like clarity, workload, caring, job satisfaction, and so on. There were nine defined sharing groups. The intent of the sharing groups was to build models specialized in a given construct. The sharing groups provided the opportunity to connect with other sharing group(s) to build models of research and measurement to more deeply understand how aspects of the work environment related to each other.

After six years, STTI decided to take a new direction and CIRC no longer was a legal entity within STTI. While significant accomplishments were derived from the work, it had run its course. I continued in my research in caring science and nurse job satisfaction with people from 30 countries still contacting me based on their interests. The last and current phase of this international collaboration ended up in my company. I was looking for a way to integrate my company's work, the work I did in caring science, RBC, and the residual work from connections made in CIRC. I ended up forming a new international division within my company, forming what is now the international collaborative that conducted the study reviewed at the beginning of this paper.

While the international work remains primarily as volunteer work, the business strategy is to use the first 70 hospitals who participate in this collaborative at no cost. Once we have 70 hospitals in the database, there will be a charge to participate for the purpose of adding to the knowledge, benchmarking, and eventual curriculum development. The number 70 was selected using a power analysis since the number 70 is large enough to use aggregate data at the hospital level to correlate concepts studied within this group. It has been found that the unit level data is very difficult to secure in most facilities, but the hospital numbers are known. For example, the fall rate for patients is not known at the unit level but is at the hospital level. A sample size of 70 will allow for studying the relationships of job satisfaction, caring, clarity and other behavioral variables with outcomes like falls, central line associated infections, readmission rates, pressure injuries, and so on. This will enable general understanding of how behavior relates to outcomes so more detailed measure models can be developed to study at the individual unit and employee level. A future goal is to use the data aggregated in the database to allow students and researchers to conduct secondary analyses to further expand scientific study through the use of this big data dataset.

The study from 2019-2020 is currently in process of being written up for several articles. Similar to the development and execution of the study by investigators from both academe and operations, the articles are being written collaboratively to unite the science and operational impacts. The articles have been conceptualized in two groups; those with technical detail related to research methods and models and operational manuscripts that detail the application of findings. It was interesting to find through the rigorous scientific testing that nurses from around the world think of job satisfaction, caring, and clarity the same way and these variables relate to one another the same. It was also interesting to note the concept of caring can vary by context and culture derived from the values and beliefs of nurses based on their country of origin.

It is hoped this international collaborative will not only help the global conversation of health but also the business plan to facilitate revenue that will allow budgeting for scholarships in developing countries that do not have the resources to participate in research studies. There is no template to use in development of this international research database and sharing, so I will rely on the collective wisdom of the participants as this emerges and unfolds as destiny determines. It is hoped this short paper provides insight and inspiration for the readers. It is also hoped that this effort will go full circle and help support primary nursing that supports what matters most – proof that the relationship between patient and nurse impacts outcomes. Our belief is that we will eventually develop a Profile of Caring™ that can be associated with outcomes that will develop into a Profile of Safety™.

REFLECTION QUESTIONS

1. Reflect on your own practice and identify the model of care delivery. Is there an aspect of the model you consider so essential to care outcomes that you would chose to study it more deeply?
2. As you consider how this international work derived from networking, what avenues do you have to meet with people and have conversations about your practice? What conferences, seminars, or social media groups might be an avenue to extend your professional circle?

REFERENCES

DiNapoli, P., Turkel, M., Nelson, J. W., & Watson, J. (2010). Measuring the caritas processes: Caring factor survey. *International Journal of Human Caring, 14*(3), 15–20. https://doi.org/10.20467/1091-5710.14.3.15

Drenkard, K. N. (2008). Integrating human caring science into a professional nursing practice model. *Critical Care Nursing Clinics of North America, 20*(4), 403–414. https://doi.org/10.1016/j.ccell.2008.08.008

Koloroutis, M. (2004). *Relationship-based care: A model for transforming practice.* Creative Health Care Management.

Koloroutis, M., & Abelson, D. (2017). *Advancing relationship-based cultures.* Springer Publishing Company.

Manthey, M. (1980). *The practice of primary nursing.* Blackwell.

Manthey, M., Ciske, K., Robertson, P., & Harris, I. (1970). Primary nursing. *Nursing Forum, 9*(1), 64–83. https://doi.org/10.1111/j.1744-6198.1970.tb00442.x

Nelson, J. W. (2000). Models of nursing care: A century of vacillation. *Journal of Nursing Administration. 30*(4), 156, 184. https://doi.org/10.1097/00005110-200004000-00001

Nelson, J. W., & Watson, J. (2011). *Measuring caring: International research on caritas as healing.* Springer Publishing Company.

CPersky, G., Nelson, J. W., Watson, J., & Bent, K. (2008). Creating a profile of a nurse effective in caring. *Nursing Administration Quarterly, 32*(1), 15–20. https://doi.org/10.1097/01.NAQ.0000305943.46440.77

Persky, G., Felgen, J., & Nelson, J. W. (2011a). Measurement of caring in a relationship-based care model of nursing. In J. W. Nelson & J. Watson (Eds.), *Measuring caring: A compilation of international research on caritas as healing intervention* (pp 125–143). Springer Publishing Company.

Persky, G., Felgen, J., & Nelson, J. W. (2011b). Measuring caring in Primary Nursing. In J. W. Nelson & J. Watson (Eds.), *Measuring caring: International research on caritas as healing* (pp. 65–86). Springer Publishing Company.

An International Partnership to Enhance Outcomes Through Academic-Practice Collaboration and Education Resulting in Redesign and Certification

Shannon Lizer, Asako Katsumata, Minami Kakuta,
Gordana Dermody, Patricia L. Thomas, K. Ninomiya,
Kiyoko Abe, Kazuko Nin, Beth Carson, and Brandie Messer

In 2012, exploration into a partnership between Saint Anthony College of Nursing (SACN) and Japanese healthcare institutions was initiated. Two SACN faculty visited the Japanese Red Cross hospitals: Kumamoto Hospital, Kyoto University Hospital, and Kyoto City Hospital. They also visited several colleges affiliated with these health systems including Toyama University Colleges of Medicine and Nursing, Kyoto University Department of Human Health Science, J. R. C. Kyushu International College of Nursing, and Kumamoto Health Science University. As part of the exploration, the Kumamoto Nurses' Association engaged in dialogue too. Organizational leaders and academic leaders and faculty from each of these institutions engaged in a conversation about nursing practice patterns in Japan and the United States to compare and contrast strengths and weaknesses to identify opportunities for collaboration. During visits to each of the organizations, faculty presented educational programs about the state of U.S. healthcare and nursing education. Focus areas related to nursing empowerment, advanced practice, clinical leadership, and the integration of evidence-based practice.

In the following year, the partnership between Japanese healthcare organizations and colleges was further expanded. Three SACN faculty and two recent BSN graduates visited Japan. During this visit, Tsukuba University Hospital and Tsukuba University College of Nursing and Saint Mary's College in Kyushu were visited. Again, multiple focus areas were identified and discussed pertaining to ways education and professional development could enhance care delivery and were discussed and shared with clinical and academic leadership at the previously visited and additional sites. The developing dialogue centered on how SACN leadership and faculty could facilitate nursing practice in Japan. Subsequently, additional visits to multiple Japanese organizations occurred in 2014 yielding similar discussions and focus. During all of the visits, faculty from the Japanese Red Cross College of Nursing, staff from the Japanese Red Cross, academic deans and faculty, students and executives, managers, and staff and from the health systems participated in workshops and seminars.

The outcome of the initial visits and from feedback from Japanese nursing leaders led to the development of an initiative aimed to present the role of the clinical nurse leader (CNL) to Japanese nurses, educators and leaders. In part, the decision was made to introduce the CNL role and practice rather than other advanced nursing practice roles because of the traditional physician leadership culture in Japan. Given the CNL role centers on the promotion of safety, quality, leadership at the point of care, and evidence-based nursing practice, the consensus of the academic and health system participants across Japan was that the CNL role had the most likelihood of acceptance.

In 2015, plans were finalized to begin formal seminars to be held in the Japanese Red Cross Kyushu International College of Nursing to present the CNL curriculum. A Japanese Red Cross grant funded and supported this work. The American Association of Colleges of Nursing (AACN) and the Commission on Nurse Certification (CNC) was engaged in this discussion and supported the project (AACN, 2020a; 2020b; CNC, 2020a). The initial seminar yielded positive evaluations. A clinical immersion at a health system in the United States that had implemented the CNL role in the United States was scheduled so participants could experience the role as a requisite expectation for CNL board certification. SACN faculty and nationally recognized CNL leaders presented the seminar and coordinated the immersion activities.

In 2016, the seminars shifted location to Tokyo and were hosted by the JRC Society and the JRC College of Nursing in Tokyo, Japan. Tsukuba University nursing faculty were also included. All seminars were presented by nationally recognized CNL leaders and SACN faculty. In addition to content related to evidence-based practices, project leadership and management, and change leadership, participants engaged in developing process maps and fishbone diagrams around concerns in their own organizations. Each seminar was followed by a visit to SACN in Rockford, Illinois and Saint Mary's Hospital in Grand Rapids, Michigan for clinical immersion experiences and board certification preparation. All participants and organizations reported positive evaluation of this program.

Groups of Japanese nursing faculty from multiple universities traveled to SACN to experience an immersion experience in graduate nursing science and clinical education. This experience also provided an opportunity for faculty to engage in conversations about advanced practice, the CNL role, curriculum design and development, and academic rigor.

In total, over 100 Japanese nurses, faculty, and organizational leaders have attended this program. Two nurse leaders have passed the CNL board certification examination (CNC, 2020b). A major difficulty with the board certification examination is the focus on the U.S. health systems that is very different from the Japanese health system. This has been a significant challenge.

As an outcome of this project, a coalition of nurses living and working across Japan has formed. These nurses have monthly study groups using distance technology to connect them to SACN and Tskuba University faculty who facilitate dialogue and additional development aimed to CNL competencies (AACN, 2020a).

An additional outcome is that AACN allowed the CNL certification examination to be taken in Japan at Kyoto University. Further, some participants of the CNL project now employ quality techniques learned through this partnership, such as microsystem analysis, fishbone analysis, Deming's PDCA (plan, do, check, act), and project management. Participants apply these techniques in their workplace and in the process of JRC international relief mission planning.

Recently, the Japanese Nursing Association leaders adopted national quality indicators, the Database for Improvement of Nursing Quality and Labor (DiNQL). Prior to adoption of the DiNQL indicators and benchmarks were set by individual health systems and not comparable (Iwasawa, 2016). Participants of the CNL seminars can now apply the knowledge they acquired from the seminars to facilitate change in their own organizations using the DiNQL national targets.

REFLECTION QUESTIONS

1. Consider your area of practice and what you understand about health-care delivery in other parts of the world. What collaboration might benefit all countries?
2. What are the accreditation or regulatory considerations you would need to explore if you started an international collaboration?
3. If you initiated collaboration for improvement, what data might you collect to demonstrate impact?

REFERENCES

American Association of Colleges of Nursing. (2020a). *About CNL.* https://www.aacnnursing.org/CNL

American Association of Colleges of Nursing. (2020b). *Competencies and curricular expectations for clinical nurse leader education and practice.* https://www.aacnnursing.org/News-Information/Position-Statements-White-Papers/CNL

Commission on Nurse Certification. (2020). *Commission on Nurse Certification.* https://www.aacnnursing.org/CNL-Certification/Commission-on-Nurse-Certification

Commission on Nurse Certification. (2020). *About the exam.* https://www.aacnnursing.org/CNL-Certification/About-the-Exam

Iwasawa, Y. (2016). *Database for improvement of Nursing Quality and Labor (DiNQL) project by Japanese Nursing Association.* https://www.jstage.jst.go.jp/article/johokanri/59/7/59_449/_article

8

Innovation, Diffusion, and Dissemination

James L. Harris

OBJECTIVES

1. Define innovation, diffusion, and dissemination as core attributes within an organization.
2. Demonstrate how the alignment of innovation, diffusion, and dissemination advance healthcare quality, safety, and value to the next level within the context of a data-driven culture.
3. Discuss ways healthcare organizations meet the triple and quadruple aims to improve quality, safety, and sustainability.
4. Propose how innovation, improvement, and data act as a catalyst for interprofessional teams to achieve continuous quality, safety, and financial outcomes.

CORE COMPETENCIES

- Understand the foundations of innovation, diffusion, and dissemination
- Approach innovation, diffusion, and dissemination from a system perspective and accept as a core value
- Adaptability to use new evidence, technology, and processes for organizational sustainability and renewal of survival
- Measure the outcomes of evidence-based practice and innovation
- Link evidence to innovations

- Transform organizations using contemporary leadership and management principles that inspire inquiry and innovation
- Use imagination as an avenue to manage innovation, change, and impending problematic situations
- Identify disruptions and create conditions of risk taking and leverage resources to support team innovation
- Develop and support formal and informal networks of innovative thought and actions

INTRODUCTION

Innovation, diffusion, and dissemination of information are present in multiple organizations when individuals are open and willing to consider different ways of thinking, accepting risk, and creating collaborative partnerships. To appreciate the impacts and outcomes of each requires testing, modification, and transparency. Innovation, diffusion, and information dissemination are the lifeblood of the 21st century organization when they are respected, valued, and linked to new ideologies of business and data-driven leadership (Kiechel, 2012; Porter-O'Grady & Malloch, 2017; Von Hippel, 2005). For purposes of this chapter, innovation, diffusion, and dissemination are defined within the context of core attributes and inherent relationships germane to advancing healthcare quality, safety, and value within a data-driven culture.

INNOVATION, DIFFUSION, AND DISSEMINATION

Many individuals have defined innovation over the decades in multiple industries and organizations (Porter-O'Grady & Malloch, 2017). For purposes here, innovation is defined as a process of learning and knowledge creation along a continuum through which problems are defined and new knowledge is accepted as alternative solutions (Fagerberg et al., 2005). Innovation requires continuous adaptation to situations and influences within the immediate and distant environments due to its random order. This notion is supported by DeloitteHealth (2019) that identifies shifts in innovation occur in seven-year cycles and underpin organizational responsiveness to future challenges.

Remaining knowledgeable of the drivers of innovation is critical in a digital and data-driven global society. Innovators rely on data and prompts from various stimuli to sustain a spirit of inquiry and innovation (Duke Nursing Magazine, 2019). Organizations associate negative occurrences as damaging to quality, safety, and financial stability. Conversely, the innovator incorporates negative occurrences into design thinking and creates positive outcomes. Risk is minimized, innovative partnerships are formed, a foundation for evidence-based practice emerges, and financial implications are addressed (Weberg & Davidson, 2019). Contemplate the example of a manager from a community mental health center that reviewed annual data of no-shows for scheduled appointments and considered various alternatives. The manager created a sense of personal space and imagined ways to reduce the trend. What followed was contact with several community leaders, businesses, and a state mental health division regarding outreach funds for a mobile clinic in order to provide services in areas where the predominance of clients for no-show appointments lived. Using data, evidence, innovative strategies, and creation of partnerships externally, funds were donated for a mobile clinic and a grant was secured for a pilot program to offer mobile services in the designated area. This example illustrates how a spirit of inquiry, creating a personal space to ponder alternatives, and stimuli can offer opportunities for an innovator to create positive outcomes and form partnerships using data from the negative outcomes. It also illustrates that when one uses imagination and different images of a situation, various insights, actions, and outcomes become reality. Morgan (1997) supported this thought and identified that imagination is a new competency required for managing turbulent times in healthcare.

Rogers (2003) stated "diffusion is the process in which innovation is communicated through certain channels over time among the members of a social system" (p. 5). He further stated that diffusion involves communication where meaning is linked to events. The idea that uncertainty and risk is involved in the process of diffusion can be moderated by seeking and attaining information that are triggering uncertainty based on other alternatives (Rogers). If information is not sought or attained, individuals have a sense of threat that limits performance and adoption of new improvement strategies. If the norm is the accepted way of doing business, organizations enter a state of operational paralysis.

When approached in a logical way and communicated widely, diffusion of new ideas and innovations can inform and reinform processes attributed to compatibility, complexity, and adoption of change within organizations. Opportunities for continuous improvement and the advancement of a data-driven culture become the norm. Clinicians and administrators attain new skills and competencies creating the potential to reduce costs, improve patient care quality and safety, and engage employees as full participants in governance and change processes. For success, clinicians and managers must possess the skills and capabilities to form improvement partnerships, be adaptive and open to innovation, effectively lead teams, and use data to inform actions. If skills and capabilities do not exist, opportunities and support must be provided by an organization. Likewise, organizations that diffuse new ideas and innovations to external stakeholders create a relative advantage where an idea or innovation is accepted and perceived as valued and superior to previous practices (Crow & DeBourgh, 2017; Rogers, 2003).

Dissemination is closely aligned to diffusion of ideas and innovations. Dissemination is defined as an action or fact of spreading something, especially information, widely (Merriam-Webster, 2001a). Information, ideas, and innovations are disseminated in a variety of ways to individuals and groups on a daily basis.

Healthcare is no exception as it is rich in data and evidence. Data and evidence guide practice, management decisions, and offer pathways for others to engage in new inquiry and test ideas before implementing. As previously discussed, diffusion of an idea or innovation in healthcare can challenge the most skilled leader. What may be a success in one setting could be slowly disseminated in another. Berwick (2003) identified three spheres of influence related to diffusion of an innovation in organizations to include: (a) innovation perceptions, (b) adopter characteristics, and (c) operating forces. Outcomes of the influences can be attributed to the value of an innovation to an organization, internal and external stakeholder support, and early adopters that possess higher levels of readiness for change.

Understanding the dynamics attributed to dissemination of ideas and innovations require a series of deliberate steps. Innovators must communicate to audiences the aims and objectives related to an innovation to spark an interest. Interest provides a platform to offer a more detail description and understanding of the innovation. These steps are pivotal for future actions by individuals and groups that will champion initiatives to disseminate the innovation within organizations, other audiences, and stakeholders (Harmsworth & Turpin, 2000).

The attributes of representative stories are also a useful technique to disseminate innovation and evidence-based outcomes to audiences (Steiner, 2007). Stories of innovation influence, inspire, and persuade others to accept and disseminate new evidence and practices. Individuals desire to hear the specifics of how an innovation was envisioned, the roadblocks to diffusing it within an area or throughout an organization, how support was garnered, and its sustainability. Any representative story should inspire a belief that the innovation offers new solutions and opportunities for future positive experiences and outcomes. The true influence or impact of any story occurs after the story has been shared and others disseminate the information, implement the innovation, and collect data to shape new stories that complement future innovations.

Innovation, diffusion, and dissemination exist synergistically. The synergy is evident when environments support innovative thought, take risk, and begin a journey of discovery that will challenge current business practices and care models. The call for change and a new journey of discovery and dissemination is now if fragmentation of care is eliminated and organizational sustainability is preserved.

ALIGNING INNOVATION, DIFFUSION, AND DISSEMINATION IN HEALTHCARE

Aligning innovation, diffusion, and dissemination in healthcare requires a series of nonlinear and purposeful actions by leaders. Contemporary leaders must include progressive processes in daily activities that advance quality, safety, and value (Rosing et al., 2011).

Processes by nature are paradoxical, yet the majority of evidence implies a gap between perceptions of occurrence and leader actions (Davidson et al., 2017). Leaders, who involve others in diverse processes, cultivate a shared meaning and value understanding of the organization and the forces that affect efficacy. What follows is a culture of data-driven decisions creating a fluid network of ideas and actions that advances healthcare to the next level. As others are included in processes, relationships form and networks are created. Mutual relationships and networks create conditions where respect, trust, and valuing the expertise of others excel. Leaders and others are more adaptive and creative emergence of ideas and information sharing is possible (Weberg & Davidson, 2019).

As innovations are diffused and disseminated, new tools and techniques become available to all stakeholders within and outside the organization. Individuals and teams begin to challenge traditional methods that lacked evidence. New skills are combined with data to shape a direction for how current and future innovation will be diffused and disseminated. Opportunities to avoid mediocrity are embraced and continuous adaptation to change and innovative thought and actions are optimized. A study by Clavelle et al. (2016) further validated the value of individual and inter-professional team contributions in identifying opportunities for innovation and the subsequent diffusion and dissemination in health practices.

Individuals, teams, and organizational leaders must ensure the equitable diffusion and dissemination of innovative evidence generated in today's turbulent healthcare environment. This is especially true when one considers the diffusion and dissemination of innovative evidence for mainstream and marginalized populations. Innovations are often diffused and disseminated in academic forums with delays to areas that provide care in underserved and minority communities (Menon et al., 2019). There continues to be no consensus for aggregating and disaggregating populations when developing new innovations (Michie et al., 2017). With the advent and advances in implementation science, the development and testing of innovative interventions for mainstream and marginalized populations are being supported and advanced (Brown et al., 2017).

As new innovations are introduced, diffused, and disseminated, a critical mass of data is being generated. The data provide a foundation for future data-driven innovations and opportunities that link quality, safety, and value-based interventions for sustainable organizational success. Multiple sources of data such as big data technologies, continuous monitoring devices, analytics, and the electronic medical record are currently disrupting existing evidential frameworks and challenging leaders to reexamine strategies and actions historically used to solve problems. However, new organizational and role capabilities must first be established where individuals understand how to collect and analyze aggregate data. Aggregate data can then be useful as meaningful predictors and forecast of the future dynamics associated with healthcare (Weberg & Davidson, 2019). Leaders must be committed to embracing innovation as a norm in the organization. This will not occur in a vacuum. It will require meaningful engagement of individuals and teams to evaluate data, its utility, and fit within an organization. It is at that point that adaption and responsiveness to innovative thought and inquiry is possible (Malloch & Porter-O'Grady, 2010).

MEETING THE TRIPLE AND QUADRUPLE AIMS IN HEALTHCARE

A triad of models and concepts contribute to the operations within any healthcare organization. These include high reliability, evidence-based practice, and process excellence. High reliability refers to a focus on mindfulness and perfection within an organization (Agency for Healthcare Research and Quality, 2008). Evidence-based practice is identified as a problem-solving approach to clinical decision-making that integrates scientific evidence with experiential evidence, incorporates an organization's culture and practice influences, supports the use of evidence to guide care, and informs continuous quality improvement (Newhouse, 2007). Process excellence is an umbrella phase used to describe various improvement methods and concentrates more on the journey than the destination when associated with improvement, sustainability, and reduction in variation.

One may ask what is the relationship of high reliability, evidence-based practice, and process excellence to the Triple and Quadruple Aims? Each of these concepts are intertwined with both the Triple and Quadruple Aims when one considers how organizations are continuously striving to transform healthcare systems as a seamless, coordinated care approach for patients.

The Triple Aim as defined by the Institute for Healthcare Improvement (IHI) is improvement of the health of populations, enhancement of patient experiences that includes quality and satisfaction, and cost reductions through continuous improvement (Stiefel & Nolan, 2012). Stiefel and Nolan further described the Triple Aim as a technique to optimize healthcare system performance by work design using five concepts to include: (a) focus on individuals and families, (b) primary care service and structure redesign, (c) population health management, (d) cost control, and (e) system integration and application. Bodenheimer and Sinsky (2014) identified the Triple Aim as a compass to enhance the performance of a healthcare system.

The Triple Aim challenges individuals and teams to champion improvement processes and use information management and technology to advance data-driven methods when responding to variations in care delivery and metrics. Understanding the value of each contributor's role in the process is vital to a successful outcome. Data components must be hardwired into management systems and the electronic medical record for data collection and analysis purposes if change occurs. Regardless of how sophisticated the information management and technology is in a healthcare organization, if individuals and teams do not understand what measures are being tracked from a strategic perspective and why, opportunities to optimize performance in terms of the Triple Aim is diminished. Three types of measurements commonly used in improvement efforts are outcome, process, and balancing measures. Outcome measures focus on how the system affects the values of patients, their well-being, and the impacts on other stakeholders. Process measures include the parts and steps to improve the system. Balancing measures seek to identify, are improvement processes and changes associated with one area introducing new problems in another area (Institute for Healthcare Improvement, n.d.).

Being mindful of the Triple Aim requires leaders and individuals to maintain a state of readiness and attentiveness to the present, rather than revisiting the past or focusing only on the future state. When individuals are mindful, they are open to ideas and input from others without discernment of right or wrong. Being mindful of the environment and others assists in coping with stresses, connecting with the patient experience, and improving the quality of life for others (Kabat-Zinn, 2012).

Mindfulness extends beyond goals of the Triple Aim with the expansion to the Quadruple Aim (Sikka et al., 2015). The Quadruple Aim underscores the value of improving work-life experiences. Improvements in work-life experiences result in an engaged workforce whose experiences are meaningful and advance the mission and goals of the organization (Bodenheimer & Sinsky, 2014; Longbrake, 2017).

The well-being of healthcare teams is a prerequisite for the Triple Aim. Without attention to improving work-life balance and the expansion of the Triple Aim to a Quadruple Aim, unintended consequences of dissatisfaction, burnout, reduction in quality and safety, and costs will intensify. If this gap persists and societal expectations widen regarding care access at a reduced costs, the unintended consequences will expand. What follows is a negative impact on patient-centered care and dissatisfied healthcare workers and patients. The compass to optimize healthcare performance proposed with the Triple Aim will therefore not point to improved care, health, lower costs, and well-being of employees.

INNOVATION, IMPROVEMENT, AND DATA AS THE CATALYST TO ACHIEVE CONTINUOUS QUALITY, SAFETY, AND FINANCIAL OUTCOMES

Imperatives to innovate, improve, and use data in healthcare offers unique challenges and opportunities for leaders and teams to achieve continuous quality, safety, and financial outcomes. But one may ask, what is the catalyst necessary to achieve success with the impending challenges and opportunities in contemporary healthcare? Initially, one must consider the definition of a catalyst and related leadership concepts. By definition, catalyst is defined as an agent that provokes change and action (Merriam-Webster, 2001b). Capability, competency, and capacity are concepts closely linked to the definition and they provide context in relation to innovative change and measurable data that represents improvement.

Capability relates to the ability to deliver innovative outputs and is measured in terms of value, improvement, and sustainability of products and services. Competency conveys the knowledge, skills, and behaviors that support innovation and its diffusion and dissemination within an organization. Capacity denotes the innovative thought and outcomes that result in shared values, understanding, and the ability to replicate innovations for continuous growth and performance (Welter, 2011). Each of the aforementioned concepts can easily be associated with actions that result in quality, safety, and financial outcomes in healthcare.

Change requires a commitment for innovation, improvement, and the use of data. When leaders commit to change and innovation, measurable outcomes will be achieved that inform healthcare environments. Before an organization makes a commitment to change, there must be an awareness that one is needed. The organization must consider what types of initiatives meet the definition of organizational innovation. Opportunities must be created and supported for innovation to occur and expand across the organization. Finally, processes to measure and quantify innovation must be identified and communicated to all stakeholders. This requires collection of data that captures the time spent on an innovation, attempts before the innovation was adopted, and techniques used, its diffusion and dissemination, and successes as documented in quality, safety, and financial return metrics (Drucker, 2018).

Drucker (2018) further posed the question of how an organization could measure an intangible such as innovation? Three steps were presented to consider when answering such a complex question. First, organizations must measure solutions that meet identified needs and foster opportunities for future ideas. Second, leading and lagging indicators associated with an innovation must also be identified. Leading indicators are easy to measure and result in rapid goal attainment. Lagging indicators on the other hand are also easy to measure, but can be difficult to influence, such as outcomes. Third, pursuits and associated outcome indicators that represent innovation in the organization must be identified. As innovation is measured, creative indicators and meaningful metrics evolve. New ideas are envisioned and their quality is improved as prior successes are diffused and disseminated. A strong correlation will become evident between quality innovations and value.

As presented in the preceding discussion, measuring innovation is a core competency in healthcare and provides acumen to guide strategy when change is needed. New methods to diffuse and disseminate innovative changes are created and others accept and recognize patterns of change more readily (Davidson et al., 2017). However, caution must be exercised in any healthcare organization due to the volume and rapidity of introducing new innovations. Otherwise, many great innovations may be dismissed, and diffusion and dissemination within and outside of organizations will be interrupted. This requires transition of the innovation to operations within an organization and integrated into each role (Malloch & Porter-O'Grady, 2017). The integration of the innovation into organizational roles does not require introduction of chaos. What it does require is mindful development and implementation of orderly methods where innovation becomes routine versus random (Davila et al., 2006). Improvements in quality, safety, and value are thus underpinned by innovations and continuous flow of data and new ideas.

Taking advantage of institutional talent and curiosity are pivotal to innovation, diffusion, and dissemination. This competitive edge has long been leveraged by organizations globally. As talent is recognized and supported, individuals become interested in what is working and ways to correct those that are not, and recognize data as a valuable asset. There is no question that innovation, improvement, and data are catalysts for the achievement of continuous quality, safety, and fiscal outcomes. Individuals who are willing to take action to achieve change and own outcomes make differences. Through innovation, sharing of new ideas, and using data to reach consensus through ongoing purposeful actions are requisites for survival and goal attainment in healthcare organizations in the 21st century.

SUMMARY

- Innovation, diffusion, and dissemination are the lifeblood of an organization when they are linked to new ideologies of business and data-driven leadership.

- Innovation is a process of learning and knowledge creation along a continuum that requires continuous adaptation due to its random order.
- Innovators require meaningful data and prompts from various stimuli to sustain a spirit of inquiry and innovation.
- Innovators incorporate negative outcomes into design thinking and create positive outcomes.
- Diffusion is a process in which innovation is communicated through channels over time among members and linked to events.
- Diffusion of ideas and innovations can inform and reinform processes associated with compatibility, complexity, and adoption of change.
- When organizations diffuse and disseminate innovations, a relative advantage is created.
- Dissemination is an action or fact of spreading something widely.
- Data and evidence guide practice, decisions, and offer pathways to test innovations.
- Representative stories are useful techniques to disseminate innovations and evidence to others.
- Innovation, diffusion, and dissemination exist synergistically.
- Processes are paradoxical in nature, yet the majority of evidence implies a gap between perceptions of occurrences and leader actions.
- Equitable diffusion and dissemination of innovations must be ensured in order to meet the needs of society.
- Innovations that are diffused and disseminated create a critical mass of data foundational for future innovations that provide quality, safety, and value within organizations.
- Meaningful engagement by others yields adoption of innovations.
- The Triple Aim focuses on improvement of the health of populations, enhancement of patient experiences, and reduction of costs and serves as the compass to enhance performance.
- The Quadruple Aim underscores the value of improving work-life experiences and is a prerequisite for the Triple Aim.
- Three types of measurements commonly used in improvement efforts are outcome, process, and balancing measures.
- Innovation, diffusion, and dissemination act as the catalyst for improvement.
- Change requires a commitment to innovation, diffusion, and use of data to achieve measurable outcomes and inform future healthcare decisions.
- Measurement of an intangible, such as innovation, requires that others recognize changes are needed, indicators are identified, and outcomes represent innovation.
- Measuring innovation is a core competency as it provides a new lens to guide strategy and future flow of ideas and information.
- Institutional talent and curiosity are essential for innovation, dissemination, and diffusion of information to occur.
- Recognizing talent and encouraging curiosity creates leverage within organizations when used properly.

REFLECTION QUESTIONS

1. Consider the healthcare organization where you are currently employed. How would you identify that change was needed? Once identified, what steps would you take to ensure innovation are supported and how new innovations are diffused and disseminated?
2. How would you define innovation, diffusion, and dissemination as the lifeblood of a 21st century healthcare organization?
3. Compare and contrast innovation, diffusion, and dissemination. How would you as a leader ensure each of these are a valuable asset in the current organization where you are employed?
4. What is the data important to survival in a global society?
5. How, as an employee, can you ensure that the Triple and Quadruple Aims add value to an organization?
6. What process, outcome, and balancing indicators are relevant to success in a healthcare organization?

REFERENCES

Agency for Healthcare Research and Quality. (2008). *Becoming a high reliability organization: Operational advice for hospital leaders.* https://psnet.ahrq.gov/issue/becoming-high-reliability-organization-operational-advice-hospital-leaders

Berwick, D. M. (2003). Disseminating innovations in health care. *Journal of the American Medical Association, 289*(15), 1969–1975. https://doi.org/10.1001/jama.289.15.1969

Bodenheimer, T., & Sinsky, C. (2014). From triple aim to quadruple aim: Care of the patient requires care of the provider. *The Annals of Family Medicine, 12*(6), 573–576. https://doi.org/10.1370/afm.1713

Brown, C. H., Curran, G., Palinkas, L. A., Aarons, G. A., Wells, K. B., & Cruden, G. (2017). An overview of research and evaluation designs for dissemination and implementation. *Annual Review of Public Health, 38*, 1–22. https://doi.org/10.1146/annurev-publhealth-031816-044215

Clavelle, J. T., Porter-O'Grady, T. P., Weston, M. J., & Verran, J. V. (2016). Evolution structural empowerment: Moving from shared to professional governance. *Journal of Nursing Administration, 46*(6), 308–312.

Crow, G. L., & DeBourgh, G. A. (2017). Shared governance: The infrastructure for innovation. In S. Davidson, D. Weberg, T. Porter-O'Grady, & K. Malloch (Eds.), *Leadership for evidence-based innovation in nursing and health professions* (pp. 401–440). Jones & Bartlett Learning.

Davidson, S., Weberg, D., Porter-O'Grady, T., & Malloch, K. (2017). *Leadership for evidence-based innovation in nursing and health professions.* Jones & Bartlett Learning.

Davila, T., Epstein, M. J., & Shelton, R. (2006). *Making innovation work: How to manage it, measure it, and profit from it.* Wharton School.

DeloitteHealth. (2019). *Perspectives: The future of health: How innovation will blur traditional health care boundaries.* https://www2.deloitte.com/us/en/pages/life-sciences-and-health-care/articles/future-of-health.html

Drucker, P. (2018). *How to measure innovation.* www.thinkhdi.com/library/supportworld.2018/how-to-measure-innovation

Duke Nursing Magazine. (2019). Creating new pathways for innovation. *Duke Nursing Magazine, 15*(2), 4–9.

Fagerberg, J., Mowrey, D. C., & Nelson, R. (2005). *The Oxford handbook of innovation.* Oxford University Press.

Harmsworth, S., & Turpin, S. (2000). *Creating an effective dissemination strategy: An expanded interactive workbook for educational development projects.* http://www.innovations.ac.uk/btg/resources/publications/dissemination.pdf

Institute for Healthcare Improvement. (n.d.). *How to improve, science of improvement: Establishing measures.* http://www.ihi.org/resources/Pages/HowtoImprove/Scienceof ImprovementEstablishingMeasures.aspx

Kabat-Zinn, J. (2012). *Mindfulness for beginners.* Sounds True.

Kiechel, W. (2012). The management century. *Harvard Business Review, 89*(11), 63–75.

Longbrake, K. (2017). Focusing on the quadruple aim of health care. *American Nurse Today, 12*(7), 44–46.

Malloch, K., & Porter-O-Grady. (2010). *Introduction to evidence-based practice in nursing and health care.* Jones & Bartlett Learning.

Malloch, K., & Porter-O'Grady, T. (2017). Complexity: Moving from static to dynamic paradigm. In S. Davidson, D. Weberg, T. Porter-O'Grady, & K. Malloch (Eds.), *Leadership for evidence-based innovation in nursing and health professions* (pp. 77–110). Jones & Bartlett Learning.

Menon, U., Cohn, E., Downs, C. A., Gephart, S. M., & Redwine, L. (2019). Precision health research and implementation reviewed through the conNECT framework. *Nursing Outlook, 67,* 302–310. https://doi.org/10.1016/j.outlook.2019.05.010

Merriam-Webster. (2001a). Dissemination. In *Merriam-Webster's new collegiate dictionary.* Random House.

Merriam-Webster. (2001b). Catalyst. In *Merriam-Webster's new collegiate dictionary.* Random House.

Michie, S., Yardley, L., West, R., Patrick, K., & Greaves, F. (2017). Developing and evaluating digital interventions to promote behavior change in health and health care: Recommendations resulting from an international workshop. *Journal of Medical Internet Research, 19*(6), e232. https://doi.org/10.2196/jmir.7126

Morgan, G. (1997). *Imagination. New mindset for seeing, organizing, and managing.* Berrett-Koehler Publications, Inc.

Newhouse, R. (2007). Diffusing confusion among evidence-based practice, quality improvement, and research. *Journal of Nursing Administration, 37*(10), 432–435. https://doi.org/10.1097/01.NNA.0000285156.58903.d3

Porter-O'Grady, T., & Malloch, K. (2017). *Quantum Leadership: Building better partnerships for better health.* Jones & Bartlett Learning.

Rogers, E. M. (2003). *Diffusion of innovations, 5th edition.* Free Press, A Division of Simon & Schuster, Inc.

Rosing, K., Frese, M., & Bausch, A. (2011). Explaining the heterogeneity of leadership-innovation relationship: Ambidextrous leadership. *The Leadership Quarterly, 22*(5), 956–974. https://doi.org/10.1016/j.leaqua.2011.07.014

Sikka, R., Morath, J. M., & Leape, L. (2015). The quadruple aim: Care, health, cost, meaning in work. *British Journal of Medicine, Quality and Safety, 24*(10), 608–610. https://doi.org/10.1136/bmjqs-2015-004160

Steiner, J. F. (2007). Using stories to disseminate research: The attributes of representative stories. *Journal of General Internal Medicine, 22*(11), 1603–1607. https://doi.org/10.1007/s11606-007-0335-9

Stiefel, M., & Nolan, K. (2012). *A guide to the Triple Aim: Population health, experience of care, and per capita cost.* Institute for Healthcare Improvement.

Von Hippel, E. (2005). *Democratizing innovation.* MIT.

Weberg, D., & Davidson, S. (2019). *Leadership for evidence-based innovation in nursing and health professions.* Jones & Bartlett Learning.

Welter, T. (2011). *A catalyst for change: The three C's of good leadership.* https://www.franchising.com/articles/a_catalyst_for_change_the_three_cs_of_good_leadership

CASE EXEMPLARS FOR APPLICATION

Real-Time Visibility of Census, Bed Status, and Discharge-Order for Better Patient Flow

Peter Sylvester

A visual display of real-time census and beds with fully integrated environmental services (EVS) management functions helped our hospital increase the % of patients discharged before 3 p.m. by 50%. Discharges home from adult med/surg units occurring before 3 p.m. went from 37% to 55% with the introduction of "Intelliflow," a homegrown application built with more effort than a traditional interface of such purchased systems, but at a fraction of the cost with the right team (Collins, 2018).

The internal team consisted of department representatives from Nursing, EVS, Registration, Admitting, Information Systems (IS), Nursing Supervisors, and Administration. Weekly meetings began and tracer exercises were conducted to document current states. Patients with an active discharge order were traced until the patient physically left the building and electronically discharged from the electronic medical record (EMR). The discharge order from the EMR triggered an alert to the EVS staff that there was a dirty bed. A "pending order" report was identified in the EMR and used for discharge orders to enable the tracer and proved to be highly valuable in a two regards. First, a small test of change during the build process led to the discharge pending order report was run manually three to five or more times a day that was sent to nurse managers. The nurse manager's awareness of these patients and pending discharge orders had an immediate impact on the percentage of patients discharged before 3 p.m., indicated by the number 1 (circle marker) in the middle of the Figure 8.1 control chart.

Second, from a design perspective, the discharge order became the start of an EVS bed request in the new system. From the electronic order, an alert and 'ticket' was created and attached as a car-avatar that appeared next to the patient and bed on the visual display. This allowed EVS staff and nursing supervisors to plan patient bed placements based on expected availability. The ticket or alert had a timing mechanism that tracked the time between the order and minutes that had lapsed. This allowed for real-time investigation into discharge barriers so corrective interventions could be made.

Once the patient was discharged, EVS staff were alerted using the new online management information system and an Apple iPads purchased as part of the project. The iPads provided a dynamic list of beds needing cleaning and beds requested for new patients. If special cleaning requirements were needed because of patient precautions, it was displayed for EVS staff. Pending bed placement requests could be reprioritized by nursing supervisors who were acutely aware of bed demand. Rooms were either displayed as assigned rooms or current status in a queued-list. When EVS staff entered a room and hit the "Start" button, the bed board status changed to indicate the room was being cleaned. Finally, once cleaned, the EVS staff hit the "Complete" button and the last visual indicator alerted everyone the bed was available for patient placement.

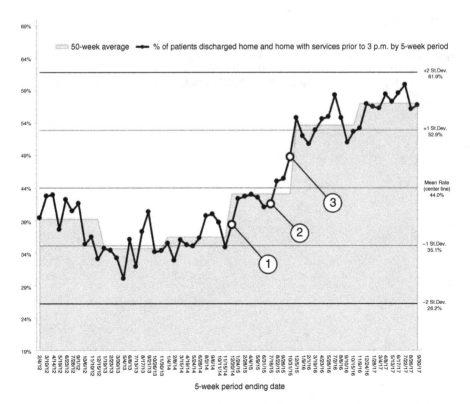

FIGURE 8.1 % Discharges home and home with services prior to 3 p.m. by 5-week period

This new process and technology supported bed turnover reporting that enabled appropriate EVS staffing to reduce the bed turnover delays. As a result, STAT bed cleaning has been decreased based on proactive prioritization, assignment, and room cleaning.

The new system was piloted on the largest nursing unit (40 beds) for eight weeks and entailed a variety of minor system and workflow changes. The pilot produced visible house-wide results indicated by the number 2 (circle marker) in Figure 8.1. House-wide go live is displayed by the number 3 (circle marker) in Figure 8.1. The impact of this interdisciplinary team project have been sustained.

REFLECTION QUESTIONS

1. Consider situations in your organization that are time dependent. What improvements might be undertaken with a visual display board to address them?
2. What is the benefit of documenting a process with members of an inter-disciplinary team?

REFERENCES

Collins, B. C. (2018). *Intelligent bed-flow and return on investment: Intelliflow. Health Information Management Systems (HIMSS) 2018 annual conference, session #295, March 9, 2018.* https://365.himss.org/sites/himss365/files/365/handouts/550235821/handout-295 .pdf

A Social Responsibility to be Innovative: Caring for Underserved Populations

Shanda Scott

Healthcare providers and educators have a social responsibility to be innovative and develop new opportunities to meet the expanding challenges presented by underserved populations (VanderWielen et al., 2015). An initial step is to understand the social determinants of health and health disparities of underserved populations. As individuals gain understanding, the development of innovative delivery models that will ultimately impact access and health outcomes evolve.

Throughout healthcare systems, underserved populations require care and are a high risk for developing multiple chronic illnesses that lead to negative outcomes. Underserved populations suffer from multiple social and physical challenges ranging from healthcare access to low health literacy, lack of or inadequate health insurance, and financial restraints perpetuating a series of poor health outcomes. Challenged to address the myriad of issues, providers and health educators can collaboratively develop and initiate community-based approaches resulting in positive outcomes for this population.

One such approach was the development of a HRSA-funded nurse-managed clinic in an economically deprived area in the southeastern United States. Staffed by registered nurses, medical assistants, and nurse practitioners, care was provided and referrals were made to other clinics for continuous and routine care regardless of health insurance or ability to pay for services. "Meeting patients where they are" became the primary motivator as care was provided in neighborhoods and surrounding communities easily accessible by walking or using public transportation. Partnerships with primary care clinics and interprofessional educational opportunities were formed that provided avenues to gain knowledge and expertise of an underserved population, while meeting their needs.

Data were continuously collected that became foundations for new patient education modalities, additions to interprofessional curricula, other available services that benefited patients and their families, and the addition of a secondary clinic providing services to homeless individuals. Medical screening and referrals, social issues, counseling, and financial concerns were addressed by physicians, nurses, and other health-related disciplines at the secondary clinic.

This innovative approach to meeting needs of underserved populations is only one example. Innovative care models create new roadmaps that culminate in inter-professional care delivery and education, and new partnerships to meet any challenge.

REFLECTION QUESTIONS

1. As a healthcare professional, what two social responsibilities can you identify that will assist underserved populations?
2. Consider a clinical situation where you are employed. What innovative approaches has a interprofessional team used to meet underserved population needs? What were the outcomes and how and where were they disseminated?
3. What is the value of an interprofessional team when tasked with advancing innovative care approaches for underserved populations? What role can you identify that will contribute to an individual successful outcome?

REFERENCE

VanderWielen, L. M., Vanderbilt, A. A., Crossman, S. A., Mayer, S. D., Enurah, A. S., Gordon, S. S., & Bradner, M. K. (2015). Health disparities and underserved populations: A potential solution, medical school partnerships with free clinics to improve curriculum. *Medical Education Online, 20,* 1–4.

9

Using Data to Build the Business Case for Change

Brian Collins and James L. Harris

OBJECTIVES

1. Discuss the evolution of a business case.
2. Identify the basic components of a business case.
3. Appreciate the value of data, analysis, and value-based purchasing in the current healthcare environment.
4. Understand how the application of publicaly reported data benefits business case development, approval, and actionable change.
5. Explore ways data support a future state of healthcare change.

CORE COMPETENCIES

- Understand the value of using data when developing a business case
- Recognize the impact of process and outcome measures on change and data generation
- Appreciate how data can drive a future state of healthcare delivery and improvement

INTRODUCTION

In the current healthcare environment, there is no immunity to the disruptive innovation occurring in the market. Adapting to disruptive market forces requires an understanding of how to use data to an organization's advantage, especially when developing a business change for actionable change. This process often requires reengineering of previous data collection methods, analysis, and data use if market competitiveness is achieved and sustained. Internal data measures and practices, external benchmarks and standards, reimbursement models, and data modeling will become the cornerstone of the business case. The ability to quantify, understand, and communicate the dollar payment value based on the value-based purchasing incentive program is requisite if any proposed change occurs and becomes a sustainable culture of quality improvement in any organization. In this chapter, an overview of the history of the business case using data; applying data, analysis, and value-based purchasing; and a future state required for healthcare change will be discussed.

MAKING THE BUSINESS CASE FOR CHANGE USING DATA: A HISTORICAL OVERVIEW

The concept of using data to make the business case is over 100 years old, literally and legally. An early example is the Eastern Rail Case of 1910 where Louis Brandeis "the people's lawyer" opposed an application to the Interstate Commerce Commission for a 10% rate increase by the rail company. Brandeis argued the rate hikes were the result of failed management and the additional associated costs should not be the burden of the general public. To make his case and at the request of the jury for a remedy, Brandeis employed the services of several individuals to testify on the value of efficiency in operations, time-motion studies, cost accounting methods that focused on standard and predictable cost of products and labor, incentives, and other management techniques (Miranti, 1999). This early example, use of experts, and supporting data to build the case for change are foundational to the development of contemporary data systems and management processes. Examples in contemporary healthcare include, but are not limited to, the following:

- Decision Support Systems (DSS)
- Science and practice of measurement
- Models and methods of efficiency
- Human factors associated with scientific management
- Efficiency reporting methods focusing on eliminating waste using measurement methods to ensure fiscal responsibility and profitability (Baumgart & Neuhauser, 2009)

THE BASICS OF A BUSINESS CASE DIRECTED AT ACTIONABLE CHANGE

The basis for a business case is an identified need based on reliable data, external forces, healthcare laws, or regulations in the current market. The business case must be designed to quantify the impact of any recommendation that will be supported by analysis and findings used to create the impetus for planned change. A convincing business case offers leaders the ability to reach conclusions based on the following:

- Comprehensive needs assessment
- Benchmarks
- Gap analysis
- Cost benefits captured using the value equation posed by Porter (2010):

$$Value = Benefits/Cost$$

- Stakeholder involvement
- The six aims posed by the Institute of Medicine (IOM) for delivering quality care: safe, effective, efficient, timely, patient-centered, and equitable (IOM, 2001)
- Organizational readiness and buy-in for change.

A comprehensive needs assessment cannot be understated and must be transparent, replicable, reliable, and supported by quantitative and qualitative data collection methods. The needs assessment should include the purpose, population, methods, instrument(s), data collection processes, analyses, and how the results will be used to assure improvements and sustainable profitability (Jones & Roussel, 2020). Once the needs assessment is completed, it becomes the source for organizing the business case.

Business cases should be concise and should not be excessive in length, as this will create a distraction for individuals reviewing and ultimately approving the proposal. A business case should include, at a minimum, the following components as presented in Box 9.1.

BOX 9.1 Business Case Components

Cover Page
Executive Summary
Background Specific to Proposed Business Case With Supporting Data
Implications for Quality, Safety, and Value Sustainability
Related Organizational and Performance Goals Linked To Proposed Metrics
Fiscal Investment to Include Start Up Cost and Recurring
Return of Investment Quarterly and per Annum With Ongoing Evaluation
Processes
Approval Signatures With Date to Implement

ACHIEVING IMPACT WITH APPLICATION OF DATA, ANALYSIS, AND VALUE-BASED PURCHASING

In the current healthcare environment, achieving impact using data is necessary for continuous improvement and fiscal stability. As more data are available, requirements for sharing persist. As data science advances, quantifying the dollar value in 2020 and beyond is paramount for improvement outcome management. This can be accomplished by calculating the dollar value of the Centers for Medicare and Medicaid Services (CMS) in fiscal year 2020 based on the value-based purchasing (VBP) incentive program using standard industry vocabulary. This however begs the question, can data provide strategies to assist in healing and does it provide an opportunity to consider how graphic representations provide a sense of direction and location? The answer is yes in an era of big data and value-based payment models that are the predominant way of reimbursement for care (Joynt et al., 2017).

Prior to discussing the VBP incentive program and its impact, an overview of VBP is necessary. VBP encompasses a broad set of performance-based strategies that standardize financial incentives to providers' performance within a set of indicators. As a demand-side strategy, VBP focuses on outcome measurement that contributes to quality improvement, healthcare spending reduction, and value for patients (National Business Coalition on Health, 2015; Zipfel et al., 2019). The value of VBP can be achieved by measuring the outcomes and costs per diagnosis while identifying variation across the cycle of care (Porter, 2008).

To quantify the dollar payment value of the Centers for Medicare and Medicaid Services (CMS) in Fiscal Year (FY) 2020 based on the Value Based Purchasing (VBP) incentive program and using standard industry vocabulary, several steps are required. With the "FY2020 VBP Adjustment Factor Correction Notice Table 16B" and the "FY2020 Inpatient Prospective Payment System Impact File" used in calculating Medicare rates, an analysis of the 2,731 hospitals with publicly reported VBP payment adjustments is necessary. For calculation purposes, the payment adjustment ranges from -1.17% of Medicare Payments to +2.9%, with an average of +0.16% (CMS, 2020a; CMS, 2020a; CMS, 2019a; CMS, 2019b).

However, this program is budget neutral and the "weighted mean" is much closer to 0.00% when factoring in size and volume of discharges among hospitals incurring a penalty or bonus, the case mix index (CMI), or acuity among the discharges included in the base DRG payment on which the penalty or bonus adjustment is applied. Larger hospitals with higher occupancy rates and CMI score lower in VBP, more likely below the 0.00% adjustment factor. Smaller hospitals, measured by the number of licensed beds with lower occupancy and CMI, score higher in VBP and above 0.00%. This observed fact is sustained in a publically issued notice stating, 55% of hospitals earned a bonus in VBP FY2020 (+0.00% Payment Adjustment %) accounting for how a program could be budget neutral (CMS, 2019a). This example uses two major sources of hospital based data and the information to quantify the dollar impact of the VBP incentive adjustment factor and other key metrics that drive hospital revenue, including occupancy of physical beds, average length of stay (ALOS), discharge volume, and case mix index (CMI). Whatever example is presented, data, analysis, and measurement are a necessity when calculating any impact for sustainability.

CMS started to withhold 1% of Medicare payments made under the Inpatient Prospective Payment System (IPPS) in FY2013 (Fiscal Year, beginning October 1, 2012 and ending September 30, 2013). Based on a linear exchange rate, hospitals could earn back their 1%, or more, or less. The program was part of the Affordable Care Act and is budget neutral, where underperforming hospital penalties fund incentive payments to the better performing.

This rate increased by 0.25% each year from FY2014 (1.25%), FY2015 (1.5%), FY2016 (1.75%), to FY2017 at 2.0% where it has remained in FY2018-2020. In FY2020, the 2,731 hospitals with a publicly reported Total Performance Score (TPS) represent over 95 billion dollars in Medicare payments with 2% or 1.9 billion dollars at-stake in VBP. That equates to a 10-digit business case (CMS, 2019a; CMS, 2019b; CMS, 2020a; CMS, 2020b).

The TPS is based-on historical performance and translated to a 10-decimal factor and used as a multiplier in calculating current year payments. The factor centers on 1.0000000000, where a hospital's Diagnostic Related Group (DRG) payment is multiplied by 1.0000000000 and hence unchanged and has earned back the 2%. Hospitals with a factor less than 1 will receive a decrease to their Medicare payments and are not earning back the 2%. Hospitals with a factor greater than 1 will receive an additional payment for performance and earn back the 2% plus a bonus payment (CMS, 2019b).

The average adjustment factor for FY2020 is 1.0016360115, representing a 0.16% increase to Medicare payments. In reality, "the average hospital" will be earning a bonus payment. What would have been a $10,000 Medicare Payment would be $10,016.36 (=$10,000 x 1.0016360115) with a hospital earning a $16.36 bonus payment for that discharge. A hospital with 3,200 Medicare Inpatient Discharges per year would earn $52,352 over the year in bonus payments (=$16.36 x 3,200), for example. In practice, this bonus payments moves with the DRG payment for any particular discharge. The higher-weighted, higher-paying discharges would carry a larger bonus payment as the same % of a higher dollar amount. This works as a bonus or penalty if the adjustment factor is above or below 1, respectively. In FY2020, 55% of hospitals have a factor greater than 1, meaning they will be receiving an additional bonus payment. Based on actual adjustment factors, estimated discharges and Medicare payments per discharge, and this analysis and estimate will build on the business case that $390,801,905 will be exchanged across the 2,731 reporting hospitals; or approximately, $1.07 million per day. The national implication of scientific management to the modern hospital industry is approximately $1,000,000 per day (CMS, 2019a; CMS, 2019b; CMS, 2020a; CMS, 2020b). This example is only one performance-based program from one insurer. There are more and more to come with more at stake. Impact can be identified with further drilldown into the FY2020 VBP results, implications, and lessons. Using this information, recommendations associated with any business case are possible and validates the value of data to drive change.

For purposes of this chapter and to further familiarize the reader with CMS VBP data for use when developing a business case, several figures and examples are provided. Exhibit 9.1 displays the CMS VBP FY2020 dollars at stake in national incentive

EXHIBIT 9.1 Centers for Medicare and Medicaid Services Value-Based Dollars in Incentive Payments

LINE	DESCRIPTION	VALUE	SOURCE
A	Hospital Beds	218	[2]
C	Days per Year	365	Actual*
D	Bed Days	79,570	= A x B
E	Patient Days	47,654.5	[2]
F	Occupancy %	59.89%	= E / D
G	Medicare %	32.0%	[2]
H	Medicare Days	15,249.4	= E x G
I	Medicare Discharges	3,210	[2]
J	Medicare ALOS	4.75	= H / I
K	Medicare CMI	1.7914	[2]
L	Medicare Base $	$6,000.00	Estimate
M	Medicare Pay/Dis	$10,748.40	= K x L
N	Medicare Payments	$34,506,734	= I x M
	VBP Hospitals	2,731	[1]
	Medicare Payments	$94,237,891,434	= N x VBP Hospitals
	VBP	2.00%	[3]
	VBP $'s at stake	$1,884,757,829	= P x Q
	VBP $'s at billions	$1.9	= R/1,000,000,000 [3]

[1] FY2020VBP Adjustment Fact or Correct ion Notice Table 168;
[2] FY2020 Inpatient Prospective Payment System Impact File contains provider data used in calculating rates.
[3] CMS Hospital Value-Based Purchasing Program Results for Fiscal Year 2020, Fact Sheet Oct 29, 2019.
*Actual Days in year = 365 for 3/4 years, as with all of the data in these data models; FY2020 = 366 Days.
†based-on discharge weighted average.
Source: Data from Centers for Medicare and Medicaid Services (CMS), CMS Value-Based Purchasing, and CMS Percentage Payment Summary Report.

payments as the last line, $1.9B. The model is built on the 2,731 hospitals with publicly reported VBP scores and data from the Inpatient Prospective Payment System (IPPS) Impact File containing beds, average daily census, Medicare discharges, and case mix index (CMI) for gauging acuity and key in the calculation of Medicare reimbursement.

Figure 9.1 displays the value-based purchasing payment adjustment % (black bar, labeled A) by standard deviations from the mean with distribution (light gray bar, labeled E), including beds (black line with square markers, labeled D), Medicare discharges (gray line with triangle markers, labeled C), and Medicare case mix index CMI (light gray line with circle markers, labeled B).

Exhibit 9.2 displays the discharge weighted average value-based adjustment factor. The provider discharge volume in the IPPS Impact File is multiplied times the provider VBP adjustment factor, then summed, and divided by the total number of Medicare discharges for the 2,731 hospitals (8,759,907 Medicare discharges). The 1.0000062551 (+0.00062551%) weighted average is more indicative of the financial reality than the 0.16% straight average over all hospitals included in the VBP program with publicly reported results. This model uses the overall (n = 2,731), average number of hospital beds (218) and weighted average daily census, occupancy %, Medicare %, Medicare ALOS and CMI as Exhibit 9.1; and the weighted average VBP adjustment factor (0.00062551%). The result is a VBP incentive payment of $215.84 (line-Q). While this seems modest, it is the center of a budget neutral linear exchange rate. It is intended to be near zero, by definition and intention.

Exhibit 9.3 holds all variables constant, but models a 1% increase in the VBP adjustment factor, from 0.0003746739% to 1.0003746739%; which is leapfrogging over 70% of hospitals in the VBP program; as 1,913 of the 2,731 (70%) of hospitals have a VBP adjustment % between -1.0 and 1.0 standard deviations from the mean ($\geq 0.49\%$ and $< 0.5\%$). This would be a monumental task involving dozens to a hundred different measures within the VBP measurement. The reward for such an accomplishment would be $345,069, or 1.0% of total Medicare payments. Exhibit 9.3 manipulates one factor (highlighted in yellow) in each of the five scenarios, resulting in a direct impact to the variables highlighted in green.

While the task of shifting the VBP by 1%, or one standard deviation may seem monumental; the same +1% shift in CMI, from 1.7914 to 1.8093; or -1% ALOS, from 4.7500 to 4.7030 days; or +1% increase in occupancy, from 59.89% to 60.49% produce the same +1% increase and nearly identical additional Medicare payments of $345,000.

As Figure 9.2 illustrates, the variables beyond the VBP adjustment factor have much larger ranges of performance. The VBP adjustment factor standard deviation of 0.0064904486 represents 0.6480% of the mean; as in, approximately 68% of hospitals have a score that falls within a range <1.0%, or, within 0.6480% to be exact. While one standard deviation for the other three measures coves a much larger range of performance: CMI 18.5%; ALOS 25.8% and occupancy 35.7%.

When reviewing Figure 9.2, one can conclude that CMI, ALOS, and occupancy are much more elastic, variable, and can be influenced through intervention with a much larger range of performance.

Medicare value based purchasing <u>incentive adjustment%</u>[1] by standard deviation from the Mean 0.16%; <u>Hospital beds</u>[2], <u>Medicare discharges</u>[2] and <u>case mix index</u>[2]

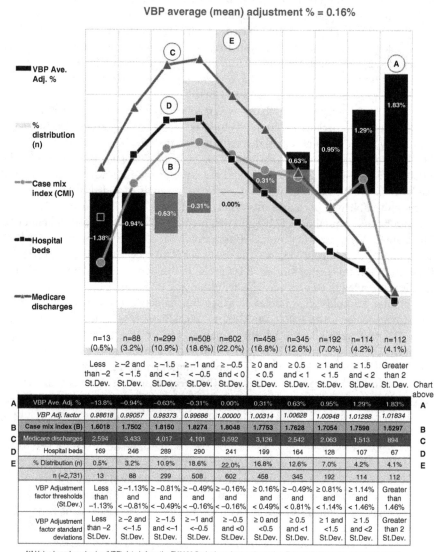

		Less than −2 St.Dev.	≥ −2 and < −1.5 St.Dev.	≥ −1.5 and < −1 St.Dev.	≥ −1 and < −0.5 St.Dev.	≥ −0.5 and < 0 St.Dev.	≥ 0 and < 0.5 St.Dev.	≥ 0.5 and < 1 St.Dev.	≥ 1 and < 1.5 St.Dev.	≥ 1.5 and < 2 St.Dev.	Greater than 2 St. Dev.	Chart above
A	VBP Ave. Adj. %	−13.8%	−0.94%	−0.63%	−0.31%	0.00%	0.31%	0.63%	0.95%	1.29%	1.83%	A
	VBP Adj. factor	0.98618	0.99057	0.99373	0.99686	1.00000	1.00314	1.00628	1.00948	1.01288	1.01834	
B	Case mix index (B)	1.6018	1.7502	1.8150	1.8274	1.8048	1.7753	1.7628	1.7054	1.7598	1.5297	B
C	Medicare discharges	2,594	3,433	4,017	4,101	3,592	3,126	2,542	2,063	1,513	894	C
D	Hospital beds	169	246	289	290	241	199	164	128	107	67	D
E	% Distribution (n)	0.5%	3.2%	10.9%	18.6%	22.0%	16.8%	12.6%	7.0%	4.2%	4.1%	E
	n (=2,731)	13	88	299	508	602	458	345	192	114	112	
	VBP Adjustment factor thresholds (St.Dev.)	Less than −1.13%	≥ −1.13% and < −0.81%	≥ −0.81% and < −0.49%	≥ −0.49% and < −0.16%	≥ −0.16% and < −0.16%	≥ 0.16% and < 0.49%	≥ −0.49% and < 0.81%	≥ 0.81% and < 1.14%	≥ 1.14% and < 1.46%	Greater than 1.46%	
	VBP Adjustment factor standard deviations	Less than −2 St.Dev.	≥ −2 and <−1.5 St.Dev.	≥ −1.5 and <−1 St.Dev.	≥ −1 and <−0.5 St.Dev.	≥ −0.5 and <0 St.Dev.	≥ 0 and <0.5 St.Dev.	≥ 0.5 and <1 St.Dev.	≥ 1 and <1.5 St.Dev.	≥ 1.5 and <2 St.Dev.	Greater than 2 St.Dev.	

[1] Value based purchasing (VBP) data is from the FY2020 final rule and correction notice, Table 16B: The value-based adjustment factors are based-on the finalized basline and perfomance period and used operating DRG payments for discharges in FY2020.

[2] FY2020 inpatient prospective payment system (IPPS) impact file, correction notice (Sep'19) contains provider data used in calculating rates.

FIGURE 9.1 Value-based purchasing incentive adjustment %.

Source: Data from Centers for Medicare and Medicaid Services (CMS), CMS Value-Based Purchasing, and CMS Percentage Payment Summary Report.

EXHIBIT 9.2 Discharge Weighted Average Value-Based Adjustment Factor

LINE	DESCRIPTION	VALUE	SOURCE
A	Hospital Beds	218	[2]
C	Days per Year	365	Actual*
D	Bed Days	79,570	= A x B
E	Patient Days	47,654.5	[2]
F	Occupancy %	59.89%	= E / D
G	Medicare %	32.0%	[2]
H	Medicare Days	15,249.4	= E x G
I	Medicare Discharges	3,210	[2]
J	Medicare ALOS	4.75	= H / I
K	Medicare CMI	1.7914	[2]
L	Medicare Base $	$6,000.00	Estimate
M	Medicare Pay/Dis	$10,748.40	= K x L
N	Medicare Payments	$34,506,734	= I x M
O	VBP Adjustment Factor	1.0000062551	[1][†]
P	Net Change in Amount	0.00062551%	= (O - 1) / 100
Q	Net Change in Payment	$215.84	= N x P
R	Medicare Payments	$34,506,950	= N + Q

[1] FY2020VBP Adjustment Fact or Correct ion Notice Table 168;
[2] FY2020 Inpatient Prospective Payment System Impact File contains provider data used in calculating rates.
[3] CMS Hospital Value-Based Purchasing Program Results for Fiscal Year 2020, Fact Sheet Oct 29, 2019.
*Actual Days in year = 365 for 3/4 years, as with all of the data in these data models; FY2020 = 366 Days.
[†]based-on discharge weighted average.
Source: Data from Centers for Medicare and Medicaid Services (CMS), CMS Value-Based Purchasing, and CMS Percentage Payment Summary Report.

EXHIBIT 9.3 Model of Medicare Payments, Scenario 1-5

MODEL OF MEDICARE PAYMENTS, SCENARIO 1-5

LINE	DESCRIPTION	SCENARIO 1 BASELINE VALUE	SCENARIO 2 +1.00% VBP ADJ. VALUE	SCENARIO 3 +1.00% CMI VALUE	SCENARIO 4 +1.00% MEDICARE ALOS VALUE	SCENARIO 5 +1.00% OCCUPANCY % VALUE
A	Hospital Beds	218	218	218	218	218
C	Days per Year	365	365	365	365	365
D	Bed Days	79,570	79,570	79,570	79,570	79,570
E	Patient Days	47,654.5	47,654.5	47,654.5	47,654.5	48,131.0
F	Occupancy %	59.89%	59.89%	59.89%	59.89%	60.40%
G	Medicare %	32.0%	32.0%	32.0%	32.0%	32.0%
H	Medicare Days	15,294.4	15,294.4	15,294.4	15,294.4	15,401.9
I	Medicare Discharges	3,210	3,210	3,210	3,243	3,243
J	Medicare ALOS	4.75	4.7500	4.7500	4.7030	4.7500
K	Medicare CMI	1.7914	1.7914	1.8093	1.7914	1.7914
L	Medicare Base $	$6,000.00	$6,000.00	$6,000.00	$6,000.00	$6,000.00

M	Medicare Pay/Dis	$10,748.40	$10,748.40	$10,855.88	$10,748.40	$10,748.40
N	Medicare Payments	$34,506,734	$34,506,734	$34,851,802	$34,851,767	$34,851,802
O	VBP Adjustment Factor	1.0000062551	1.01000053176	1.0000037467	1.0000037467	1.0000037467
P	Net Change in Amount	0.00062551%	1.00063176%	0.00037467%	0.00037467%	0.00037467%
Q	Net Change in Payment	$215.84	$345,285,34	$130.58	$130.58	$130.58
R	Medicare Payments	$34,506,950	$34,852,020	$34,851,932	$34,851,897	$34,851,932
	$ Change (Δ) from Baseline		$345,070	$344,982	$344,947	$344,982
	% Change (Δ) from Baseline	1.00%	1.00%	1.00%	1.00%	1.00%

Source: Data from Centers for Medicare and Medicaid Services (CMS), CMS Value-Based Purchasing, and CMS Percentage Payment Summary Report.

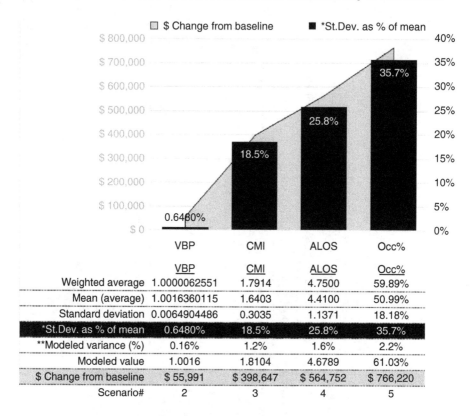

	VBP	CMI	ALOS	Occ%
Weighted average	1.0000062551	1.7914	4.7500	59.89%
Mean (average)	1.0016360115	1.6403	4.4100	50.99%
Standard deviation	0.0064904486	0.3035	1.1371	18.18%
*St.Dev. as % of mean	0.6480%	18.5%	25.8%	35.7%
**Modeled variance (%)	0.16%	1.2%	1.6%	2.2%
Modeled value	1.0016	1.8104	4.6789	61.03%
$ Change from baseline	$ 55,991	$ 398,647	$ 564,752	$ 766,220
Scenario#	2	3	4	5

* Standard deviation as % of Mean, by measure (VBP, CMI, ALOS, Occ%).
**Modeled variance % = (standard deviation as % of mean/4) for VBP and
(standard deviation as % of mean / 16) for CMI, ALOS, and occupancy %

FIGURE 9.2 Average financial impact of standard deviance by measure.

Source: Data from Centers for Medicare and Medicaid Services (CMS), CMS Value-Based Purchasing, and CMS Percentage Payment Summary Report.

For a conservative estimate of increased Medicare payments and potential performance across interventions to improve from baseline (Scenario #1 in Exhibit 9.4), the range of performance for VBP was divided by four; so 0.6480% / 4 = 0.16%; and this factor was used to model VBP incentive payments if a hospital went from the weighted average score of 0.00062551% to 0.16288672%; for +$56,209.89 in Medicare Payments. To be extremely conservative, the other three variables performance range (one standard deviation as a % of the mean) is divided by 16; so the CMI standard deviation of 0.3035 divided by 1.6403 = 18.5%; which is then divided by 16 to model a 1.2% increase in CMI, from 1.7914 to 1.8121; for +$342,647 in Medicare payments.

Value-based purchasing has much potential for developing effectiveness of care where the patient is a valued consumer. Throughout this section of the chapter,

EXHIBIT 9.4 Model of Medicare Payments, Scenario #1

MODEL OF MEDICARE PAYMENTS, SCENARIO 1–5

LINE	DESCRIPTION	SCENARIO 1 BASELINE VALUE	SCENARIO 2 +0.16% VBP ADJ. VALUE	SCENARIO 3 +1.06% CMI VALUE	SCENARIO 4 -1.50% MEDICARE ALOS VALUE	SCENARIO 5 +1.90% OCCUPANCY % VALUE
A	Hospital Beds	218	218	218	218	218
C	Days per Year	365	365	365	365	365
D	Bed Days	79,570	79,570	79,570	79,570	79,570
E	Patient Days	47,654.5	47,654.5	47,654.5	47,654.5	48,712.8
F	Occupancy %	59.89%	59.89%	59.89%	59.89%	61.22%
G	Medicare %	32.0%	32.0%	32.0%	32.0%	32.0%
H	Medicare Days	15,249.4	15,249.4	15,249.4	15,249.4	15,588.1
I	Medicare Discharges	3,210	3,210	3,210	3,263	3,282
J	Medicare ALOS	4.75	4.75	4.75	4.6735	4.75
K	Medicare CMI	1.7914	1.7914	1.8121	1.7914	1.7914
L	Medicare Base $	$6,000.00	$6,000.00	$6,000.00	$6,000.00	$6,000.00

(continued)

EXHIBIT 9.4 Model of Medicare Payments, Scenario #1 (continued)

MODEL OF MEDICARE PAYMENTS, SCENARIO 1–5

LINE	DESCRIPTION	SCENARIO 1 BASELINE VALUE	SCENARIO 2 +0.16% VBP ADJ. VALUE	SCENARIO 3 +1.06% CMI VALUE	SCENARIO 4 -1.50% MEDICARE ALOS VALUE	SCENARIO 5 +1.90% OCCUPANCY % VALUE
M	Medicare Pay/Dis	$10,748.40	$10,748.40	$10,872.60	$10,748.40	$10,748.40
N	Medicare Payments	$34,506,734	$34,506,734	$34,905,467	$35,071,571	$35,273,038
O	VBP Adjustment Factor	1.0000062551	1.0016288672	1.0000037467	1.0000037467	1.0000037467
P	Net Change in Amount	0.000062551%	0.162886729%	0.00037467%	0.00037467%	0.00037467%
Q	Net Change in Payment	$215.84	$56,206.89	$130.78	$131.40	$132.16
R	Medicare Payments	$34,506,950	$34,562,941	$34,905,598	$35,071,703	$35,273,171
	$ Change () from Baseline		$55,991	$398,647	$564,752	$766,220
	% Change () from Baseline		0.2%	1.2%	1.6%	2.2%
			$55,991	$342,656	$508,761	$710,229

Source: Data from Centers for Medicare and Medicaid Services (CMS), CMS Value-Based Purchasing, and CMS Percentage Payment Summary Report.

achieving impact through data application, analysis, and VBP was discussed. The information and examples provide a useful tool when building any business case for change.

CREATING A FUTURE STATE OF CHANGE UNDERPINNED BY A DATA-DRIVEN BUSINESS CASE

Change in healthcare is constant and dependent on valid and reliable data. Without useable data that is understandable and readily available, the future state of any organization is at stake. As individuals are tasked with developing business cases, data can raise awareness of organizational accomplishments, variances, and plant the seed for innovative change that will guide improvement and evidence sustainable outcomes.

The strategy behind the strategy of any business case is a solid platform based on understanding and using data toward an envisioned desired outcome. This will require fluidity and accommodation in order to assimilate information, select metrics that will drive change, and understand that staff are increasingly invested in quality outcomes. Each of these factors offers opportunities to develop a business case that encompasses the uniqueness of the digital age and forge innovative thought and action. Viewing the landscape of healthcare and envisioning a new vision for change will provide foundational direction to develop and achieve outcomes proposed in any business case. As the fourth industrial revolution of data explosion evolves, healthcare organizations are poised to transition into a new age with a different set of parameters where the value of work and data are a function of the outcome.

SUMMARY

- The concept of using data to make the business case dates to over 100 years, literally and legally. The Eastern Rail Case of 1910 is one example that shaped contemporary data and management systems.
- Business cases rely on valid and reliable data and include a series of purposeful steps when developing and presenting for approval.
- Value is mathematically defined as Value = Benefits/Cost.
- The business case executive summary should be concise, factual, and void of extraneous information.
- Impacts associated with improvement can be achieved using data, analysis, and VBP components.
- VBP encompasses a broad set of performance-based strategies that standardize financial incentives to providers' performance within a set of indicators.
- The dollar payment value of the Centers for Medicare and Medicaid Services (CMS) in Fiscal Year (FY) 2020 based on the Value-Based Purchasing (VBP) incentive program and standard industry vocabulary can be easily quantified.
- Figures 9.1 to 9.3 and Exhibit 9.1 to 9.4 in the text provide data related to VBP and reimbursement.

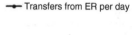

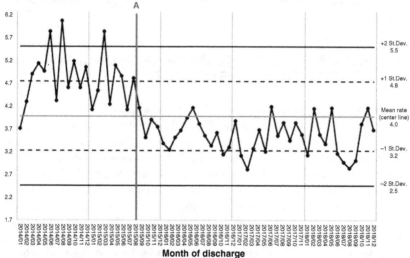

Month of discharge

FIGURE 9.3 Emergency room (ER) transfers to other acute care hospitals, Lawrence General Hospital, Lawrence, Massachusetts

- Without useable data that is understandable and readily available, the future state of any organization is at stake.
- Viewing the landscape of healthcare and envisioning a new vision for change will provide foundational direction to develop and achieve outcomes proposed in a business case.
- As the fourth industrial revolution of data explosion evolves, healthcare organizations are poised to transition into a new age with a different set of parameters where the value of work and data are a function of the outcome.

REFLECTION QUESTIONS

1. From the figures (9.1 to 9.3) and Exhibit (9.1 to 9.4) provided in this chapter, how can you use the data to develop a business case for improvement?
2. You are tasked with developing a business case for improvement due to declining revenues imposed by CMS penalties. What steps would you take, and who would be involved and why?

REFERENCES

Baumgart, A., & Neuhauser, D. (2009). Frank and Lillian Gilbreth: Scientific management in the operating room. *Quality and Safety in Health Care*, *18*(5), 413–415. https://doi.org/10.1136/qshc.2009.032409

Centers for Medicare and Medicaid Services. (2019a). *CMS hospital value-based purchasing program results for fiscal year 2020. Fact sheet, CMS Newsroom,* October 29, 2019. https://www.cms.gov/newsroom/fact-sheets/cms-hospital-value-based-purchasing -program-results-fiscal-year-2020

Centers for Medicare and Medicaid Services. (2019b). *How to read your fiscal year (FY) 2020 hospital value-based purchasing (VBP) program percentage payment summary report (PPSR).* Provided by the Inpatient Value, Incentives, and Quality Reporting (VIQR) Outreach and Education Support Contractor (SC), July 2019. https://www .qualityreportingcenter.com/globalassets/iqr_resources/july-2019/fy2020-ppsr-release -help-guide-gs-ec_07252019_vfinal508.pdf

Centers for Medicare and Medicaid Services. (2020a). *FY 2020 final rule and correction notice impact file.* https://www.cms.gov/Medicare/Medicare-Fee-for-Service-Payment/ AcuteInpatientPPS/FY2020-IPPS-Final-Rule-Home-Page-Items/FY2020-IPPS -Final-Rule-Data-Files

Centers for Medicare and Medicaid Services. (2020b). *FY 2020 final rule and correction notice tables, hospital value-based purchasing program, table 16B, adjustment factor.* https://www.cms.gov/Medicare/Medicare-Fee-for-Service-Payment/AcuteInpatientPPS/ FY2020-IPPS-Final-Rule-Home-Page-Items/FY2020-IPPS-Final-Rule-Tables

Institute of Medicine. (2001). *Crossing the quality chasm: A new health system for the 21st century.* National Academies Press.

Jones, C. T., & Roussel, L. (2020) Making the case for a project: Needs assessment. In J. L. Harris, L. Roussel, C. Dearman, & P. L. Thomas, *Project planning and management. A guide for nurses and interprofessional teams* (pp. 137–149). Jones & Bartlett Learning.

Joynt, K. E., De Lew, N., Sheingold, S. H., Conway, P. H., Goodrich, K., & Epstein, A. M. (2017). Should Medicare value-based purchasing take social risk into account? *New England Journal of Medicine, 376*(6), 510–513. https://doi.org/10.1056/NEJMp1616278

Miranti, P. J. (1996). Louis D. Brandeis and standard cost accounting: A study of the construction of historical agency. *Accounting, Organizations and Society, 21*(6), 569–586. https://doi. org/10.1016/0361-3682(95)00033-X

National Business Coalition on Health. (2015). *Value-based purchasing: A definition.* http:// www.nbch.org/Value-based-Purchasing-A-Definition

Porter, M. E. (2008). Value-based health care delivery. *Annals of Surgery, 248*(4), 503–509.

Porter, M. E. (2010). What is value in health care? *New England Journal of Medicine, 363*(26), 2477–2481. https://doi.org/10.1056/NEJMp1011024

Zipfel, N., van der Nat, P. B., Rensign, B. J. W., Daeter, E. J., Westert, G. P., & Groenewoud, A. S. (2019). The implementation of change model adds value to value-based healthcare: A qualitative study. *BMC Health Services Research, 19*(643), 1–12. https://doi.org/10.1186/ s12913-019-4498-y

CASE EXEMPLARS FOR APPLICATION

Sustainability and Value Over Volume in a Community Hospital

Teresa Pazdral

Our community hospital is 30 minutes north of Boston, Massachusetts. We are a medium-sized inpatient acute care hospital with 186 licensed beds. Our emergency room (ER) is very busy with over 68,000 annual visits. When the hospital reaches capacity, a trickle-down effect happens and severely hinders hospital profitability. Starting with patient's having basic conditions, such as chest pain, spending two to three days between the ER and a med/surg unit, these patients were occupying inpatient beds that cannot be used for patients ready to be transferred out of the Intensive Care Unit (ICU). If the ICU was at full capacity and a bed could not be made available, the next patient arriving in the ER needing critical care services was transferred out of the ER to another local hospital within two hours. The patients were in the clinical reach of our hospital, we merely lacked the physical capacity to keep the care local. Often these patients were transferred to urban, higher cost care settings. This type of transfer was a subset of the four to six transfers to other acute care hospitals per day from the ER, shown to the left of graph with the vertical line labeled 'A' in Figure 9.4.

In late 2015, the Transformation Steering Committee (TSC) identified this a major system failure of the hospital and several interventions were put into place (Collins et al., 2017). Rounding on the ICU was standardized to identify opportunities for transfer of patients from the ICU to medical-surgical units and several initiatives to expedite the discharge process, communication, and bed management helped as well.

Among the TSC key initiatives was the Emergency Department Observation Unit (EDOU), which started with a chest pain protocol and has now expanded to more than a dozen condition-specific protocols. Where an inpatient discharge for

"Chest Pain" (MSDRG 313) with a case weight of <0.70 or "Syncope & Collapse" (MSDRG 312) with a case weight <0.80 that has an expected stay between 1.8 to 2.4 days respectively, now observation protocols have been developed in conjunction with specialists who had patients discharged within 15 to 24 versus 43 to 57 hours. In approximately 20% of the cases the observation patients would "test-out" of the protocol with a high troponin result or alarming stress or exercise tolerance test (ETT). In those instances, the patient would then be admitted as an npatient and an MS-DRG such as "Heart Failure" or "Other Circulatory System Diagnoses with case weights in the higher ranges from 0.95 to 1.90. (Centers for Medicare and Medicaid Services [CMS], 2017)

More important was the quality of patient care and providing two or more days of care within 15 to 24 hours with definitive diagnostic results and rule-outs. This and other interventions led to increased capacity and was used to prevent transfers and retain patients at our hospital for no other reason than bed availability. With ER transfers to other acute care hospitals decreasing from four to six per day to three to four per day, this is noted in the vertical line A in Figure 9.4. Fewer "Chest Pain" and "Syncope" discharges were replaced by higher case weight DRG inpatients because more complex patient care needs were identified earlier through the "rule out" protocol process.

This transformation is symbolic of value versus volume as fewer inpatient discharges were offset by the higher CMI that resulted in an annual net impact of greater than $1.25million for Medicare patients representing one-third of our hospitals discharges (Collins et al., 2017). Shown in Figure 9.4 with the vertical line A, the housewide CMI based on MSDRG weights by month increased 10%. The beginning of

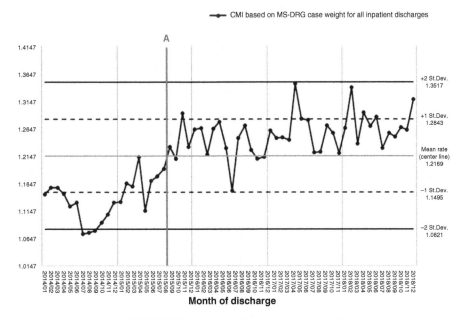

FIGURE 9.4 House-wide case mix index (CMI)

a transformation paradigm at our hospital was achieved by keeping care local and patient-centered for the community and healthcare system.

REFERENCES

Centers for Medicare and Medicaid Services. (2017). *Final rule and correction notice, table 5. List of Medicare Severity Diagnosis Related Groups (MS-DRG's) relative weighting factors, geometric and arithmetic mean length of stay for FY 2017.* https://www.cms.gov/medicaremedicare-fee-service-paymentacuteinpatientppsacute-inpatient-files-download/files-fy-2017-final-rule-and-correction-notice

Collins, B., Kondylis, G., Kunupakaphun, S., & Eamranond, P. (2017). Raising CMI through a multidisciplinary approach in the community hospital setting. *Healthcare Financial Management Journal.* https://www.hfma.org/topics/article/54574.html

Influences and Processes Guiding Redesign of Employee Orientation Programs and Competency Validation

Lonnie K. Williams

As medical science and technology have rapidly advanced, considerable attention has been focused on ensuring that healthcare providers are prepared to meet the increasing care demands across the lifespan. Multiple mandates, regulations, performance indicators, and landmark reports have equally reinforced the attention that healthcare systems redesign employee orientation processes to ensure staffs possess the ability to translate knowledge into practice and respond to changes with the current healthcare environment.

Prior to redesigning any process requires reflection and a series of steps that include, but are not limited to:

- Assessment of readiness of the environment for change
- Management and stakeholder buy-in
- Skills and knowledge of staff regarding adult learning principles, use of evidence, and technology savvy within the education department
- Availability of evidence to guide content and competency validation redesign
- Available supporting data, resources, and technology
- What is working and areas that require updates?

The six core domains identified by the Institute of Medicine (IOM) in 2001 (safe, effective, patient-centered, timely, efficient, and equitable care) can provide a starting point for the process. Asking the question, how can the six domains underpin redesign and inform the process using this information? Will using this information inform the process? A solid understanding of information resources, tools, and software to access current evidence as presented in Chapter 12 of this textbook will also prove useful as the process progresses. As the redesign progresses and evidence from the literature is collected, a repository of information becomes readily available to frame orientation content and competency validation experiences.

A successful redesign of an orientation and skills validation program was successfully completed and implemented in a healthcare system. The program became a prototype for redesigning programs for a multilevel system with positive outcomes. Use of the IOM aims, supporting data, and available evidence were identified as the rationale for spreading the program throughout the entire healthcare entity. While this is one example, updates are consistently required for any program based on the rapidity of change, new evidence, and innovative practices occurring daily.

REFLECTION QUESTIONS

1. Consider that you are assigned to an improvement team tasked with redesigning an employee orientation and skills validation program. What steps should the team include to guide the process and what data, evidence, and/or tools can guide the improvement activity?
2. What evaluation tools could be used to validate the effectiveness of a redesigned employee orientation and skills validation program? How could this data be disseminated and in what format?

REFERENCE

Institute of Medicine. (2001). *Crossing the quality chasm. A new health system for the 21st century.* National Academy Press.

10

How Consumer Demands and Data Are Driving Change

Megan Williams, Lauran Hardin,
Niranjani Radhakrishnan, and Patricia L. Thomas

CHAPTER OBJECTIVES

1. Identify primary causes of escalating healthcare costs.
2. Discuss how Social Determinants of Health (SDOH) and health literacy provide impetus for care redesign.
3. List how data, data sharing, and assessment tools assist in understanding problems and create opportunities for change.
4. Describe the impact of health literacy in society.
5. Discuss the issues associated with inoperability of data systems.

CORE COMPETENCIES

- Knowledge of healthcare, costs, and strategies to reduce escalating care cost
- Consumer demand knowledge and their value in managing SDOH
- Management of use of data and evidence to guide change
- Recognize the impact of health literacy
- Understand how health literacy impacts care delivery and society

INTRODUCTION

Rising costs have fueled development of new fields of study and innovation in models of healthcare delivery. According to Kaiser Health News, the United States spent $10,224 per person on healthcare in 2017 and currently spends 28% more than any other comparable nation (Sawyer & Cox, 2018). The expenditure is not resulting in improved quality or health outcomes. The United States has experienced lower improvements in life expectancy and disease burden compared to other countries. Spending on healthcare has risen 40% in the last 25 years and has risen to 17.9% of gross domestic product or $3.3 trillion (Peterson-Kaiser Health System Tracker, n.d.).

An important study by Bradley and Taylor (2014) also revealed that, compared to other nations, the United States spends the least amount on social services (Avendano & Kawachi, 2014) as illustrated in Figure 10.1.

Consumers experience a cascade of effects from this cost conundrum. Rising healthcare costs place pressure on the economy and limit job growth. Healthcare costs impact affordability for consumers and an increasing number of bankruptcies have occurred directly related to these costs (Claxton et al., 2018; Krulick, 2019; Kaiser Health News, n.d.).

A lack of investment in the social services infrastructure impacts access for consumers to needed services such as behavioral health treatment or supportive

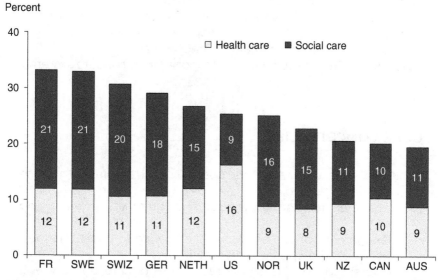

FIGURE 10.1 Health and social care spending as a percentage of gross domestic product.

Source: From Bradley, E. H., & Taylor, L. A. (2014). The American health care paradox: Why spending more is getting us less. *Choice Reviews Online, 51*(09), 51–5127. https://doi.org/10.5860/choice.51-5127, copyright © 2013, 2015. Reprinted by permission of PublicAffairs, an imprint of Hachette Book Group, Inc.

housing. Growing economic impact has incentivized an entire field of study to understand what is underneath high cost care and what can be done to reduce costs in the U.S. healthcare system. In 2016, 5% of the population utilized 50% of healthcare costs. The National Academy of Science, Engineering, and Medicine (NASEM) convened a national analysis of the population and coined the phrase "high cost, high needs" to describe a group of individuals driving costs that often have a combination of medical and social complexity (Long et al., 2017; Sawyer & Claxton, 2019).

Root causes for high-cost, high-needs patients include lack of housing, food security, behavioral health and addiction treatment, transportation, and access to care. Understanding these social determinants of health (SDOH) is a key focus area for delivery system re-design and a driver for care integration of multiple disciplines at the table to improve outcomes for complex patients (Long et al., 2017).

TRENDS IN THE POPULATION

One of the earliest innovators in care models for this population is the Camden Coalition of Healthcare Providers, which focuses solely on serving people facing the most complex medical and social challenges. Beginning with a breakfast group of physicians interested in how to improve the healthcare system on behalf of their patients, the Camden Coalition has evolved over time to become a coalition of hospitals, primary care and social service providers, and community representatives. Founded by Dr. Jeffrey Brenner, the Camden Coalition's early internal data analysis revealed that, much like what is seen across the country, 1% of patients in Camden represented 30% of the hospital costs. Based on these data and clinical observation, the Camden Coalition created a care management approach, called the Camden Core Model, to intervene with the population, and work with the community to address improvements in delivery based on what they were learning from the people they served. The model is based on utilizing data and building authentic healing relationships with patients to understand their needs and goals. The intervention is deeply focused on addressing medical as well as nonmedical barriers, such as housing, to health and stabilization. The COACH framework of engagement was created from the lessons they learned and creates respect and engagement with patients by developing an authentic healing relationship.

Knowing that caring for this population is community-specific, and wanting to both teach and learn from others, in 2016 the Camden Coalition launched the National Center for Complex Health and Social Needs with funding from AARP, the Robert Wood Johnson Foundation (RWJF), and Atlantic Philanthropies. The National Center for Complex Health and Social Needs convenes stakeholders and translates lessons into a national movement to improve care for complex populations. The approach is informed directly by the voices of people with lived experience of complexity and includes understanding change requires addressing an ecosystem approach with community collaborations and diverse partners to truly change the healthcare system.

The Blueprint for Complex Care, collaboratively developed by the National Center, IHI and CHCS in 2018, lays out the current state of complex care and provides 11 recommendations for building a field centered around serving people with complex needs. Key trends have emerged in understanding and effectively providing care to complex populations (Camden Coalition, n.d.).

SOCIAL DETERMINANTS OF HEALTH

As payment models have moved from a fee-for-service system to value-based payment, the incentive to understand the needs and characteristics of complex patients has grown. Social determinants of health (SDOH), which include social, behavioral, and environmental factors that influence health outcomes, have taken center stage in the national dialogue. McGinnis and colleagues describe the impact of SDOH as up to 60% of what actually determines health outcomes. Despite the evidence related to identifying the importance of these factors, clinicians and health systems have been slow to integrate assessment and delivery interventions into standard of care across settings (McGinnis et al., 2002; Taylor et al., 2016).

The impact of homelessness and safe, stable housing has risen to the top as one of the strongest evidence-based drivers of health outcomes. Numerous studies have demonstrated the negative health aspects of homelessness and a range of partners from payers to health systems to government have begun to invest in housing as a health intervention (Taylor, 2018).

Food security is another area that has emerged as a driver of health outcomes. Evidence reveals the clear impact of nutrition on health and disease management and leading edge health systems have begun to partner with food pantries for improved access and are offering medically tailored meals as a health intervention (Berkowitz & Waters, n.d.; Mason, 2020). has emerged as a driver of complexity and negative health outcomes. The AARP Foundation found that nearly 50% of adults over 45 report experiencing loneliness and social isolation is associated with an additional $6.7 billion in Medicare spending. Assessment of depression, anxiety, and/or loneliness is increasingly integrated in value-based payment outcomes and there is increasing investment internationally in interventions to address loneliness (Berkowitz & Waters, n.d.; Thayer & Anderson, 2018).

The impact of behavioral health and addiction treatment has been shown to be a key driver in stabilizing complex populations and reducing cost. The epidemic of opioid deaths has turned the attention of the nation to comprehensive assessment and treatment of substance misuse and the integration of comprehensive behavioral health assessment and treatment is foundational to addressing this issue for complex populations (NIDA, 2019; Thomas-Henkel, Hamblin, & Hendricks, 2015).

THE IMPACT OF HEALTH LITERACY

Health literacy is the degree to which individuals have the capacity to obtain, process, and understand basic health information and services (Institute of Medicine, 2004).

In 2003, the U.S. Department of Education commissioned for a health literacy assessment study, (Kutner et al., 2003) which was conducted by the National Assessment of Adult Literacy (NAAL). They found that 36%, or approximately 80 million of the U.S. adult population have a basic or below basic health literacy and face significant challenges understanding health information which can lead to poor health outcomes (Kutner et al., 2003).

In 2012, a cyclical, large-scale study called The Program for the International Assessment of Adult Competencies (PIAAC) was developed under the Organization of Economic Cooperation and Development (OECD) (States et al., 2013). This study surveyed 24 countries around literacy, numeracy, and problem solving skills. They concluded, larger proportions of adults in the United States than in other countries have poor literacy, numeracy skills, and problem solving than in other countries despite the relatively high educational systems. They also concluded that socioeconomic backgrounds have a stronger impact on adult literacy skills in the United States than in other countries. Black and Hispanic adults are substantially overrepresented in the low-skilled population. The link between literacy skills are connected not only to employment outcomes, but also to personal and social well-being. In the United States the odds of being in poor health are four times greater for low-skilled adults than for those with the highest proficiency, which is double the average across participating countries. Further studies have confirmed limited health literacy is common among vulnerable populations such as older adults, those living in poverty, and minority groups. Furthermore, these groups have drastically increased healthcare costs, patient safety, higher rates of hospitalizations, overutilization of Emergency Departments for non-emergency services, a greater number of chronic medical conditions, and decreased compliance with medications (Haun et al., 2015; Hersh et al., 2015; Ylitalo et al., 2018).

Low health literacy is directly affecting our national healthcare costs and should be assessed and addressed in communities that treat these individuals. Many of the underserved patients live in communities that have Federally Qualified Health Centers (FQHCs), which are health clinics that provide primary care services to underserved areas funded by Health Resources & Services Administration (HRSA). According to HRSA, (U.S. Department of Health and Human Services Health Resources and Services Administration, 2018) their role in healthcare is to promote health literacy by helping those that are poor and medically underserved navigate through complex health systems. In some instances patients with low health literacy may have difficulty in locating providers and services, filling out complex health forms, sharing their medical story with providers, seeking preventive healthcare, knowing the connection between risky behaviors and health, managing chronic health conditions and understanding directions on medications.

Health Literacy Assessment Tools

Various screening tools exist that measure health literacy. The gold standard tools are the Test of Functional Health Literacy in Adults (TOFHLA) and the Rapid Estimate of Adult Literacy in Medicine (REALM) (Collins, 2013). Two additional valid tools are the Newest Vital Sign (NVS) and the eHealth Literacy scale (eHEALS) (Collins, 2013).

The TOFHLA looks at comprehension and the ability to read and correctly pronounce words. This tool can take up to 22 minutes, but is very comprehensive in its assessment of health literacy. The REALM and NVS are shorter tests that take 2 to 3 minutes to complete. The NVS measures reading and applying information after answering six questions about a nutritional label. The REALM consists of word recognition and pronunciation of 66 medical terms read aloud (Hersh et al., 2015). Many providers have little time to complete lengthy assessments because of limited time with patients in the clinical setting. A shorter form resulted in an increased likelihood of completion. The type of assessment and benefits of completion have varying benefits based on their use, which is determined by the organization and provider (Collins, 2013; Ylitalo et al., 2018).

Improving Health Literacy

According to the U.S. Department of Health and Human Services National Action plan, everyone has the right to health information that helps them make informed decisions and to have health services delivered in ways that are understandable and beneficial to health, longevity, and quality of life. Goals to achieve health literacy and strategies for achieving them include:

- Develop and disseminate health and safety information that is accurate, accessible, and actionable
- Promote changes in the healthcare system that improve health information, communication, informed decision-making, and access to health services
- Incorporate accurate, standards-based, and developmentally appropriate health and science information and curricula in child care and education through the university level
- Support and expand local efforts to provide adult education, English language instruction, and culturally and linguistically appropriate health information services in the community
- Build partnerships, develop guidance, and change policies
- Increase basic research and the development, implementation, and evaluation of practices and interventions to improve health literacy
- Increase the dissemination and use of evidence-based health literacy practices and interventions (Thompson, 2014)

Routinely screening patients for health literacy will not improve long-term health outcomes and regular screening is not recommended due to inconsistency of results (Hersh et al., 2015). Organizations should provide understandable and accessible information to all patients to ensure everyone benefits from clear communication. This includes using plain, nonmedical language, limiting content, and easy-to-read materials. Also, recommendations for enhancing communications with patients, which includes verbal, written, and the use of visual aids (Hersh et al., 2015). Within communities that have vulnerable populations, there is research around the use of peer-support programs and the importance of patient empowerment, self-management, and patient activation. (Batterham et al., 2016).

There are many tools and resources that measure and increase health. It will take every one working together to help to improve the care of patients. By creating a universal health literacy language, everyone is treated equally and is assessed in a way that will improve accessibility, provide safety, reduce cost, and improve healthcare to all patients.

UNDERSTANDING THE PROBLEM: SHARING DATA

The current healthcare system in the United States is fragmented and patients receive care from various medical providers across multiple settings and health systems. This results in a patient's medical history being spread across the many locations they receive care and the multiple computer technologies utilized by these locations. As a result, medical providers are forced to make decisions from insufficient information which can lead to many negative unintended consequences such as overlooked diagnoses, superfluous labs, toxic mixing of medications, medical errors, and increased medical costs (Adjerid et al., 2016). There is a need to improve care coordination, and the sharing of medical data across information technologies or the *interoperability* of data which is the innovative practice that can improve patient care across the United States (American Hospital Association, 2019).

Data Sharing Among Hospitals and Community Organizations

In January of 2019, America's Essential Hospitals, American Hospital Association, Association of American Medical Colleges, Catholic Health Association of the United States, Children's Hospital Association, Federation of American Hospitals, and the National Association for Behavioral Healthcare released an assessment called *Sharing Data, Saving Lives: The Hospital Agenda for Interoperability* that described the benefits of a fully interoperable data system for healthcare providers and their patients and the need to "enlist and expand public and private stakeholder support around this goal (interoperability among health IT systems) to benefit all individuals, their families and caregivers" (American Hospital Association, 2019). They describe benefits such as efficient care coordination from current patient data in the hands of patients and providers that equips everyone to make the best decisions from up-to-date and comprehensive information, improved patient safety from the reduction of repetitive or concluding tests and medications, improved patient empowerment from expanded access to personal and comprehensive medical records and the ability to provide knowledge play an active role in their own medical care, reduced medical costs from reduction in financial resources and time from avoiding duplication of services and tracking down medical histories, improved public health efforts from the availability of in-depth data that can be used for disease prevention and population-level health initiatives (American Hospital Association, 2019).

Data interoperability is critical among hospitals and community-based organizations that provide healthcare services. However, the technical incompatibilities across computer systems makes it challenging to create a seamless system to transfer data easily. For example, information needs to essentially be "translated" so that data correlates correctly. Semantics in one system are completely different in another. Building these translation channels from scratch or creating one-off solutions when a problem arises is costly in terms of financial resources and staff time and could lead to gaps in the systems that make them vulnerable to hacking. Other challenges include unequal adoption of technologies where some locations cannot send or receive digital information in standardized formats, various regulations around data sharing and patient privacy for health systems compared to IT companies, health plans, or protocols that prohibit claims data sharing or only allow partial data set transferring for specific populations such as children or populations with behavioral or mental health issues (American Hospital Association, 2019).

Health Information Exchanges (HIEs) are an innovative solution that aims to join health technologies across healthcare systems. HIEs are agreements established among a variety of health-related stakeholders and act as a channel to pull information out of health silos and "facilitate the exchange of patient health information between hospitals belonging to different health systems or distinct physician practices" resulting in health records to digitally follow a patient as they move across settings (Adjerid et al., 2016). Many states have created HIEs which have allowed healthcare providers such as doctors, nurses, pharmacists, and more to securely access and share critical medical information digitally across systems, which has improved the "quality, safety, speed, and cost of patient care" (American Hospital Association, 2019). Studies have projected that full implementation of HIEs "could yield approximately $78 billion in annual savings from administrative efficienciences and redundant utilization" and by reducing medical errors (such as administering incorrect or conflicting medications or redundant testing) from accessing comprehensive medical histories would save over $24 billion per year in the United States (Adjerid et al., 2016). However, there are challenges associated with HIEs. HIEs still cannot reliably transfer data across different technologies or across ambulatory or post-acute settings, and they may still prohibit patients from accessing their own medical data (American Hospital Association, 2019). One of the biggest challenges is that exchangeable data is defined by and limited to a region or a state based on their state regulations (Adjerid et al., 2016; American Hospital Association, 2019).

Many states have enacted laws that provide incentives for HIEs and define privacy and patient consent requirements around sharing a patient's health record (Adjerid et al., 2016). A study conducted in 2015 showed that states with strict privacy and consent laws decreased the operationalizing and implementation of HIEs; however, when enacted alongside incentives (i.e., provided funding) for implementation, HIEs operation increased (Adjerid et al., 2016). The conversation around patient privacy and consent has sparked a debate around HIEs implementation. On one hand, patients find it increasingly important to actively provide consent and opt-in rather than an opt-out system due to the increase in access to personal information in this digital age; on the other hand, others advocate that privacy laws (i.e., HIPAA) are critical but costly and too restrictive as digital technology now provides the opportunity to improve patient care with access to comprehensive information (Adjerid et al., 2016).

As of 2016, 25 states (as well as the District of Columbia) have enacted legislation around HIEs that either provide incentives that fund HIE efforts and address privacy and consent concerns; however, policy makers have enacted different types of privacy protections and incentives or a variety of combinations (incentives plus privacy, only privacy, only incentives) across states (Adjerid et al., 2016). Eleven states explicitly designated funds to support HIE efforts, and seven states had incentives that focused on creating statewide HIEs instead of disjointed regional efforts. In addition to incentive differences, states have a variety of funding and sustainability models. For example, some states have HIE stakeholder participants pay for the exchange through participant fees; however, a study from 2015 indicated that only 33% of operational exchanges in their dataset covered their entire operational HIE costs solely from participant fees (Adjerid et al., 2016). There are challenges associated with identifying revenue streams for HIEs because of different gains and losses for each stakeholder: high administrative and technical costs, duplicative and redundant services translates into revenue under fee-for-service healthcare reimbursement models. HIEs alleviate the burden of switching among providers and systems that results in healthcare entities losing patients. Providers may lose revenue while payers and patients accrue savings. Therefore, these concerns have led to some states treating HIEs as a "public good with support from the government." States have enacted legislation to reduce costs in legal, managerial, and coordination of services associated with pursuing HIE efforts (Adjerid et al., 2016).

LATEST TRENDS IN DATA INTEROPERABILITY

Federally, there has been movement towards advocating for extensive and efficient health data interoperability. The Office of the National Coordinator for Health IT (ONC) funds a State HIE Cooperative Agreement Program that "promotes innovative approaches to the secure exchange of health information within and across states and ensures that healthcare providers and hospitals meet national standards and meaningful use requirements" and promotes "using electronic health records in a meaningful way to qualify for the Medicare and Medicaid EHR Incentive Programs" (HealthIT. gov, n.d.). In 2010, ONC awarded $548 million through 56 rewards to assist states and territories to facilitate HIE implementation, and in 2011 they awarded an additional $1 and $2 million to the above grantees to develop additional "innovative and scalable solutions in five key areas: achieving health goals through health information exchange, improving long-term and post-acute care transitions, consumer-mediated information exchange, enabling enhanced query for patient care, and fostering distributed population-level analytics" (HealthIT.gov, n.d.). In 2018, the Department of Health and Human Services drafted the "Trusted Exchange Framework and Common Agreement" that proposed standards across all HIEs including a goal of "establishing nonproprietary, vendor-neutral data exchange platform[s] with hospitals playing a key governance role" (American Hospital Association, 2019). In 2019, the Centers for Medicare and Medicaid Services (CMS) proposed a national rule change (The Interoperability and Patient Access proposed rule) that would "break down existing barriers to important data exchanged needed to empower patients by giving them access to their health data" and would provide expanded access to health information to approximately 125 million Americans (Proposals & Services, 2019). This rule is currently no longer accepting new comments and is under review by the current administration (Centers for Medicare & Medicaid Services, 2019).

Nationally, organizations and companies are inventing new ways to connect and access data and break down barriers. In 2018, CommenWell and Carequality paved the way for more than 15,000 health-related entities to connect with each other and share data across two major EHR vendors, Epic and Cerner, new phone apps provide patients with real-time and up-to-date information, and health systems are contributing information that can assist in translating technical information across systems and data formatting for exchanging EHRs (American Hospital Association, 2019). Statewide and organizational initiatives are proving to be successful from small rural hospitals reducing readmissions (Nemaha County Hospital, Nebraska), to connecting hospitals statewide and exchanging real-time admission/discharge/transfer data to coordinate care (Tennessee Hospital Association) to closing surgical referral loops (HCA Healthcare) to reducing Hurricane Harvey's death toll by treating evacuees with up-to-date comprehensive health information to inform better provider decisions (Greater Houston Healthconnect). For more success stories, read the full report *Sharing Data, Saving Lives: The Hospital Agenda for Interoperability* (American Hospital Association, 2019).

Interoperability of Social Determinants of Health Patient Data

One of the advancements in data interoperability is the availability of digital platforms that screen patients for social determinants of health, link patients to health-entities in their communities, close referral loops, and share data across these entities. These systems support the idea of patient-centered care and empowering patients to be partners in healthcare decisions that affect them. There are many benefits of these interoperable information systems: individual health data exists in one platform, both medical/clinical data (i.e., devices, labs, billing, EHRs) and user-generated (i.e., fitness and socioeconomic data): data seamlessly moves across care settings, and data is accumulated and stored to provide a warehouse of information for population health research and innovation (American Hospital Association, 2019). Additionally, by integrating SDOH screening into a platform where clinical data exists, physicians can relieve the burden of having to extend beyond their practice and expertise and quickly refer to information collected through a team-based or community-based effort; the workflow of patient care gets redistributed to multiple entities and stakeholders (i.e., nurses, medical assistants and support staff, care coordinators, health coaches, social workers, community health workers), including the patient (O'Gurek & Henke, 2018).

As with interoperability of data in general, there are challenges associated with SDOH platforms: the social service sector has not been provided the same financial and technological support compared to the medical sector to meet the data and security standards of sharing patient information, some social sectors or community-based organizations may not have the same privacy standards (i.e., HIPAA) making patient data vulnerable, the social care workforce may be in need of more advanced data and technology training, patients may feel uncomfortable with physicians knowing social or economic details such as homelessness or hunger, SDOH platforms can help track and monitor individual social issues but should not be seen as a solution to a systemic population-level problem, digitizing information could lead to inequitable to access and unintended consequences, and smart technologies (i.e., artificial intelligence and modeling) could potentially replicate social biases that could perpetuate health disparities and inequitable outcomes (SGIM reports). To combat these challenges, the American Hospital Association has defined best practices of interoperability platforms and models: prioritize security and privacy, create efficient and usable solutions that utilize cost-effective and enhanced infrastructure, define standards that work across systems and settings, explore data connections beyond EHRs to include SDOH and personal medical devices, and share best practices among stakeholders (hospitals and health systems, consumers, clinicians and other care settings, EHR vendors and other IT companies, insurers, HIEs, medical device companies, and government) (American Hospital Association, 2019).

CONCLUSION

As the conversation around interoperability continues and expands, companies are creating digital platforms that aim to implement these best practices. The largest contributor to this field is Aunt Bertha, which includes SDOH screening tools, seamless EHR integration, free open access to the public, a database of community and clinical resources and partners, and a referral loop workflow (Aunt Bertha, n.d.). Duet Health, another large digital platform, tracks referrals, captures charges, includes rounding tools, and organizes care coordination (Duet Health, n.d.). Eccovia Solutions is another large competitor that integrates with state, county, and community HIEs, gives Medicaid providers access to real-time EHR progress notes, medical histories, and SDOH screening results, and creates a document that pulls from social and medical health assessments that is accessible to multidisciplinary care team members (Eccovia Solutions, n.d.). Along with large competitors are smaller projects in their infancy. All of these platforms aim to increase data sharing among patients, providers, and community partners while empowering patients to be the center of the care they receive.

As interoperability expands, integrated data sets are emerging to help understand and visualize population level information. The University of Missouri founded the Center for Applied Research and Engagement Systems in 1992 with the purpose of developing reports, mapping and collaboration systems that enable the public, policymakers, and nonprofit organizations to visual data and make informed decisions. The site allows a participant to map key population indicators for their specific region and build reports to identify opportunities and map outcomes for initiatives for vulnerable populations (Center for Applied Research and Engagement Systems, n.d.). AARP developed the Livability Index interactive tool to allow people to map key indicators regarding the health of their neighborhoods (AARP Public Policy Institute, 2017). The Robert Wood Johnson Foundation has funded development of additional tools and resources that can be used to inform population initiatives to create a culture of health (Robert Wood Johnson Foundation [RWJF], n.d.). As collaboration and data-sharing advances, so too do questions about overcoming structural and policy barriers to sharing health, social system, and other data such as criminal justice data, across the community. Data Across Sectors for Health (DASH) is an organization that was established to facilitate dissemination and scale of data sharing across communities and offers many tools and resources to overcome barriers to developing these networks (Data Across Sectors for Health, n.d.). The emergence of these big data set interactive tools is changing the dialogue on broad sector problems by allowing diverse constituents to have access to key data to inform initiatives and track outcomes of interest.

SUMMARY

- The impact of healthcare costs has led to rapid investment in understanding populations, visualizing data, understanding consumer needs, and designing interprofessional models of care delivery to impact cost and quality of care delivery.
- The rise of interoperability of data and the interest in collaborating across communities is fueling innovation in new structures and new ways of viewing delivery for complex populations and redesigning care to meet consumer needs.

REFLECTION QUESTIONS

1. What big data sets have you accessed as part of your role in population intervention?
2. What data sources have you analyzed in defining a problem you are trying to solve?
3. What impact will understanding about social determinants of health have on your assessment and delivery of care to vulnerable patients?
4. What is an example of a collaborative you have participated in to solve a complex problem? Who were the partners? What were facilitators and barriers to the success of the collaborative?
5. What resources exists in your community to meet the needs of complex consumers?
6. How do you assess for health literacy in your current practice? What might you change in your practice to comprehensively assess health literacy?
7. Who might you collaborate with in the future to address social determinants of health issues for your patient population?

REFERENCES

AARP Public Policy Institute. (2017). *AARP livability Iindex - Great neighborhoods for all ages.* https://livabilityindex.aarp.org

Adjerid, I., Acquisti, A., Telang, R., & Padman, R. (2016). The impact of privacy regulation and technology incentives: The case of health information exchanges. *Julia Adler-Milstein, 62*(4), 1042–1063. https://doi.org/10.1287/mnsc.2015.2194

American Hospital Association. (2019). *Sharing data, saving lives: The hospital agenda for interoperability.* https://www.aha.org/system/files/2019-01/Report01_18_19-Sharing-Data-Saving-Lives_FINAL.pdf

Aunt Bertha. (n.d.). *The Social Care Network.* https://company.auntbertha.com

Avendano, M., & Kawachi, I. (2014). Why do Americans have shorter life expectancy and worse health than do people in other high-income countries? *Annual Review of Public Health, 35*(1), 307–325. https://doi.org/10.1146/annurev-publhealth-032013-182411

Batterham, R. W., Hawkins, M., Collins, P. A., Buchbinder, R., & Osborne, R. H. (2016). Health literacy: Applying current concepts to improve health services and reduce health inequalities. *Public Health, 132,* 3–12. https://doi.org/10.1016/j.puhe.2016.01.001

Bradley, E. H., & Taylor, L. A. (2014). The American health care paradox: why spending more is getting us less. *Choice Reviews Online, 51*(09), 51–5127. https://doi.org/10.5860/choice.51-5127

Berkowitz, S., & Waters, D. B. (n.d.). *The impact of medically tailored meals: An innovative model for reducing healthcare costs and improving health.* Community Servings. https://www.servings.org/wp-content/uploads/2018/06/MTM_Community-Servings-Final_Web-Friendly.pdf

Camden Coalition. (n.d.). *Blueprint for complex care.* https://camdenhealth.org/resources/blueprint-for-complex-care

Center for Applied Research and Engagement Systems. (n.d.). *CARES Engagement Network.* https://engagementnetwork.org

Centers for Medicare & Medicaid Services. (2019). *Medicare and Medicaid Programs; Patient Protection and Affordable Care Act; Interoperability and Patient Access for Medicare Advantage Organization and Medicaid Managed Care Plans, State Medicaid Agencies, CHIP Agencies and CHIP Managed Care Entities, Iss.* https://www.federalregister.gov/documents/2019/03/04/2019-02200/medicare-and-medicaid-programs-patient-protection-and-affordable-care-act-interoperability-and

Claxton, G., Levitt, L., Rae, M., & Sawyer, B. (2018). *Increases in cost-sharing payments continue to outpace wage growth.* Peterson-Kaiser Health System Tracker. https://www.healthsystemtracker.org/brief/increases-in-cost-sharing-payments-have-far-outpaced-wage-growth

Collins, S. A., Currie, L. M., Bakken, S., Vawdrey, D. K., & Stone, P. W. (2013). Health literacy screening instruments for eHealth applications: A systematic review. *Journal of Biomedical Informatics, 45*(3), 598–607. https://doi.org/10.1016/j.jbi.2012.04.001

Data Across Sectors for Health. (n.d.). *Empowering communities through shared information.* https://dashconnect.org

Duet Health. (n.d.). *Patient engagement software.* https://www.duethealth.com

Eccovia Solutions. (n.d.). *Leading SDoH care coordination solution.* https://eccoviasolutions.com

Haun, J. N., Patel, N. R., French, D. D., Campbell, R. R., Bradham, D. D., & Lapcevic, W. A. (2015). Association between health literacy and medical care costs in an integrated healthcare system: A regional population based study. *BMC Health Services Research, 15,* Article 249. https://doi.org/10.1186/s12913-015-0887-z

HealthIT.gov. (n.d.). *Health information exchange challenge grant program.* https://www.healthit. gov/topic/grants-contracts/health-information-exchange-challenge-grant-program

Hersh, L., Salzman, B., & Snyderman, D. (2015). Health literacy in primary care practice. *Am Fam Physician, 92*(2), 118–124. https://www.aafp.org/afp

Institute of Medicine. (2004). *Health literacy: A prescription to end confusion.* The National Academies Press. https://doi.org/10.17226/10883

Kaiser Health News. (n.d.). *Paying it forward: 'Bill of the month' series, a vital toolkit for patients, wraps year 2.* https://khn.org/news/paying-it-forward-bill-of -the-month-series-a-vital-toolkit-for-patients-wraps-year-2

Krulick, A. (2019). *Medical bankruptcy statistics.* https://www.thebalance.com/ medical-bankruptcy-statistics-4154729

Kutner, M., Greenberg, E., Jin, Y., & Paulsen, C. (2003). *The health literacy of America's adults: Results from the 2003 national assessment of adult literacy.* U.S. Department of Education.

Long, P., Abrams, M., Milstein, A., Anderson, G., Lewis Apton, K., Lund Dahlberg, M., and Whicher, D. (Eds.). (2017). *Effective care for high-need patients: Opportunities for improving outcomes, value, and health.* National Academy of Medicine. https://lccn.loc.gov/ 2017041343

Mason, D. J. (2020). JAMA Forum: Food insecurity and a threatened safety net. *JAMA, 323*(5), 406–407. https://doi.org/10.1001/jama.2019.22150

McGinnis, J. M., Williams-Russo, P., & Knickman, J. R. (2002). The case for more active policy attention to health promotion. *Health Affairs, 21*(2), 78–93. https://doi.org/10.1377/ hlthaff.21.2.78

National Institute on Drug Abuse. (2019). *Overdose death rates* https://www.drugabuse.gov/ related-topics/trends-statistics/overdose-death-rates

O'Gurek, D. T., & Henke, C. (2018). A practical approach to screening for social determinants of health. *Family Practice Management, 25*, 7–11. https://www.aafp.org/fpm

Peterson-Kaiser Health System Tracker. (n.d.). *Health spending and the economy.* https://www .healthsystemtracker.org/indicator/spending/health-expenditure-gdp

Proposals, N., & Services, M. (2019). *CMS advances interoperability & patient access to health data through new proposals.* https://edit.cms.gov/newsroom/fact-sheets/ cms-advances-interoperability-patient-access-health-data-through-new-proposals

Robert Wood Johnson Foundation. (n.d.). *Health data: Resources for public health and community action.* https://www.rwjf.org/en/library/collections/better-data-for-better -health.html

Sawyer, B., & Claxton, G. (2019). *How do health expenditures vary across the population?* Peterson-KFF Health System Tracker. https://www.healthsystemtracker.org/chart -collection/health-expenditures-vary-across-population/#item-start

Sawyer, B., & Cox, C. (2018). *How does health spending in the U.S. compare to other countries?* Peterson-Kaiser Health System Tracker. https://www.healthsystemtracker.org/chart -collection/health-spending-u-s-compare-countries/#item-relative-size-wealth-u-s -spends-disproportionate-amount-health

States, U., Survey, T., & Skills, A. (2013). United States key issues. *Oecd,* (March 2012), 1–15. https://doi.org/10.1787/9789264204904-en

Taylor, L. (2018). "Housing and health: An overview of the literature." Health Affairs health policy brief. *Health Affairs.* https://doi.org/10.1377/hpb20180313.396577

Taylor, L. A., Tan, A. X., Coyle, C. E., Ndumele, C., Rogan, E., Canavan, M., Curry, L. A., & Bradley, E. H. (2016). Leveraging the social determinants of health: What works? *PLoS ONE, 11*(8), e0160217. https://doi.org/10.1371/journal.pone.0160217

Thayer, C., & Anderson, G. O. (2018). *Loneliness and social connections: A national survey of adults 45 and older*. https://doi.org/10.26419/res.00246.001

Thomas-Henkel, C., Hamblin, A., & Hendricks, T. (2015). *Supporting a culture of health for high-need, high-cost populations: Opportunities to improve models of care for people with complex needs: Literature review*. The Robert Wood Johnson Foundation and the Center for Health Care Strategies. http://www.chcs.org/media/HNHC_CHCS_Report_Final.pdf

Thompson, T. (2014). National action plan to improve health literacy. *Encyclopedia of health communication*. https://doi.org/10.4135/9781483346427.n360

U.S. Department of Health and Human Services Health Resources and Services Administration. (2018). *Health equity report 2017*. U.S. Department of Health and Human Services. https://www.hrsa.gov/sites/default/files/hrsa/health-equity/2017-HRSA-health-equity -report.pdf

Ylitalo, K. R., Meyer, M. R. U., Lanning, B. A., During, C., Laschober, R., & Griggs, J. O. (2018). Simple screening tools to identify limited health literacy in a low-income patient population. *Medicine (United States)*, *97*(10), e0110. https://doi.org/10.1097/MD.0000000000010110

CASE EXEMPLARS FOR APPLICATION

Mercy Health Saint Mary's, Grand Rapids, MI

Complex Care Center Model

Megan Williams, Lauran Hardin, Michael Sims, and Cyrus Batheja

BACKGROUND AND PROBLEM

Mercy Health Saint Mary's is a regional nonprofit teaching health center located in Grand Rapids, MI. With specializations in neurology, cancer care, kidney transplants, diabetes, and behavioral healthcare, and a location in the urban core, the health system provides care for a concentration of diverse complex populations. In 2010, the system embarked on a journey to understand the characteristics of their most complex patients and design a model of intervention to meet their needs.

Led by a clinical nurse leader, the work began with analyzing population data from the EMR and claims systems to understand the characteristics of people who had frequent access to the healthcare system, their root cause drivers, and the financial impact this was having on the health system. Prior to this investigation, the health system had analyzed data indicating the volume of services provided in different specialties such as cardiac surgery, but had not done a deep analysis of the characteristics of their most frequent customers through the lens of the patient experience. The analysis uncovered a small group of 600 patients who represented over 10% of the business of the health system with more than 7,000 annual visits. Root cause analysis revealed unexpected characteristics including 70% being less than 60 years old, with prevalence of chronic pain, substance use disorder, behavioral health and social issues driving high-frequency access (ancc.confex.com/ancc/ANCCMagnet2015/webprogram/Handout/Session1754/c932.pdf). Using data to understand and target the opportunity created support to develop a model of care focused on complex and high-frequency access patients.

METHODS AND OUTCOMES

The Complex Care Center model was created in response to the needs of the population. With a nurse-led intervention, the Center built a response system for high-frequency and complex patients accessing the health network. Core components of the model include:

- Using data to case find the most vulnerable populations and create business intelligence on the population.
- Comprehensive root cause assessment and capture of the patient story including medical, behavioral, social and system root causes of instability in the patient's plan of care.
- A cross continuum case conference including all providers intersecting with the patient to develop a shared plan of care across systems that is integrated in the electronic health record.
- Translating lessons learned from patient intervention into process improvements to impact populations and communities.
- Convening community collaborative to address broader systems problems and impact populations.

The Center staff operate as facilitators and accelerators of improved care for patients. Rather than becoming a new case manager, the Complex Care Center convenes existing care providers and enhances their collaborative understanding of patient needs. Root cause needs are addressed for the patients and services initiated to improve outcomes. The shared care plan was developed into a succinct one-page summary called a Complex Care Map integrated in the electronic health record attached to an alert. This equipped providers at the point of care across systems with targeted information to improve delivery for vulnerable populations (Hardin et al., 2017).

People with high-frequency access to the healthcare system often have a combination of medical and social complexity driving their instability. These root causes are not often solved by one system. The Complex Care Center convened process improvement groups to work on root causes for populations, such as an evidence-based pathway for treating gastroparesis across inpatient and outpatient systems. Community collaboratives were also convened to address broader systems issues such as an ED collaborative creating standardized pathways for treating chronic pain across the city or a community wide group working on care of chronic homeless alcoholics who were intersecting with multiple systems.

Using data to target populations and addressing whole person care needs including social and behavioral root cause drivers, resulted in greater than 40% reduction in emergency room visits and inpatient hospitalizations, 47% reduction in direct expenses, and a 73% improvement in operating margin for the health system. By providing the right care in a coordinated interprofessional manner, quality and cost improved for very vulnerable populations. The success of the model led to adaptation across the Trinity Health system and in other States such as the Vermont SIM initiative (Blueprint for Health, n.d.; Hardin et al., 2017).

REFERENCES

Blueprint for Health. (n.d.). *Integrated Communities Care Management*. https://blueprintforhealth. vermont.gov/about-blueprint/integrated-communities-care-management

Hardin, L., Kilian, A., Muller, L., Callison, K., & Olgren, M. (2017). Cross-continuum tool is associated with reduced utilization and cost for frequent high-need users. *Western Journal of Emergency Medicine, 18*(2), 189–200. https://doi.org/10.5811/westjem.2016.11.31916

Regional One Health, Memphis, TN

One Health Model: Data-Driven Intervention for the Uninsured

Megan Williams, Lauran Hardin,
Michael Sims, and Cyrus Batheja

BACKGROUND AND PROBLEM

Memphis, Tennessee, is a city where crime and poverty are amongst the highest in the country (Delavega, 2017; Federal Bureau of Investigation's Uniform Crime Reporting Program, 2018). Tennessee is a state that did not expand Medicaid and according to the United Stated Census Bureau, approximately 675,000 individuals are without insurance in the state of Tennessee (Berchick et al., 2019).

Access to care and other resources can be difficult to obtain for those without insurance. Regional One Health (ROH) is a level one trauma center, level one burn center, and high-risk perinatal hospital. ROH also provides services to the uninsured and serves as the safety net facility for multiple counties in a tristate area that includes Tennessee, Mississippi, and Arkansas. In a recent look at financial data, ROH provided $83 million in uncompensated care, net of all subsidies, during fiscal year 2018.

The leadership at ROH began to look for ways to improve health and decrease the cost and utilization of this group of uninsured patients. They sought out the consultative model of the Camden Coalition's National Center for Complex Health and Social Needs in Camden New Jersey. In a codesign framework, the consultants partnered with ROH to analyze data to find trends and patterns of healthcare utilization and apply understanding of the population to design models for complex populations. The model utilizes an ecosystem approach in developing programs including asset mapping community resources to serve the population, codesigning evidence-based intervention models, and building process improvements and community collaborations to address root causes influencing the population. Within each healthcare system, there is small group of patients, 5%, that contribute to over 50% of total costs

(Mitchell, 2001). Often a combination of medical and social complexity drives this population to frequent utilization of services. Many patients lack ways to seek appropriate levels of care as well as trying to seek help for social issues such as homelessness and food insecurity. ROH, created a focused program called ONE Health to identify, understand, implement strategies to address the reasons for over utilization, and create better health and social outcomes for the uninsured.

METHODS AND OUTCOMES

ROH began with analysis of the data utilizing a combination of information from the electronic health record and data from the hospital financial system. From July 2016 to June 2018, ROH's ED saw 34,499 patients, of whom 47% were uninsured. Among them, 774 patients used the ED 10 to 210 times, collectively costing $20.2 million (Vaida, 2019). Extensive patient chart reviews were completed to determine trends and patterns of access. Medical diagnoses of each visit were reviewed for trends in patterns of access. This revealed end stage renal disease, sickle cell, seizures, and diabetes. Many of these diseases are chronic conditions that are better managed in the outpatient area. Also, the chart reviewed revealed untreated behavioral health, substance use disorders, and a lack of social determinants of health being met, which included homelessness, lack of income, and food insecurity. Similar to complex patients across the country, the ROH population had a combination of medical and social complexities drives their high utilization of the healthcare system.

Regional One chose an interprofessional, nurse led model of care delivery called ONE Health that includes teams of nurses and social workers collaborating in delivery of care. Data analysis is used to identify uninsured patients with a pattern of high frequency access to the health system including 10 or more ED visits and/or two or more inpatient admissions in the prior two years who may qualify for the intervention. The team conducts a comprehensive assessment (Hardin et al., 2017) to identify root cause drivers in the medical, behavioral, social, and system realms that may be contributing to increased utilization. Patients are engaged in the emergency room, hospital, outpatient clinic, or the community and offered a person-centered intervention model with a systems approach focused on building self-sustainability and independence. The team meets patients where they are in a trauma-informed care approach and helps to build authentic healing relationships.

Upon entering the program, each patient completes an Arizona Self-Sufficiency Matrix tool (Self-SuffiencyTaskforce, 2010). The Matrix focuses on 18 social determinants of health factors and is an effective and efficient tool for documenting the progress or maintenance of client skills and abilities by providing a clear illustration of where a client has strengths, as well as where to focus additional energy to generate improvement. Based on the patient's response to the Matrix, links are made with existing resources in the community to cultivate strong, cohesive partnerships.

Case conferencing may occur with community partners, the patient, and other organizations to create a cohesive care plan that encompasses all aspects of the patient's care (Hardin, Kilian, and Spykerman, 2017). The intervention with

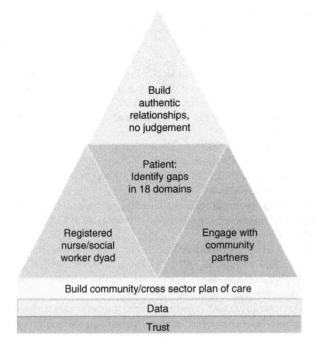

FIGURE 10.2 Quantitative and qualitative successes of both patients and community.

the patient has a focus on resolving root cause issues and linking them when stable to a permanent medical home. ONE Health has used data on patient needs from the root cause assessment and Matrix to identify process improvements and community partnerships to address broader systems issues impacting the populations. Additional resources such as an on-site food pantry, transportation services, meal delivery services, housing services, extensive mental health and substance use treatment have been built to support the needs of the population. All social determinants and improvements are examined to measure both quantitative and qualitative successes of the patients and the community as displayed in Figure 10.2.

Monthly cost and utilization data has shown a consistent decrease in utilization and cost. In 18 months, outcomes for the 300 individuals enrolled show an $8.5 million reduction in total cost of care, 71% reduction in inpatient admissions, and 61% reduction in emergency department visits. Monthly and annual reporting of outcomes data and population data has helped to continuously build momentum for investment in resources and intervention for the population.

REFERENCES

Berchick, E. R., Barnett, J. C., & Upton, R. D. (2019). *Health insurance coverage in the United States: 2018 current population reports.* U.S. Government Printing Office. https://www.census.gov/content/dam/Census/library/publications/2019/demo/p60-267.pdf

Delavega, E. (2017). *Memphis poverty fact sheet: 2017 update.* Department of Social Work in the School of Urban Affairs and Public Policy at the University of Memphis; Benjamin L. Hooks Institute for Social Change. https://www.memphis.edu/socialwork/research/2017 povertyfactsheetwebversion.pdf

Federal Bureau of Investigation's Uniform Crime Reporting Program. (2018). *Federal Crime Data 2018: 2018 Crime in the United States.* U.S. Department of Justice; Federal Bureau of Investigation; Criminal Justice Information Services Division. https://ucr.fbi.gov/crime -in-the-u.s/2018/crime-in-the-u.s.-2018/additional-data-collections/federal-crime-data/ federal-crime-data.pdf

Hardin, L., Kilian, A., Muller, L., Callison, K., & Olgren, M. (2017). Cross-continuum tool is associated with reduced utilization and cost for frequent high-need users. *Western Journal of Emergency Medicine, XVIII*(2), 189–200. https://doi.org/10.5811/westjem.2016.11.31916

Hardin, L., Kilian, A., & Spykerman, K. (2017). Competing health care systems and complex patients: An inter-professional collaboration to improve outcomes and reduce health care costs. *Journal of Interprofessional Education & Practice, 7,* 5–10. https://doi.org/10.1016/ j.xjep.2017.01.002

Mitchell, E. M. (2001). Concentration of health expenditures in the U.S. civilian noninstitutionalized population, 2014. In: *Statistical brief (medical expenditure panel survey (US)) [Internet]* (pp. 1–6). Agency for Healthcare Research and Quality (US). http://www.ncbi.nlm.nih.gov/pubmed/28422468

Self-SuffiencyTaskforce. (2010). *Self-suffiency matrix: An assessment and measurement tool.* http://www.selfsufficiencystandard.org/sites/default/files/selfsuff/docs/SelfSufficiency Matrix2010.pdf

Vaida, B. L. (2019). For the uninsured in Memphis, a stronger safety net: A new model moves high-need patients out of the emergency department and into a rich network of social supports. *Health Affairs, 38*(9), 1420–1424. https://doi.org/10.1377/hlthaff.2019.00999

Alliance Healthcare Services, Memphis, Tennessee

Pre-Arrest Diversion Model Initiative

Megan Williams, Lauran Hardin,
Michael Sims, and Cyrus Batheja

BACKGROUND AND PROBLEM

For more than 35 years, Alliance Healthcare Services (AHS) has served Shelby County's mental health residents. With a staff of more than 400 caring professionals at 18 locations, AHS is the largest provider of outpatient mental health services in the Memphis area. AHS is a nonprofit organization, offering a full range of services including outpatient, housing, and crisis intervention. AHS serves more than 22,000 individuals yearly with over 16,000 being served through Crisis Continuum and Pre-Arrest Diversion Services. AHS Crisis Continuum and Pre-Arrest Diversion Services provides crisis care for more than double the amount of individuals than of any other mental health agency in the state of Tennessee.

In 2017 Governor Haslam and the Tennessee General Assembly provided $15 million in funding for the prearrest diversion infrastructure (PADI) across the state of Tennessee. The goal of the PADI program is to reduce or eliminate the time individuals with mental illness, substance use, or co-occurring disorders spend incarcerated. This occurs by redirecting them from the criminal justice system to community-based treatment. The Pre-Arrest Diversion and Infrastructure grant was awarded to AHS by the Tennessee Department of Mental Health and Substance Abuse Services. AHS collaborated with the Memphis Fire Department, Memphis Police Department, and Shelby County Government including the Mental Health Court and Public Defenders Office. The project's goals were created and designed to divert individuals with behavioral health needs away from jail and emergency departments to appropriate community-based treatment. This will also result in alleviating jail overcrowding, reducing costs of incarceration, and developing a coordinated system between health providers, law enforcement and the judicial system (Tennessee Department of Mental Health and Substance Abuse Services, n.d.).

Data for this project was collected using information from the AHS Crisis Program, Shelby County Sheriff's Office Jail Report Card (Jail et al., 2019), Memphis Fire Department, and Memphis Police Department. The Memphis Police Department receives an average of 15,000 calls annually with approximately 2,500 of those being individuals with a serious or persistent mental illness through the Emergency Medical Services (EMS) System. Memphis Fire Department reports having 278 high-frequency individuals utilizing the Memphis Fire EMS system; with 111 having a mental health diagnosis. After numerous meeting between Alliance Healthcare Services, Memphis Fire, Memphis Police, Shelby County government officials, and mental health court, it was determined that these same individuals were over utilizing all of the systems without linkage to appropriate follow-up services.

A cross community collaborative was created to address this problem by creating the Crisis Assessment and Response to Emergencies Team (CARE Team) which is a collaboration between AHS, Memphis Fire and Memphis Police. This unique partnership is an approach that consists of a Crisis Intervention Team (CIT) police officer, paramedic, and a licensed mental health professional. Two specific programs that have been created from this collaborative are the Enhanced Follow-Up Team, and CARE Team which are patterned after the Colorado Springs Mobile Integrated Healthcare program and the Bexar County Model SAMHSA Jail Diversion Tool Kit. These teams use Motivational Interviewing, Illness Management Recovery, Cognitive Behavioral Therapy (CBT), and Cognitive Processing Therapy (CPT) for trauma, and refer to quality services not provided at the Crisis Center. The Enhanced Follow-Up Team also uses Cognitive Adaptive Training (CAT) to prevent rehospitalizations (Evans, n.d.; Bronsky, Johnson, & Giordano, 2016).

The goal of the team is to decrease nonemergency calls to the 911 communications line, decrease overuse of the local emergency departments, and educate individuals to other ways of accessing mental health services. By dispatching the CARE Team, individuals with a history of treatment for mental health are given an on-site minor medical screening, mental health assessment, and are connected to community resources based on the results of the assessment. The mental health screening used to assess the severity of the mental illness is the Columbia-Suicide Screening tool (Posner et al., 2011). This tool associates risk of the client's suicidal ideation and mental health behavior to the appropriate level of care. For example, if a client is suicidal and has a plan, the client would be referred to inpatient mental health services. Another example is if a client is depressed, has no plan for suicide, and is in the care of their family, a referral to outpatient mental health services may be an appropriate referral. This response allows the CARE team to triage calls that are nonemergencies and frees up first responders to respond to true medical emergencies in the community.

The CARE Team has responded to over 967 calls from September 24, 2018 to October 31, 2019. The median age range of the individuals is 43 with 51.7% males and 48.3% females. Of the calls made 26% (256) went to the crisis assessment center,

14% (132) went to the local hospital emergency room, and 2% (19) went to an inpatient mental health facility. Leaving 58% (560) of all calls successfully treated in the community with the CARE team. The collaboration has been essential in ensuring individuals are receiving adequate mental health services and are connected to other resources unknown to them and their family members.

Once the CARE Team makes contact with the client, they are triaged and then referred to AHS Enhanced Follow-Up Team, which was created based upon the Assertive Community Treatment (ACT) model (Scott & Dixon, 1995). The Enhanced Follow-Up Team provides intensive treatment and case management support services to individuals who have severe and persistent mental illness and have been identified to have high recidivism rates and poor compliance rates with appointment and medication follow through. The clients participate in individual & Illness Management and Recovery (IMR) group therapy, case management, medication evaluation, and other support services.

The Enhanced Follow-Up Team consists of a psychiatrist, clinical supervisor, four licensed therapists, a peer support specialist, and two case managers. The Enhanced Follow-up Team will offer these services with the individual and family to ensure a warm appropriate handoff to outpatient mental health services. These services are individually tailored for each client to address needs, goals, and preferences of the individual. Admissions to this team are made through direct referrals from inpatient psychiatric facilities, outpatient programs, and other partners in the community. Clients are referred to the Follow-Up Team by the following three criteria:

1. Excessive use (two or more visits in a 30-day period) of crisis/emergency services with failed linkages
2. Repeated (two or more in a 90-day period) arrests and incarceration for offenses related to mental illness such as trespassing, vagrancy, or other minor offenses
3. Severe homelessness that leads to overuse of ED Departments (Mobile Crisis Response)

To highlight some of the success of the Enhanced Follow-Up Team, data was reviewed using pre- and postmental health crisis hospitalization admissions for clients served since the inception of the enhanced follow-up program, April 1, 2018. The data was collected over a two-year period between April 1, 2018 and October 31, 2019, on 137 clients. The total crisis admissions Pre-PADIP were approximately 514 with an average of 7.138 admissions per consumer. The total crisis admissions Post-PADIP were approximately 153 with an average of 2.125 admissions per consumer. The total hospital admissions Pre-PADIP were approximately 177 with an average of 2.458 admissions per consumer. The total hospital admissions Post-PADIP were approximately 53 with an average of 0.736 admissions per consumer. Based on the data, the crisis and hospital admissions collectively show a significant decrease Post-PADIP intervention. There was a 70% decrease of crisis admissions and a 70% decrease of hospital admissions with the individuals serviced by the Enhanced Follow-Up Team.

REFERENCES

Bronsky, S., Johnson, R., & Giordano, K. (2016). Mobile integrated healthcare program changing how EMS responds to behavioral health crises. *Journal of Emergency Medical Services*, *41*(10). https://www.jems.com/2016/09/30/mobile-integrated-healthcare -program-changing-how-ems-responds-to-behavioral-health-crises

Evans, L. (n.d.). *Blueprint for success: The Bexar County Model: How to set up a jail diversion program in your community*. https://www.naco.org/sites/default/files/documents/Bexar -County-Model-report.pdf

Jail, D., East, J., & Services, J. D. (2019). *Shelby County Sheriff's Office | Jail Division February 2019 jail report card*. (February).

Posner, K., Brown, G. K., Stanley, B., Brent, D. A., Yershova, K. V., Oquendo, M. A., Currier, G. W., Melvin, G. A., Greenhill, L., Shen, S., & Mann, J. J. (2011). The Columbia-suicide severity rating scale: Initial validity and internal consistency findings from three multisite studies with adolescents and adults. *American Journal of Psychiatry, 168*(12), 1266–1277. https://doi.org/10.1176/appi.ajp.2011.10111704

Scott, J. E., & Dixon, L. B. (1995). Assertive community treatment and case management for schizophrenia. *Schizophrenia Bulletin, 21*(4), 657–668. https://doi.org/10.1093/ schbul/21.4.657

Tennessee Department of Mental Health and Substance Abuse Services. (n.d.). *Pre-arrest diversion infrastructure program*. https://www.tn.gov/behavioral-health/mental-health -services/adults/pre-arrest-diversion-infrastructure-program.html

Adventist Health, Clearlake, CA

Project Restoration Model: A System Wide Approach to Complex Populations

Megan Williams, Lauran Hardin,
Michael Sims, and Cyrus Batheja

BACKGROUND AND PROBLEM

Adventist Health Clear Lake is located in one of the poorest counties in Northern California, with health rankings in the lowest decile of the state. Challenged by wildfire devastation, lack of affordable housing, limited employment opportunities, and widespread addiction, the community was at capacity for addressing the complex needs of the rural population. An innovative approach to solve this crisis was taken by convening a cross-sector, interprofessional collaborative including healthcare, social services, criminal justice, emergency response services, the mayor, and other community agencies interested in improving outcomes for vulnerable populations.

METHODS AND OUTCOMES

The initiative was led by the Community Wellness Director for Adventist Health. Individual meetings occurred with community stakeholders to invite them to participate in a new approach to addressing community challenges. The project kicked off with a summit that included presentations from successful programs such as the Camden Coalition and homeless initiatives from neighboring counties. Community members participated in activities to map the existing assets for complex populations and identified the top three priorities of focus for the collaborative: housing, transportation, and access to behavioral health and addiction services.

The collaborative, named Project Restoration, began their work with these focus areas in mind and created a charter to identify shared goals and initiatives. In partnership with Camden Coalition's National Center for Complex Health and Social Needs, they analyzed data from a range of service providers including the health system, EMS system and criminal justice system, to understand the population. A business associates agreement (BAA) and memorandum of understanding (MOU) were completed by members to describe the parameters and principles of sharing data between organizations. Shared metrics were created across sectors to measure success in a way that mattered to each stakeholder (Hardin et al., 2019).

Using a data informed approach, the health, EMS and criminal justice systems identified the people in the community with the highest utilization of services. A shared intervention model was created in collaboration with multiple agencies to reach out to these community members and offer a different kind of support. They began by simply asking the person to tell their story and what mattered most to them. As trust was established, an intervention plan was created that was informed by the values of the person. In partnership, the community provided needed services such as access to benefits, addiction treatment, transportation, food, and safe housing.

The collaborative quickly learned from intervention with individuals that there were significant gaps in access to services. They developed a centralized infrastructure to translate lessons learned from intervention into process improvements for the community. Monthly case conferences were convened to develop shared care plans across agencies for vulnerable individuals. A coordinated point of contact was created for behavioral health access. The community partnered to open a 10-bed transitional housing unit called Restoration House to fill a gap in homeless services. Success of their efforts led to a $1.3 million grant from a benefactor to finance the opening of a collaborative center for the county where agencies will colocate and deliver services together.

An analysis of the first 28 patients served by Restoration House was completed and found that the collaborative approach was associated with a 44% reduction in hospital utilization, an 83% reduction in community response system usage, and a 71% reduction in costs for the population. The success of the model generated interest at a systems level in the potential for community collaboration to impact broader health outcomes. The Adventist Health system serves over 80 communities in California, Oregon, Washington, and Hawaii. The Project Restoration model will be incorporated in the Adventist community well-being strategy and financed by community benefit in multiple markets. Targeting populations with data analysis, identifying shared metrics, translating consumer needs into process improvements, and collaborating across the community created an effective way to address broad systems change and improve outcomes (Hardin et al., 2019).

REFERENCES

Hardin, L., Trumbo, S., & Wiest, D. (2019). Cross-sector collaboration for vulnerable populations reduces utilization and strengthens community partnerships. *Journal of Interprofessional Education and Practice, 18*, 100291. https://doi.org/10.1016/j.xjep.2019.100291

United Healthcare

A National Application to Data Analysis and Consumer Needs

Megan Williams, Lauran Hardin,
Michael Sims, and Cyrus Batheja

BACKGROUND AND PROBLEM

The United States spends substantially more than other industrialized countries on healthcare, but have poorer outcomes. This is particularly true for people living within the lowest socioeconomic bracket of society. People living in poverty face greater risk of adverse childhood experiences (ACEs) and trauma throughout life (Tilson, 2018).

Through a rigorous study of Medicaid patients, it became clear that social determinant challenges deeply interfere with patients' safety, health, and well-being. As a result of this population health analysis, it was determined that unsafe and unstable housing leads to poor health outcomes, drives extreme health system cost, and creates significant patient-provider disruptions. Using a hypothesis, that safe housing improves health, a team of experts worked together to develop a transitional housing model to support the highest cost, chronically homeless patients. The program provided transitional housing connected to trauma-informed wrap-around supports (Substance Abuse and Mental Health Services Administration [SAMHSA], n.d.). Patients in the program averaged a year of support, during which they stabilized medically and began healing from the traumas they had encountered. As a result, a large majority were able to gain a sense of agency and identity. This has led many to self-sufficiency, finding life purpose, reuniting with family, and gaining access to essential social supports (i.e., housing vouchers, waivers, SNAP, SSI/SSDI).

METHODS AND OUTCOMES: PROGRAM DESCRIPTION

Using a blend of medical claims data that included ICD-10 social determinant of health codes (i.e., Z59.0), along with social service data (i.e., HMIS), we identified a cohort of roughly 5,000 target patients. These patients had used the ER and/or been admitted to the hospital enough to have an annual total cost of care of at least $50,000. Also, they were all identified as experiencing homelessness, addiction, recent release from incarceration, and/or aging out of system supports like foster care. The identified cohort was spread across 30 states, in urban, suburban, and rural settings.

Based on the identified cohort, patients were physically located through a referral from a community-based organization, health plan, or medical system when they arrived for services. The cohort aligned with other studies of at risk populations (The National Child Traumatic Stress Network [NCTSN], 2019). Based on common needs the program developed support networks made up of high-quality housing and supportive services, starting with the communities identified as having the greatest amount of target patients. The network partners were able to deliver high-fidelity services. The model that removes traditional barriers to housing such as addiction, rental history, and finances. Fundamentally, the program uses a harm reduction model that targets patients with significant mental health and addiction issues. In some cases, if the partner was new to the Housing First concept, the field teams provided training and ongoing technical assistance. Partners were paid a monthly per patient per month fee, which usually included funds for both the housing and wrap-around trauma-informed services (SAMHSA, n.d.). In addition, in some states, government agencies provided collaborative support which includes vouchers for the housing units.

Using a national medical network, the program connected patients to dignified housing and trauma-informed wrap-around services while they were being discharged from the ER or inpatient, improving health system service delivery (SAMHSA, n.d.). Moreover, the program leveraged interdisciplinary teams that included community health workers, nurses, and social workers as first line supports and medical staff as secondary.

The program demonstrated a number of factors that contributed to communication, collaboration, and engagement. It recognized that poor physical or mental health leads to a breakdown in communication between patients seeking treatment and the person providing care. The team understood comfort gestures and that a patient experiencing illness or distress may grow tired of communicating issues to one healthcare professional after another or find it difficult to describe a particular issue, and this become a barrier to high-quality care (NCTSN, 2019).

The team was trained on communication strategies to determine whether one's communication style adequately conveys one's thoughts, needs, and goals. Using motivational interviewing, a therapeutic, evidence-based approach, individuals who found themselves often engaged in misunderstandings were able to explore what causes them to misinterpret the viewpoints of others or inaccurately convey their own ideas. Moreover, the program aligned with partners that provided therapy and facilitated the improvement of interpersonal and intergroup skills by helping individuals to improve the quality, nature, and frequency of their communications.

Program goals included:

- Reduce ED, inpatient hospital, SNF utilization; reducing system cost
- Improve patient health outcomes
- Support patients' sense of agency, self-purpose, and contribution
- Enhance patient and provider experiences
- Generate innovative demonstrations to influence policy for the most complex patients
- Connect homeless patients to dignified, affordable housing

Quantitatively, over a yearlong study, the model demonstrated total cost of care savings in Arizona of 10% and Nevada of 22%. Qualitatively, a survey of patients reported the following results:

- 93% rating that staff care for you like a person
- 94% rating that staff earned your trust
- 95% rating that this has helped you to live a healthier life
- 93% that this program understands your personal needs
- 94% that this program is able to help the patient with other's needs
- 95% of the time the program is easy to interact with
- 90% of the time it was easy to get care
- 92% staff gave information that was needed and/or helpful

The program used several evidence-based approaches to support patient success. The program was built using principles of trauma-informed care, adverse childhood experiences (ACES), and Housing First.

TRAUMA-INFORMED CARE

Exposure to violence and trauma can have a significant impact on functioning, interpersonal relationships, and physical and mental health. Coping strategies such as substance use and aggression may lead to criminal justice involvement. The field staff was trained to recognize historic trauma. Within the population served, incarceration further intensified problems and symptomology. The prevalence of trauma and posttraumatic stress disorder (PTSD) was higher among individuals in the program than in the general population. As such, the field staff was trained to utilize trauma-informed practices like harm reduction and positive psychology to minimize retraumatization and reduce PTSD symptoms (SAMHSA, n.d.).

ADVERSE CHILDHOOD EXPERIENCES (ACES)

Screening and supporting patients based on ACEs assessments were central in the program (Tilson, 2018). Studies, including the Texas Institute for Child and Family

Well-being, recognize that "Adverse Childhood Experiences (ACEs) include child abuse (emotional, physical and/or sexual abuse); household challenges (family violence, substance use, mental illness, divorce, and/or incarceration of a family member); and neglect (emotional and/or physical)" (Faulkner et al., 2018). ACEs cause health difficulties; the field-based teams were trained on ACEs and equipped with assessments to support (Tilson, 2018).

HOUSING FIRST

Housing First was an evidence-based model which helped our patients access housing and alignment with services including care management, counseling, medication-assisted treatment (MAT), advocacy, and social service assistance. The approach was used to achieve stability in permanent housing directly from homelessness and offer stable housing as the foundation for pursuing other health and social service goals. Implementing Housing First involved tenant screening practices that promoted the acceptance of an applicant regardless of sobriety status, completion of treatment, and participation in services. The program addressed the homelessness crisis with a response system that obtained safe, supportive, dignified housing as quickly and simply as possible.

A key driving force of the program was the commitment to community and patient-oriented collaboration while improving whole-person health. By allocating human and financial resources to address the broader social determinants of health, and through the Housing First strategy, it achieved deeper collaborations and engagements. A community partner described this as, "A game-changer in care, reflecting the only partnership of its kind on Long Island." In all, the program was also dedicated to ensuring better care at lower costs for complex populations, one individual at a time (UnitedHealth Group, n.d. a; UnitedHealth Group, n.d. b).

REFERENCES

Faulkner, M., Belseth, T., Adkins, T., & Perez, A. (2018). *Authentic Relationships Matter Most: A new model for permanency.* https://txicfw.socialwork.utexas.edu/wp-content/uploads/2018/03/TYPS-Pilot-Study-Report_3.6.18.pdf

The National Child Traumatic Stress Network. (2019). *What is child trauma? Populations at risk.* https://www.nctsn.org/what-is-child-trauma/populations-at-risk

Substance Abuse and Mental Health Services Administration. (n.d.). *TIP 57 Trauma-Informed Care in Behavioral Health Services.* http://store.samhsa.gov

Tilson, E. C. (2018). Adverse Childhood Experiences (ACEs). *North Carolina Medical Journal, 79*(3), 166–169. https://doi.org/10.18043/ncm.79.3.166

UnitedHealth Group. (n.d. a). *Jobs and company culture.* https://www.themuse.com/profiles/unitedhealthgroup

UnitedHealth Group. (n.d. b). *Working with UnitedHealthcare team.* https://www.themuse.com/profiles/unitedhealthgroup/team/unitedhealthcare

11

Data-Mining Techniques and Tools for Sustainable Outcomes

Brian Collins

OBJECTIVES

1. Define systems theory and its link to quality and data mining in healthcare.
2. Discuss the culture and components of continuous quality improvement.
3. Define data mining in relationship to continuous improvement and sustaining outcomes.
4. Explore data mining tools and techniques unique to healthcare.
5. Discuss how data mining will influence a cost effective and sustainable organization in the 21st century.

CORE COMPETENCIES

- Understand systems theory and statistical process control (SPC)
- Recognize the importance of performance measurement in continuous quality improvement
- Appreciate how knowledge of performance can identify opportunities and drive improvement in a modern healthcare system

INTRODUCTION

This chapter is an introduction to the tools, techniques, and culture necessary for interdisciplinary teams tasked with improvement initiatives. The emphasis is on data-driven, sustainable, and manageable change with measureable results in time sensitive and dynamic environments. Beginning with a brief history of systems theory and the link to quality and data mining, the chapter includes a focus on measurement, components and culture of systems theory and continuous quality improvement (CQI), data-mining tools and techniques, and how future directions of how data mining will influence a cost-effective and sustainable organization in the 21st century.

SYSTEMS THEORY: THE LINK TO CONTINUOUS QUALITY IMPROVEMENT AND DATA MINING

Walter Shewhart introduced statistical process control (SPC) to manage the quality of a manufactured product (Shewhart, 1923). Contrary to popular industrial and management philosophies of the time, Shewhart likened the output of a complex production process to that of natural phenomena. Instead of holding to rigid assumptions and management desire for flawless output of the highest quality, the end products of a system will vary for no assignable reason, simply by chance. Variations introduced by raw materials, environment, and humans are a constant system of chance causes effecting the end product. Instead of forcing the issue of flawless production or managing to goals, it is more important to understand the variation and determine an acceptable range of output. The goal is to make a prediction of future performance. For example, if a factory owner can assume that 4% of products will be defective and that is within a reasonable cost, an additional 4% can be produced to make-up for defective products. Over time and with sufficient volume, a mean (average) and standard deviation will develop and "a phenomenon will be said to be controlled when, through the use of past experience, we can predict, at least within limits, how the phenomenon may be expected to vary in the future" (Shewhart, 1923, p. 6). In a normal distribution, performance is split evenly about the mean and 99.7% of observed outcomes will fall within three (>-3 and <3) standard deviations of the mean, 95.4% fall within two (>-2 and <2), and 68.2% fall within one (>-1 and <1). The latter consists of two sigmas, consisting of one standard deviation above the mean and one standard deviation below the mean. The former (+/-3) is the namesake of six sigma, a set of quality improvement tools aptly named after the measurement foundation. From waiting times to mortality rates, these measurements are characteristics of the system (Berwick, 1996).

Outcomes will vary over time by nature. Measurement is the means to know when variance is more than desirable. Constant systems of chance causes are inevitable and unknown within a degree of variation from an average performance. Alternatively, "assignable cause" (special cause) of variation can be identified and addressed so the process can be put back in control (Shewhart, 1923).

Shewhart was an influence on two other recognized improvement pioneers. Joseph Juran worked in the same factory where SPC was introduced from 1924 to 1941 (Best & Neuhauser, 2006). W. Edward Deming interned with Shewhart in 1925 and 1926, continued to be mentored, and won the Shewhart Medal from the American Society for Quality (ASQ) in 1955. ASQ also awards the Juran Medal for executive leadership and the Deming Medal for statistical thinking and management contributions. Shewhart, Juran, and Deming are often considered the three founders of quality improvement (Best & Neuhauser, 2005). With the latter, Deming referred to the PDSA model as the Shewhart cycle as it is rooted in measurement and systems theory. Measuring variation is one of the key elements of CQI, including variance over time, compared to like systems, or to assess a test of change.

Understanding that improvement is change, but not all change is improvement, the central law of CQI is that "every system is perfectly designed to achieve the results it achieves" (Berwick, 1996, p. 619). Problems are system issues and rarely caused by lack of will, skill, or ill intent. "Even when people were at the root of defects, they (Juran and Deming) learned, the problem was generally not one of motivation or effort, but rather of poor job design, failure of leadership, or unclear purpose" (Berwick, 1989, p. 54). Instead, people involved in the process are the most valuable participants in CQI, closest to the point of care, and will likely have the best ideas for improvement through small changes introduced and observed over time.

COMPONENTS AND CULTURE OF SYSTEMS THEORY AND CONTINUOUS QUALITY IMPROVEMENT

For CQI to be successful within an organization, four dimensions have proven instrumental. Complete absence of any dimension will limit the potential of CQI, which is demanding but extremely impactful, and best enabled by four organizational dimensions: (a) strategic, (b) technical, (c) structural, and (d) cultural (Shortell et al., 1998).

The strategic dimension is having aim and knowing which processes are most important to the organization achieving its mission. It is knowledge of current performance compared to expectations in measureable terms. The technical dimension is the training, data, and information systems necessary to succeed. This includes the hardware, software, network, processing, and human resources necessary to provide analysis for improvement teams. The combination of the first two dimensions are best exemplified in performance dashboards. At least at the highest level of the organization, a dashboard ensures a clear aim through specific measures and outcomes data to relative to predicted or benchmark targets. The effectiveness of dashboards and CQI are still dependent on the remaining two dimensions and the data mining skills described later in the chapter. The structural dimension is the ability to facilitate learning and disseminate information; including teams, task forces, committees, work groups, electronic communication, and other methods. And the cultural dimension refers to the values, norms, and behavior of the organization that either inhibit or support CQI work.

All four dimensions must be present in some degree for CQI to be effective. From 0.01 to 0.1, or 1% to 10% respectively, the impact of each dimension is similar to that an equation where anything multiplied by 0 is equal to 0. Ideally, each dimension is 100% present with a factor of 1. To illustrate the impact of each dimension on CQI efforts, the following equation represents the likelihood of improvement, or positive change: $p\Delta$ = strategic x technical x structural x cultural, or, $p\Delta = 1 \times 1 \times 1 \times 1$. Any factor being equal to zero would mathematically render the equation zero as well and produce the following hypothesized results. Organizations missing the strategic dimension ($0 \times 1 \times 1 \times 1 = 0$) will not have significant results on anything really important. Absent the technical dimension ($1 \times 0 \times 1 \times 1 = 0$) will lead to frustration and false starts. Lack of the structural dimension ($1 \times 1 \times 0 \times 1 = 0$) will end with the inability to capture the learning and spread it throughout the organization. CQI without the cultural dimension ($1 \times 1 \times 1 \times 0 = 0$) will result in small, temporary effects with no lasting impact. Any dimension being in question, where there is a 50% chance of its impact on CQI, essentially flipping a coin with a factor of 0.5 would render the equation equal to 0.5 with a 50% probability of CQI being effective ($1 \times 1 \times 1 \times 0.5 = 0.5$). Most ideal, all four dimensions are fully present in an organization, represented by a factor of 1 ($1 \times 1 \times 1 \times 1 = 1$) where CQI will be 100% effective, producing lasting organization-wide impact (Shortell et al., 1998). It is difficult but rewarding work and as systems theory suggests, it is a living thing. For CQI to flourish

It must be carefully cultivated in a rich soil bed (e.g., a receptive organization), given constant attention (e.g., sustained leadership), assured of appropriate amount of light (e.g., training and support) and water (e.g., measurement and data systems), and protected from damaging pests (e.g., overly burdensome regulation and parochial views) (Shortell et al., 1998, p. 605).

CONTINUOUS QUALITY IMPROVEMENT IN HEALTHCARE

The Institute of Medicine (IOM) defines quality as the "degree to which health services for individuals and populations increase the likelihood of desired health outcomes and are consistent with current professional knowledge" (IOM, 1990, p. 4). Healthcare services provided are expected to have a net benefit and should reflect appropriate use of the most current knowledge about scientific, clinical, technical, interpersonal, manual, cognitive, organizational, and management elements of healthcare. Benefit is measureable and expected to reflect considerations of patient satisfaction, well-being, health status, and quality-of-life outcomes (IOM, 1990).

Improving and delivering patient-centered care requires improvement teams that are dedicated to evidence-based practice, quality improvement approaches and informatics (IOM, 2003). As presented in Chapter 6, the **Data Information Knowledge Wisdom (DIKW) hierarchy** provides context for the necessary for improvement approaches that include:

- Continually understand and measure quality of care in terms of structure, inputs, process, interactions, evidence, and outcomes. **Data > Information.**

- Assess current practices and compare with practices elsewhere as a means of identifying opportunities for improvement. ***Information > Knowledge.***
- Design and test interventions to change the process of care, with the objective of improving quality. ***Knowledge > Wisdom.***

Informatics skills necessary to perform the CQI functions include abilities to:

- Manage knowledge and information: employ word processing, presentation, and data analysis software
- Support decision-making: manage, search, retrieve, and make decisions using electronic data from internal databases and external online databases
- Communicate: effectively use IT such as e-mail, internet and intranet, and file transfers; and understand data security standards (Institute of Medicine [IOM], 2003)

Regardless of the improvement team or healthcare system, the skills by audience are important for continuous quality successes and performance-based measurement. Figure 11.1 illustrates this notion along a continuum from and audience of many to few.

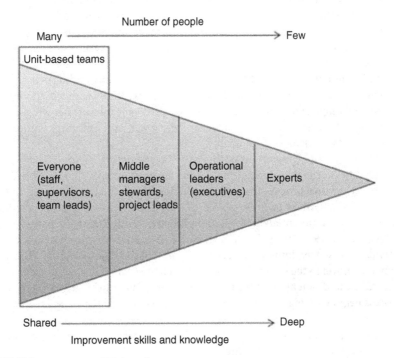

FIGURE 11.1 Improvement skills by audience.

Source: Reprinted from Schilling, L., Chase, A., Kehrli, S., Liu, A. Y., Stiefel, M., & Brentari, R. (2010). Kaiser Permanente's performance improvement system, part 1: From Benchmarking to executing on strategic priorities. *The Joint Commission Journal on Quality and Patient Safety, 36*(11), 484–498, with permission from Elsevier. Copyright © 2011 The Joint Commission.

As various audiences understand and use CQI, successes will be visually available within the system and through open access. For example, consider a cohort of 83 among the 2731 value-based purchasing (VBP) acute hospitals where CQI/Baldrige represents two healthcare systems where data are rich and available illustrating successes and potential processes. The (VBP) adjustment factors for the Mayo Clinic (Kamath et al., 2017) ranged from 0.31% to 1.79% versus the national average of 0.16 (Centers for Medicare and Medicaid Services [CMS], 2020a). Kaiser Permanente's "Big Q" or quality dashboard is another example that provides context for continuous improvement (Schilling et al., 2010) as presented in Table 11.1.

The Malcolm Baldrige National Quality Award recognizes organizations that have implemented successful quality management systems. Among the criteria are measurement, analysis, and knowledge management; including how the organization uses data to support key processes and manage performance (Baldrige, 2019).

DATA MINING FOR SUSTAINABLE OUTCOMES

Every process produces data, from electronic environments to tally sheets and manual checklists that may be facilitating a test of change. This includes outcomes data and performance indicators, such as CMS VBP factors discussed in Chapter 9 with $1.9B at stake basedon achievement, improvement, and consistency in 19 publicly reported measures in four domains. Improvement in quality depends on understanding and revising the process on the basis of data about the process itself (Berwick, 1989). When data are turned into information, applied to trend or benchmark performance to create indicators and knowledge, and presented with variance that defies a predicted range of outcomes, an engaged inquisitive team member will ask, "Why?" Questions, discussion, assessment, planning, action, and reflection will create wisdom around performance and quality.

Data mining refers to tasks that are a combination of tools and techniques intended to accelerate learning, build knowledge, and drive change. This is the last step of an iterative process that mirrors the five Vs of big data discussed in Chapter 6. "Knowledge Discovery in Databases (KDD) is the non-trivial process of identifying valid, novel, potentially useful, and ultimately understandable patterns in data" (Fayyad et al., 1996, p. 6). This nontrivial process assumes a level of autonomy and intends to discover knowledge versus report data and information. The patterns should be novel to the system with respect to changes in the data, expected or normative values, and potentially lead to useful actions. The proceeding steps in the KDD process begin with big data as discussed in Chapter 6 with the associated five Vs:

1. Develop an understanding of the goals of the organization or project and relevant prior knowledge (*Value*)
2. Select a data set or focus on a subset of variables to mine (*Variety*)
3. Clean and reprocess data, remove noise and outliers if appropriate, identify and decide how to handle missing data fields, account for time sequence information, and known changes or considerations (*Veracity*)

TABLE 11.1 Kaiser Permanente's Measures in "Big Q" Data Dashboard

DOMAIN	MEASURE	DEFINITION
Clinical Effectiveness	Hospital Standardized Mortality Ratio	Ratio of observed to expected mortality, after adjustment for selected patient-mix and community variables, among Medicare patients with diagnoses accounting for 80% of inpatient mortality
	HEDIS composite	An averaged aggregation of 33 HEDIS outpatient measures into a single measure that spans conditions and types of care.
	The Joint Commission composite	An averaged aggregation of 21 Joint Commission indicator measures into a single measure that spans conditions and populations
Safety	SRE composite	Mean number of days elapsed between SREs, charted quarterly, program-wide for Kaiser Permanente. It is comprised of 12 serious reportable event incident types.
Resource Stewardship	Total care delivery costs	Year-to-date percentage change in total costs of care delivery per member per month, program wide
Service	Health plan rating	Program-wide assessment of health plan by commercial HMO members using the CAHPS 4.0 H questionnaire. The numerator reflects overall ratings of 9 or 10 on a scale of 0–10.
	Healthcare rating	Program-wide assessment of healthcare by commercial HMO members using the CAHPS 4.0 H questionnaire.30 The numerator reflects overall ratings of 9 or 10 on a scale of 0–10.
	Hospital rating	Program-wide assessment of hospitals by patients on the HCAHPS survey.31 The numerator reflects overall ratings of 9 or 10 on a scale of 0 to 10.

CAHPS, consumer assessment of healthcare providers and systems; HCAHPS, hospital consumer assessment of healthcare providers and systems; HEDIS, healthcare effectiveness data and information set; HMO, health maintenance organization; SRE, serious reportable event.

Source: The Joint Commission Journal on Quality and Patient Safety 36(11), page 485, Table 1; Reprinted from Schilling, L., Chase, A., Kehrli, S., Liu, A. Y., Stiefel, M., & Brentari, R. (2010). Kaiser Permanente's performance improvement system, part 1: From Benchmarking to Executing on Strategic Priorities. *The Joint Commission Journal on Quality and Patient Safety, 36*(11), 484–498, with permission from Elsevier. Copyright © 2011 The Joint Commission.

4. Reduce, combine, and transform data to reduce the effective number of variables by finding useful features to represent the goal (*Volume*)
5. Data mine to accelerate the pace of making informed decisions by understanding what is relevant, valuable, and actionable and assess (*Velocity*)

Data mining is a step in the KDD process, combining tools and techniques that produce a particular enumeration of patterns and find anomalies and correlations to predict outcomes. This KDD process ends or continues with data mining to identify interesting patterns and make them understandable to humans in order to facilitate better understanding of underlying data (Fayyad et al., 1996). At the conclusion of step 5, an analyst interprets patterns and possibly returns to any of the previous steps, performs other data mining tasks, or communicates findings to other members of the team. Within that cycle and using the following tools and techniques (tasks), data mining provides a continuous stream of information to improvement teams for evaluation and knowledge building. Success will depend on how quickly insights can be discovered and used to drive better actions across the organization (SAS, 2016).

DATA-MINING TASKS

A data-mining task is a combination of tools and techniques and intended to describe or predict (Fayyad et al., 1996), including: (a) summarization, (b) classification, (c) clustering, (d) dependency modeling, (e) change and deviation.

Summarization tasks search for a compact description for a subset of data. This includes a multivariate visualization intended to uncover functional relationships between variables, such as Figure 9.1 in Chapter 9, "Medicare Value-Based Purchasing Incentive Adjustment % by Standard Deviation from the Mean, Hospital Beds, Medicare Discharges, and Case Mix Index." Charting 2731 acute care hospitals according to increasing VBP performance indicated that larger (# beds), busier (discharge volume), and higher acuity (CMI) hospitals seem to perform worse. Another technique is calculating the mean and standard deviation for all fields in a data set. This is similar to the last task described in this section and illustrates this point, data mining may be a combination of tasks in addition to each task being a combination of tool and technique. Knowledge discovery is an iterative process and involves exercises in judgment, interpretation, collaboration, and creativity. The goal is to learn something new that moves the organization towards action. Let the data take you to the next question and lesson.

Classification tasks generalize known structure to apply new data and describe, or learn functions that map items into predefined classes. Machine learning uses algorithms to automate anything that can be programmed in the KDD process. An example of automating part of the KDD process is having the ability to report outcomes by structural elements, such as department, nursing unit, medical service, and other organizational levels within overall top-level performance. That detail may not be relevant in every analysis, but addressing slight variations in overall performance may be as simple as drilling down to sub-levels representing a fraction of overall volume but having major variance that is disproportionately driving aggregate performance. Having an awareness of outcomes across structural factors builds knowledge around organizational performance and develops wisdom over time and through experience. Data mining the structure of VBP acute care hospitals reveals nine ownership structures and eight provider types for 17 overlapping structural variables and 47 mutually exclusive combinations of both structural elements as presented in Table 11.2.

The next data-mining task will help reduce the variables in this analysis for understanding as to how structure may influence VBP outcomes.

Clustering is a data-mining task where a finite set of categories are used to describe data. The categories may be mutually exclusive and exhaustive, or consist of hierarchical or overlapping categories. Instead of 17 or 47 different structural variables with sample size ranging from 1 to 1,823, the 2,731 acute care hospitals are mapped into eight categories with sample sizes ranging from 138 to 864 that combine provider type and ownership structure: Rural Referral Center (RRC), Inpatient Prospective Payment System (IPPS) Proprietary and Physician, IPPS Government, IPPS Non-Profit Private, IPPS Non-profit Church and Other, Sole Community Hospital (SCH) and RRC, SCH, and Other; which includes Medicare Dependent Hospitals (MDH), Essential Access Community Hospital (EACH), Indian Health Services (IHS), MDH/RCC, and EACH/RRC. The eight categories are color coded and displayed as a scatter plot (Figure 11.2).

Locate clusters around VBP Payment Adjustment % on the Y-axis and the number of licensed hospital beds on the X-axis. Occupancy % of beds is indicated by size of the marker. A vertical line at 100 beds and a horizontal line at 0.25% VBP Adjustment helps parse the cluster and reveal that Sole Community Hospitals (SCH) and other are most typically under 100 beds with VBP bonus adjustments in excess of 0.25%. SCH and other hospitals with VBP < 0.25% are busier with higher occupancy indicated by larger markers. Similarly, hospitals with more than 100 beds fall below 0.25%, increasingly the cases move to the right and the occupancy appears higher; perhaps larger busier hospitals are less likely to fare well in VBP, regardless of provider type and ownership structure. Maintaining the color scheme associated with the eight categories, the size reflecting occupancy %, and focusing on the upper right section of the scatter plot where hospitals have more than 100 beds and a VBP bonus in excess of 0.25%. Changing the shapes to reflect a CQI classification for 83 among the 2,731 hospitals (3%) provides more context and understanding of the larger hospitals with the highest VBP performance along the upper-right perimeter of the scatter plot. Including a hospital with almost 1,100 beds and a VBP adjustment over 1.10% which represents an estimated FY2020 VBP bonus payment in excess of $3M (Figure 11.3; CMS, 2019).

Figure 11.4 illustrates a different and final view of clustered data splits of each hospital category into the eight types and ownership-based groups alongside the CQI group, which is a combination of the former but clustered here as a group due to their system improvement attributes versus structural dimension. While analysts and teams can make their own judgment as to the validity of the charted results, the goal of data mining was to create observable patterns that are understandable to humans and provide enough information to learn something new.

TABLE 11.2. Acute Care Hospital Ownership Structure

ACUTE CARE HOSPITAL BY PROVIDER TYPE SORTED BY VOLUME OF THE FAR RIGHT↓	← ACUTE CARE HOSPITAL OWNERSHIP STRUCTURE →									TOTAL BY PROVIDER TYPE →
	GOV'T - DISTRICT OR AUTHORITY	GOV'T LOCAL	GOV'T STATE	GOV'T FEDERAL	PHYSICIAN	PROPRIETARY	VOLUNTARY NONPROFIT PRIVATE	VOLUNTARY NONPROFIT OTHER	VOLUNTARY NONPROFIT CHURCH	
IPPS	125	72	28	5	15	373	864	176	165	1823
RRC	21	18	3		2	59	190	38	42	373
SCH	30	27	3	2		34	112	29	17	254
SCH/RRC	14	15		1		25	65	18	5	143
MDH	10	11			1	24	41	14	6	107
MDH/RRC		2				3	10	2	2	19
IHS				5				4		9
EACH/RRC							3			3
Total by Ownership	200	145	34	13	18	518	1285	280	237	**2731**

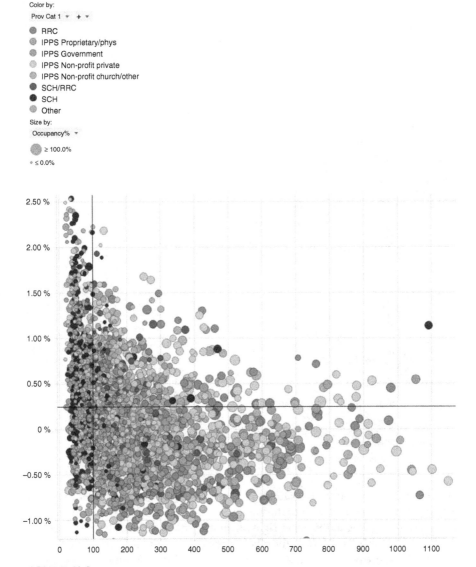

FIGURE 11.2 Scatter plot clusters.

IPPS, inpatient prospective payment system; RRC, rural referral center; SCH, sole community hospital.

Source: Data from Centers for Medicare and Medicaid Services (CMS), CMS Value-Based Purchasing, and CMS Percentage Payment Summary Report.

Dependency Modeling is tasks for finding a model that describes significant dependencies between variables. Similar to summarization, but two levels of analysis model evolve the information into evidence. The structural level specifies which variables are dependent on each other and the quantitative level gauges the strength of the dependencies using a numerical scale, such as a p value. Looking at the previous

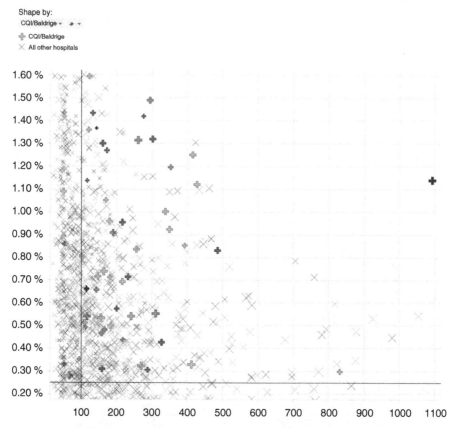

FIGURE 11.3 Continuous quality improvement/Baldrige cohort (n = 83) among all other value-based purchasing hospitals (n = 2648).

CQI, continuous quality improvement.

example, there are clear visual patterns of a relationship between provider type ownership, hospital size, and VBP performance. Also, CQI (n = 83) is only cohort with more hospitals falling in the upper right quadrant, with more than 100 beds and better than a 0.25% VBP bonus and the mix of structures within that cohort further suggests CQI is more of an influence. Dependency modeling techniques are essential in the discovery of evidence based medicine for example, they are not the focus of CQI. System improvements do not require perfect inference, randomization, and power calculations, just enough information for an organization to take the next step in learning. "In measurement for improvement the best is often the enemy of the good" (Berwick, 1996, p. 621)

Change and Deviation tasks focus on discovering significant changes in the data from previously measured or normative values. An example of this task may be seen in the control charts from Chapter 3 measuring the mean and standard deviation over 25+ time periods to search for significant patterns that indicate a system

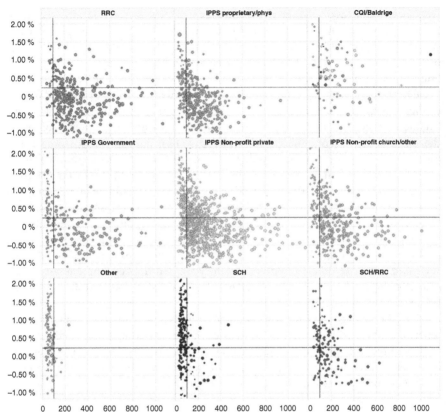

FIGURE 11.4 Clustered data splits of hospital categories.

CQI, continuous quality improvement.

change. If the most recent time period is exactly the average of the past 24 time periods reported, the standard deviation from the mean, or z-score will be 0.000; indicating there is no variance to predicted outcomes based on past performance. The other example is discovering variance from normative performance to identify opportunity, as with Kaiser's "Big Q" dashboard and SPC in general, combines with the summarization task to report the mean and standard deviation for the eight structural-based groups. Using those values, the z-score is also created to create a uniform measure of variance that has been normalized across all measures. In this instance, a z-score of 0.000 indicates that system performance in that measure is the same as the average or mean hospital performance; there is no variance and therefore no opportunity for improvement.

DATA MINING FOR A COST EFFECTIVE AND SUSTAINABLE ORGANIZATION IN THE 21ST CENTURY

Approaches and tasks such as those presented in this chapter are essential in an increasingly competitive healthcare market. Whether or not variance in performance suggests an opportunity depends on the potential for an intervention to produce better outcomes. Turning data into information and knowledge to create a shared understanding of performance, brainstorm ideas, and test change are critical. The likelihood of an intervention being successful is combined with the projected impact of the intervention to find the most interesting opportunities in calculable terms (Matheus & McNeill, 1996). For example, the business case in Chapter 9 compared the impact of moving one standard deviation in VBP, occupancy, ALOS, and CMI to each other; but the VBP impact was divided by 4 (x0.25 or 25%) while the other three scenarios were divided by 16 (x0.0625 or 6.25%). In terms of the four dimensions of CQI discussed earlier in this chapter, the former example would be questioning two dimensions, where structural and cultural factors are each 50% and the probability of success, $p\Delta = 1 \times 1 \times 0.5 \times 0.5 = 0.25$, or 25%. And the latter example would be questions of all four dimensions, including strategic and technical are 50% and the probability of success, $p\Delta = 0.5 \times 0.5 \times 0.5 \times 0.5 = 0.0625$, or 6.25%. Using dimensions and factors or others multiplied by the projected impact, "the interestingness of a deviation is related to the estimated benefit achievable through available actions" (Matheus & McNeill, 1996, p. 498).

Healthcare organizations will continue to be required to collect, analyze, and report data. This will require that systems be in place to compile accurate data collection, mining, analysis, and dissemination for sustainability. Data transformed into information, presented in such a way to build knowledge, and used to gain wisdom of current performance will drive improvement into the future.

SUMMARY

- A production process can be complex and outcomes may vary by chance, which is more similar to a natural phenomenon versus straight probability, such as flipping a coin.
- Outcomes will vary over time by nature and measurement as the means to know when variance is more than desirable; statistical process control (SPC) provide a best estimate and observed range of future performance, with predictable variance.
- Average performance and the degree of variation about the average over time are characteristics of the system. And every system is perfectly designed to achieve the results it achieves.
- CQI centers on understanding and revising of processes based on data about the processes themselves.
- CQI and measurement for improvement needs the cultural, strategic, technical, and structure to be successful, otherwise, the results are unlikely to be sustained.

- Awareness of current performance, over time and compared to peers, develops knowledge of the system and the wisdom to ask, "Why?"
- KDD is the nontrivial process of identifying valid, novel, potentially useful, and ultimately understandable patterns in data.
- Data-mining tasks are a combination of tools and techniques and intended to describe or predict, including: a) summarization, b) classification, c) clustering, d) dependency modeling, and e) change and deviation.
- Dashboards created with SPC and systems thinking allow for measures to be aggregated into composites and variance within one measure to be compared to variance of all other measures, identifying which is the most significant and presenting the biggest opportunity.

REFLECTION QUESTIONS

1. Thinking of systems and performance as characteristics, how would you describe the place you work now or recently worked in terms of process and outcomes, not physical characteristics?
2. Using the data presented in this chapter, what ways will you improve efficiency and use of data for continuous improvement?

REFERENCES

Baldrige, M (2019). *Performance excellence program 2019–2020. Baldrige excellence framework: Proven leadership and management practices for high performance (health care).* U.S. Department of Commerce, National Institute of Standards and Technology. https://www.nist.gov/baldrige

Berwick, D. M. (1989). Sounding board, continuous improvement as an ideal in health care. *The New England Journal of Medicine, 320*(1), 53–56. https://doi.org/10.1056/NEJM198901053200110

Berwick, D. M. (1996). A primer on leading the improvement of systems. *British Medical Journal, 312,* 619–622. https://doi.org/10.1136/bmj.312.7031.619

Best, M., & Neuhauser, D. (2005). W. Edwards Deming: Father of quality management, patient and composer. *Quality and Safety in Health Care 2005, 14,* 310-312. https://doi.org/10.1136/qshc.2005.015289

Best, M., & Neuhauser, D. (2006). Walter A. Shewhart, 1924, and the Hawthorne factory. *Quality and Safety in Health Care 2006, 15,* 142–143. https://doi.org/10.1136/qshc.2006.018093

Centers for Medicare and Medicaid Services. (2019). *How to read your fiscal year (FY) 2020 hospital value-based purchasing (VBP) program percentage payment summary report (PPSR).* Inpatient Value, Incentives, and Quality Reporting (VIQR) Outreach and Education Support Contractor (SC). https://www.qualityreportingcenter.com/globalassets/iqr_resources/july-2019/fy2020-ppsr-release-help-guide-gs-ec_07252019_vfinal508.pdf

Centers for Medicare and Medicaid Services. (2020a). *FY 2020 final rule and correction notice data files.* https://www.cms.gov/Medicare/Medicare-Fee-for-Service-Payment/AcuteInpatientPPS/FY2020-IPPS-Final-Rule-Home-Page-Items/FY2020-IPPS-Final-Rule-Data-Files

Centers for Medicare and Medicaid Services. (2020b). *FY 2020 final rule and correction notice tables, hospital value-based purchasing (VBP) program. Table 16B.* https://www.cms.gov/Medicare/Medicare-Fee-for-Service-Payment/AcuteInpatientPPS/FY2020-IPPS-Final-Rule-Home-Page-Items/FY2020-IPPS-Final-Rule-Tables

Fayyad, U. M., Piatetsky-Shapiro, G., & Smyth, P. (1996). *From data mining to knowledge discover. Advances in knowledge discovery and data mining.* AAAI Press /The MIT Press.

Institute of Medicine Committee to Design a Strategy for Quality Review and Assurance in Medicare, Lohr, K. N. (Eds.). (1990). *Medicare: A strategy for quality assurance.* National Academies Press. https://pubmed.ncbi.nlm.nih.gov/25144047/

Institute of Medicine. (2003). *Health professions education: A bridge to quality.* Committee on the Health Professions Education Summit, Board on Health Care Services, Institute of Medicine. National Academy Press. http://www.nap.edu/catalog/10681.html

Kamath, J. R., Peavler, O. P., Steffens, F. L., Dankbar, G. C., & Donahoe-Anshus, A. L. (2017). Seventy years of management engineering and consulting: Integrating health care delivery for an enduring mission. *Mayo Clinic Proceedings, 92*(10), 139–145. https://doi.org/10.1016/j.mayocp.2017.08.001

Matheus, C. J., & McNeill, D. (1996). *Selecting and reporting what is interesting. Advances in knowledge discovery and data mining.* AAAI Press /MIT Press.

SAS. (2016). *Data Mining from A to Z: How to Discover Insights and Drive Better Opportunities.* SAS Institute Inc. https://www.sas.com/content/dam/SAS/en_us/doc/whitepaper1/data-mining-from-a-z-104937.pdf

Schilling, L., Chase A., Kehrli, S., Liu, A.Y., Stiefel, M., & Brentari, R. (2010). Kaiser Permanente's performance improvement system, Part 1: From benchmarking to executing on strategic priorities. *The Joint Commission Journal on Quality and Patient Safety, 36*(11), 484–498. https://doi.org/10.1016/S1553-7250(10)36072-7

Shewhart, W. A. (1923). *Economic control of quality of manufactured product.* D. Van Nostrand Company, Inc.

Shortell, S. M., Bennett, C. L., & Byck, G. R. (1998). Assessing the impact of continuous quality improvement on clinical practice: What it will take to accelerate progress. *The Millbank Quarterly, 76*(4) 593–624. https://doi.org/10.1111/1468-0009.00107

CASE EXEMPLARS FOR APPLICATION

Re-Discovering Success Through Data Mining

Christina Wolf

As a new clinical nurse leader (CNL) in a hospital that had an established CNL program, I wanted leverage opportunities that had been identified from past projects. While there were different quality improvement activities underway, no work was centered on interdisciplinary bedside rounds as the vehicle to improve communication. Based on historic HCAHPS patient satisfaction survey results, there was an opportunity to improve physician/nurse communication.

HCAHPS surveys are sent to patients after discharge to measure perceptions of the hospital experience. The survey contains 19 core questions that center on communication with doctors and nurses, responsiveness of hospital staff, cleanliness and quietness of the hospital, discharge information, understanding medications, and whether they would recommend the hospital (Centers for Medicare and Medicaid Services [CMS], 2020).

Working with an interprofessional team comprised of nurses, decision support analysts, and information services, it was decided that a data visualization tool that integrated Hospital Consumer Assessment of Healthcare Providers and Systems (HCAHPS) data and displayed the "top-box" or percent of "Always" responses would enhance interdisciplinary bedside report. The two HCAHPS questions most relevant to this work were:

1. "How often did nurses explain things in a way you could understand?"
   And
2. "How often did doctors explain things in a way you could understand?"

In creating the data visualization tool, the improvement team first needed to learn how to navigate HCAHPS data, registration information data, and nursing unit admission data. Initially the team looked at six months of data and had facilitated discussions

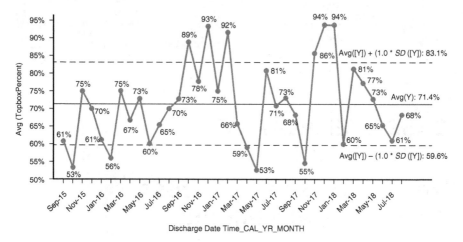

FIGURE 11.5 Hospital consumer assessment of healthcare providers and systems top box % by month.

by a CNL and physician. This process generated unit specific questions that were specific and meaningful because they were based on previous documentation practices during interdisciplinary rounds. Instead of looking at HCAHPS data reported and presented in Hospital Compare, the team could look at hospital specific information like admission or discharge date to better align the interventions documented. A report was generated to display a three-year top-box percent average a baseline of 71.4% related to two communication questions. The focus of the interdisciplinary team communications jumped-off the screen as we recognized the need for specific improvements. The six-month period data starting the first month was 73%, the lowest average percentage of satisfaction with communication. The highest month was 93% with an average during the six-month period of 83%. (Figure 11.5). When the interdisciplinary team members saw the data and improvements, the rationale for interdisciplinary patient bedside rounds spoke for itself and trying to establish "buy-in" was no longer a focus.

REFLECTION QUESTIONS

1. Consider an area for improvement in your workplace that staff do not readily embrace. What data would you need to generate a visual depiction that makes the case for improvement?
2. What are the advantages and disadvantages of using retrospective data in improvement?
3. What data is already collected and used for reporting that might have a different use?

REFERENCE

Centers for Medicare and Medicaid Services. (2020). *HCAHPS: Patients' perspectives of care survey*. https://www.cms.gov/Medicare/Quality-Initiatives-Patient-Assessment -Instruments/HospitalQualityInits/HospitalHCAHPS

Increasing Bed Capacity To Meet Demand

Peter Sylvester and Mark Morreo

Members of Infectious Disease and Information Systems (IS) teamed up to create a process to improve bed capacity and save time. Nurses from the Infectious Disease (ID) department were spending between two to four hours reviewing 120 adult inpatient medical records on five medical-surgical units to identify whether or not patients with similar infection precautions could be cohorted in semi-private rooms. Patients who were hospitalized with diagnoses that included clostridium difficile (C. Diff) or Methicillin-resistant Staphylococcus aureus (MRSA) infections and others, were often placed in a semi-private rooms. This resulted in a bed that was taken off-line and not occupied thereby decreasing overall bed capacity for the hospital. Quite often, the opportunity to identify patients who could be transferred into a cohort room was missed because patients were within a day of discharge. At this point, moving a patient was deemed disruptive and not worthwhile.

To save time in identifying potential patients to cohort, a collaborative team comprised of team members from Infectious Disease (ID), Information Systems (IS) and Decision Support (DS) came together to review process flow and develop an on-demand report. The report would include all patients in the hospital that had an order for precaution alerts. The design meeting took less than one hour and screens and fields from the Electronic Medical Record (EMR) were identified with pictures, or "screenshots" from the ID nurses that made compiling the report very straight forward because the request was very specific.

The report elements were sorted by precaution alert, gender, age, and location and instantly drew attention to opportunities for cohorting patients resulting in the ability to have semi-private rooms occupied by two patients thereby increasing hospital bed capacity. While clinical judgement and decision-making is still required, the ID nurses were not spending time identifying where the possibilities existed.

The online and on-demand report had an immediate impact of aggregating like patients throughout by alert type and location. This generated a net increase of three beds per unit on the five busiest nursing units going from less than 118 beds to over 121 beds representing a 2.5% increase in capacity (Figure 11.6). More importantly,

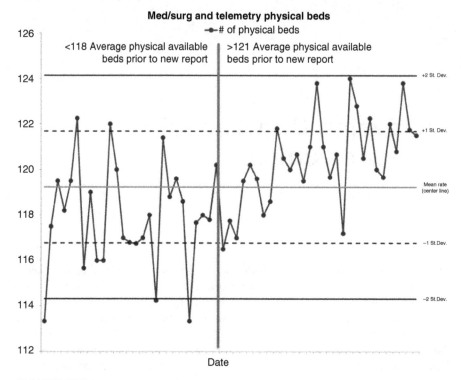

FIGURE 11.6 Medical-surgical and telemetry physical beds.

the range of available beds was much more predictable, with a range of nine beds (113–122) to five (119–124), representing a higher ceiling and higher floor or narrower central tendency.

REFLECTION QUESTIONS

1. Identify areas in your practice where the manual and visual review of data occurs. How much time is spent by members of your team doing this review on a daily, weekly or monthly basis? Calculate the expense.
2. How would you convince your colleagues who invest in this manual review that automating the process is beneficial? Would you stress the accuracy, time, or consistency as you make the case that their time and knowledge would be better served in other activities?

12

Techniques to Extract Evidence That Guide Quality and Safety

Clista Clanton

OBJECTIVES

1. Discuss how to use information systems and technology.
2. Explore appraisal tools for evaluating evidence and reference management software for collection and organization of information sources.
3. Describe how evidence guides outcomes that contribute to systems efficiency and creation of large data sets that inform change.

CORE COMPETENCIES

- Knowledge and use of information systems, technology, and reference management software
- Understand how appraisal tools and evidence guides outcomes and informs change, efficiency, and evidence generation

INTRODUCTION

Interprofessional teams are tasked with information and outcomes management as part of their daily practice. This chapter focuses on an overview of the use of information systems and technology, appraisal tools for evaluating evidence, reference management software for collection and organization of information sources, and how evidence guides outcomes that contribute to systems efficiency and creation of large data sets that inform change and evidence generation.

EVIDENCE-BASED PRACTICE

Evidence-based practice (EBP) is widely recognized as being necessary to improve the quality of healthcare and patient outcomes. As EBP has evolved and matured from the seminal evidence-based medicine (EBM) definition of the 1990's, the core elements of combining the best available research evidence with clinical expertise and patients' values and preferences to influence healthcare continue as defining features (Sackett et al., 1996; Straus et al., 2018).

Health science curricula introduce students to the concepts and various models of EBP in order to prepare them for the implementation of the best evidence in their future practice settings. For those who have been in practice for years and may not have received formal training on EBP or need a refresher, continuing education opportunities through professional associations as well as projects and activities at the organizational level may help to fill those gaps in knowledge (Andrew & Theiss, 2015; Copeland et al., 2020; Laibhen-Parkes et al., 2015). The current state of EBP competencies among healthcare professionals around the world continues to warrant concern, however, as there is still confusion among significant numbers of healthcare professionals about the commonly accepted definitions of EBP as well as the meanings of basic EBP concepts. While self-reported attitudes toward and beliefs in the importance and value of EBP are generally positive across health disciplines, these attitudes and beliefs are not necessarily translating into practice on a regular basis or in a way that positively impacts patient outcomes (Saunders et al., 2019). Inconsistencies in the content of EBP teaching and learning programs has recently led to the development of minimum core competencies in EBP for health professionals (Albarqouni et al., 2018), which help to ensure benchmark standards for EBP teaching and learning programs. Starting with an introductory section, the EBP core competencies are grouped by the five domains of Ask, Acquire, Appraise and Interpret, Apply, and Evaluate (Table 12.1).

BARRIERS TO INTEGRATION OF EVIDENCE INTO PRACTICE

As healthcare practitioners grapple with increasing their EBP knowledge and skills, and lack of time, knowledge, and access to resources continue to be significant barriers to the integration of research evidence into practice (Sadeghi-Bazargani et al., 2014; Williams et al., 2015), the importance of becoming skilled managers of information is increasingly apparent (Slawson & Shaughnessy, 2005). These barriers have influenced the design of databases used to access the research literature and have led to models, decision support systems, point-of-care databases, and other tools to help

TABLE 12.1 Evidence-Based Practice Core Competencies Grouped by Main Evidence-Based Practice Domains

EBP CORE COMPETENCIES		RATING
1.	**Introductory**	
0.1	EBP defined as the integration of the best research evidence with clinical expertise and patient's unique values and circumstances	E
0.2	Recognize the rationale for EBP	M
	This competency includes the need to recognize:	
	The daily clinical need for valid information to inform decision-making, and the inadequacy of traditional sources for this information	M
	The disparity between diagnostic skills and clinical judgment, which increase with experience, and up-to-date knowledge and clinical performance, which decline with age and experience	M
	Lack of time to find and assimilate evidence as a clinician	M
	The gaps between evidence and practice can lead to suboptimal practice and quality of care	M
	The potential discordance between a pathophysiological and empirical approach to thinking about whether something is effective	M
0.3	For each type of clinical question, identify the preferred order of study designs, including the pros and cons of the major study designs	E
	This competency includes:	
	Classify the major study designs for each type of clinical question	E
0.4	Practice the five steps of EBP: ask, acquire, appraise and interpret, apply, and evaluate	P
0.5	Understand the distinction between using research to inform clinical-decision making vs. conducting research	M
1.	**Ask**	
1.1	Explain the difference between the types of questions that cannot typically be answered by research (background questions) and those that can (foreground questions)	E

(continued)

TABLE 12.1 Evidence-Based Practice Core Competencies Grouped by Main Evidence-Based Practice Domains (continued)

EBP CORE COMPETENCIES		RATING
1.2	Identify different types of clinical questions, such as questions about treatment, diagnosis, prognosis, and etiology	P
1.3	Convert clinical questions into structured, answerable clinical questions using PICO	P
	This competency includes:	
	Recognize the importance of and strategies for identifying and prioritizing uncertainties or knowledge gaps in practice	M
	Understand the rationale for using structured clinical questions	E
	Identify the elements of PICO questions and use variations of it when appropriate (e.g., PICOT, PO, PECO-Exposure) to structure answerable clinical questions	P
2.	**Acquire**	
2.1	Outline the different major categories of sources of research information, including biomedical research databases or databases of filtered or preappraised evidence or resources	E
	The competency includes:	
	Outline the advantages of using filtered or preappraised evidence sources and recognize relevant resources	E
	Indicate the differences between the hierarchy of evidence, level of processing of evidence, and types of evidence-based medicine resources	E
2.2	Construct and carry out an appropriate search strategy for clinical questions	P
	This competency includes:	
	Know where to look first to address a clinical question	P
	When necessary, construct a search strategy that reflects the purpose of the search	P
	Apply a general search strategy including the use of search terms, and the role of Boolean operators; truncation; and search filters for more efficient searches	E

(continued)

TABLE 12.1 Evidence-Based Practice Core Competencies Grouped by Main Evidence-Based Practice Domains (continued)	
EBP CORE COMPETENCIES	**RATING**
2.3 State the differences in broad topics covered by the major research databases	M
2.4 Outline strategies to obtain the full text of articles and other evidence resources	E
3. **Appraise and Interpret**	
3.1 Identify key competencies relevant to the critical evaluation of the integrity, reliability, and applicability of health-related research	E
This competency includes:	
Understand the difference between random error and systematic error (bias)	E
Identify the major categories of bias and the impact of these biases on the results	E
Interpret commonly used measures of uncertainty, in particular, confidence intervals	P
Recognize that association does not imply causation and explain why	E
Recognize the importance of considering conflict of interest and funding sources	M
Recognize the uses and limitations of subgroup analysis and how to interpret its results	M
3.2 Interpret different types of measures of association and effect, including key graphical presentations	P
This competency includes:	
Identify the basic types of data such as categorical and continuous	E
Recognize the meaning of some basic frequency measures	M
Identify the difference between "statistical significance" and "importance," and between a lack of evidence of an effect and "evidence of no effect"	E

(continued)

TABLE 12.1 Evidence-Based Practice Core Competencies Grouped by Main Evidence-Based Practice Domains (continued)

EBP CORE COMPETENCIES		RATING
3.3	Critically appraise and interpret a systematic review	P
	This competency includes:	
	Recognize the difference between systematic reviews, meta-analyses, and nonsystematic reviews	M
	Identify and critically appraise key elements of a systematic review	P
	Interpret presentations of the pooling of studies such as a forest plot and summary of findings table	P
3.4	Critically appraise and interpret a treatment study	P
	This competency includes:	
	Identify and appraise key features of a controlled trial	P
	Interpret the results, including measures of effect	P
	Identify the limitations of observational studies as treatment studies, and recognize the basics of adjustment methods and their limitations	E
3.5	Critically appraise and interpret a diagnostic accuracy study	P
	This competency includes:	
	Identify and appraise key features of a diagnostic accuracy study	P
	Interpret the results, including interpret measures to evaluate diagnostic accuracy	P
	Recognize the purpose and use of clinical prediction rules	M
3.6	Distinguish evidence-based from opinion-based clinical practice guidelines	P
3.7	Identify the key features of, and be able to interpret, a prognostic study	E
	This competency includes:	
	Identify and appraise key features of a prognostic study	E
	Interpret the results including measures of effect (e.g., Kaplan-Meier survival curves) and uncertainty	E

(continued)

TABLE 12.1 Evidence-Based Practice Core Competencies Grouped by Main Evidence-Based Practice Domains (continued)

EBP CORE COMPETENCIES		RATING
Recognize the purpose and use of clinical prediction rules		M
3.8	Explain the use of harm and etiologies study for (rare) adverse effects of interventions	E
	This competency includes:	
	Indicate that common treatment harms can usually be observed in controlled trials, but some rare or late harms will only be seen in observational studies	E
3.9	Explain the purpose and processes of a qualitative study	E
	The competency includes:	
	Recognize how qualitative research can inform the decision-making process	M
4.	**Apply**	
4.1	Engage patients in the decision making process, using shared decisionmaking, including explaining the evidence and integrating their preferences	P
	This competency includes:	
	Recognize the nature of the patient's dilemma, hopes, expectations, fears, and values and preferences	M
	Understand and practice shared decision-making	P
	Recognize how decision support tools such as patient decision aids can assist in shared decision-making	M
4.2	Outline different strategies to manage uncertainty in clinical decision-making in practice	E
	This competency includes:	
	Recognize professional, ethical, and legal components and dimensions of clinical decision-making, and the role of clinical reasoning	M
4.3	Explain the importance of the baseline risk of individual patients when estimating individual expected benefit	E
	This competency includes:	

(continued)

TABLE 12.1 Evidence-Based Practice Core Competencies Grouped by Main Evidence-Based Practice Domains (continued)

EBP CORE COMPETENCIES		RATING
	Recognize different types of outcome measures (surrogate vs. composite endpoints measures)	M
4.4	Interpret the grading of the certainty in evidence and the strength of recommendations in healthcare	E
5.	**Evaluate**	
5.1	Recognize potential individual-level barriers to knowledge translation and strategies to overcome these	M
	This competency includes:	
	Recognize the process of reflective clinical practice	M
5.2	Recognize the role of personal clinical audit in facilitating EBP	M

E, explained; EBP, evidence-based practice; M, mentioned; P, practiced with exercises; PECO, population, exposure, comparison, outcome; PICO, patient, intervention, comparison, outcome; PICOT, population, intervention, comparison, outcome, time; P, population, outcome.

Source: Adapted from Albarqouni, L., Hoffmann, T., Straus, S., Olsen, N. R., Young, T., Ilic, D., Shaneyfelt, T., Haynes, R. B., Guyatt, G., & Glasziou, P. (2018). Core competencies in evidence-based practice for health professionals: Consensus statement based on a systematic review and Delphi survey. *JAMA Network Open, 1*(2), e180281. https://doi.org/10.1001/jamanetworkopen.2018.0281. Copyright 2018 by the JAMA Network Open.

streamline the process of finding relevant information quickly and effectively. They are also resulting in calls for a shift from the more traditional approach where clinicians are expected to be fully competent in all of the five EBP domains and focus instead on providing clinicians with the skills to critically interpret synthesized or preappraised evidence, such as systematic reviews and clinical practice guidelines (Djulbegovic & Guyatt, 2017; Guyatt et al., 2000).

CLASSIFICATION OF INFORMATION RESOURCES

The 6S hierarchy of preappraised evidence is one way of classifying and approaching the various information resources available (Dicenso et al., 2009; Table 12.2). This model is a six-level pyramid of information resource categories that prompts users to better understand what types of information are available in the different categories and which resources are best for different information needs. The bottom level of the pyramid contains original studies from the journal literature, which are indexed in databases such as PubMed, CINAHL, Scopus, and PsycINFO. Google Scholar also falls into this category, as journal articles will be retrieved while excluding less scholarly forms of information. The next level starts the preappraised evidence and

TABLE 12.2	6S Hierarchy of Information Resources	
HAYNES' PYRAMID LEVELS	**FREE RESOURCES**	**SUBSCRIPTION RESOURCES**
Systems	None	Institutional electronic health records with decision support link out to evidence-based resources
Summaries	ECRI Institutes Guidelines Trust guidelines.ecri.org/ Trip Database www.tripdatabase.com/	ACP PIER www.acponline.org/clinical-information BMJ Best Practice bestpractice.bmj.com/ Clinical Key www.clinicalkey.com Clinical Key for Nursing www.clinicalkey.com/nursing Dynamed www.dynamed.com/home/ Joanna Briggs Institute know.lww.com/JBI-resources.html UptoDate www.uptodate.com/home
Synopses of syntheses	Epistemonikos www.epistemonikos.org	ACP Journal Club acpjc.acponline.org/ BMJ Evidence-Based Nursing ebn.bmj.com/ BMJ Evidence-Based Mental Health ebmh.bmj.com BMJ Evidence-Based Medicine ebm.bmj.com
Syntheses	AHRQ EPC Evidence-Based Reports www.ahrq.gov/research/findings/evidence-based-reports/index.html Epistemonikos www.epistemonikos.org Nursing +plus. mcmaster.ca/NP/ PubMed Clinical Queries for Systematic Reviews www.ncbi.nlm.nih.gov/pubmed/clinical TRIP Database www.tripdatabase.com/	Cochrane Library: Cochrane Reviews cochranelibrary.com/ Joanna Briggs Institute know.lww.com/JBI-resources.html

(continued)

TABLE 12.2 6S Hierarchy of Information Resources (continued)		
HAYNES' PYRAMID LEVELS	**FREE RESOURCES**	**SUBSCRIPTION RESOURCES**

Synopses of Single Studies	Evidence Updates
	  plus.mcmaster.ca/
	  evidenceupdates/
	PubMed Clinical Queries
	  www.ncbi.nlm.nih.gov/
	  pubmed/clinical
	TRIP Database
	  www.tripdatabase.com/
		ACP Journal Club
		  annals.org/aim/journal-club
		Evidence-Based Nursing
		  ebn.bmj.com/
		Evidence-Based Mental Health
		  ebmh.bmj.com
		Evidence-Based Medicine
		  ebm.bmj.com

Studies	PubMed
	  pubmed.ncbi.nlm.nih.
	  gov/
	TRIP Database
	  www.tripdatabase.com/
	Google Scholar
	  scholar.google.com/
		CINAHL Plus Full Text
		  www.ebsco.com/products/
		  research-databases/cinahl-plus-
		  full-text
		PsycINFO
		  www.apa.org/pubs/databases/
		  psycinfo/
		Scopus
		  www.scopus.com

contains synopses of studies, which provide a brief summary of a high-quality study that can inform clinical practice and that contains value-added commentaries that address the clinical applicability of study findings. These can be found in evidence-based journals such as *ACP Journal Club, Evidence-Based Medicine, Evidence-Based Mental Health*, and *Evidence-Based Nursing*. The third lowest level is syntheses, which contains systematic reviews such as those found in the Cochrane Library, the Joanna Briggs Institute EBP Database, or Epistemonikos.org. PubMed, CINAHL, and Scopus also contain systematic reviews that are published in the various journals indexed in these databases. After syntheses comes the synopses of syntheses level, which summarizes the findings of a high-quality systematic review to provide sufficient information to support clinical action. The advantage of this level is that it provides a convenient summary of the corresponding systematic review and is accompanied by a commentary that addresses the methodological quality of the systematic review and the clinical applicability of its findings. These syntheses can be found in journals such as the *ACP Journal Club, Evidence-Based Medicine, Evidence-Based Mental Health,* and *Evidence-Based Nursing*.

Next is the summaries level, which integrates the best available evidence from the lower levels to provide a full range of evidence concerning management options for a particular health condition. These include clinical pathways, textbook summaries, and point-of-care databases that integrate evidence-based information about specific clinical problems and provide regular updating. Resources such as BMJ Best

Practice, DynaMed Plus, Lippincott Procedures, UptoDate, and current evidence-based clinical practice guidelines fall into this category. The top level is systems, or electronic health records (EHRs), which contains individual patient information and link out capability to the current best evidence to support that patient's care. The goal in using the 6S model is to start at the highest level and work downward if evidence is not available from the upper-level resources. Starting at the top levels of the hierarchy saves the clinician time because the resources within these levels have already identified, filtered, critically appraised, and often graded the most relevant research on a particular topic.

TOOLS TO ASSIST WITH CREATION AND APPRAISAL OF RESOURCES

Multiple tools have been developed to help with the creation and appraisal of pre-appraised resources such as clinical practice guidelines and systematic reviews. The Appraisal of Guidelines Research and Evaluation (AGREE) II is an international instrument that provides a framework to assess the quality of clinical practice guidelines, including the confidence that potential biases have been addressed and that the recommendations are both valid and feasible for practice (Brouwers et al., 2010). The instrument also provides a methodological strategy for developing guidelines and informs on what information and how that information should be reported. Composed of 23 items within six domains, AGREE II allows developers or reviewers of a guideline a way to assign numeric values to the scope and purpose, stakeholder involvement, rigor of development, clarity of presentation, applicability, and editorial independence. Available in both print and electronic formats, AGREE II as well as training materials are available for use at www.agreetrust.org/agree-ii.

A tool that assists with the implementation of guidelines is the Guideline Implementability Appraisal (GLIA) 2.0. Implementability in this context refers to the guideline characteristics that may indicate potential challenges to effective implementation. GLIA focuses primarily on factors such as executability, decidability, validity, flexibility, effect on process of care, measurability, novelty/innovation, and computability and consists of 30 questions spread across these domains. When using GLIA, users should select the guideline recommendations for which implementation is planned, as the unit of implementation is the individual recommendation, as opposed to the whole guideline. GLIA 2.0 is available in .pdf format at http://nutmeg.med.yale.edu/glia/login.htm, and a web-based version (eGLIA) is available through request.

The GRADE (Grading of Recommendations Assessment, Development and Evaluation) Working Group developed the GRADE approach for grading the quality of evidence and strength of recommendations, and is applicable to different types of evidence including evidence on intervention effects, test accuracy, prognosis, resources, and values and preference (Alonso-Coello et al., 2016). GRADE-CERQual can be used to assess the confidence in findings from qualitative data for systematic reviews of qualitative evidence. GRADE is currently used by over 100 organizations such as the World Health Organization (WHO) and the

Cochrane Collaboration, with many of these organizations having provided input into the development of the tool. GRADE is considered to be a standard in guideline development, as it provides an approach that assesses the certainty or quality of a body of evidence by outcome(s) while also providing an approach to moving evidence to a decision using Evidence to Decision (EtD) frameworks (GRADE, 2019; Zhang et al., 2019). The GRADE Working Group (www.gradeworkinggroup. org) also wanted to reduce unnecessary confusion arising from multiple systems for grading evidence and recommendations, and to that end the suggested criteria for using the GRADE approach to assess evidence or develop recommendations are:

1. The certainty in the evidence (also known as quality of evidence or confidence in the estimates) should be defined consistently with the definitions used by the GRADE Working Group.
2. Explicit consideration should be given to each of the GRADE domains for assessing the certainty in the evidence (although different terminology may be used).
3. The overall certainty in the evidence should be assessed for each important outcome using three or four categories (such as high, moderate, low and/or very low) and definitions for each category that are consistent with the definitions used by the GRADE Working Group.
4. Evidence summaries and evidence to decision criteria should be used as the basis for judgments about the certainty in the evidence and the strength of recommendations. Ideally, evidence profiles should be used to assess the certainty in the evidence and these should be based on systematic reviews. At a minimum, the evidence that was assessed and the methods that were used to identify and appraise that evidence should be clearly described.
5. Explicit consideration should be given to each of the GRADE criteria for determining the direction and strength of a recommendation or decision. Ideally, GRADE evidence to decision frameworks should be used to document the considered research evidence, additional considerations and judgments transparently.
6. The strength of recommendations should be assessed using two categories (for or against an option) and definitions for each category such as strong and weak/conditional that are consistent with the definitions used by the GRADE Working Group (although different terminology may be used), such as strong (GRADE, 2019).

The Preferred Reporting Items for Systematic Reviews and Meta-Analyses (PRISMA) is an evidence-based minimum set of 27 items for reporting in systematic reviews and meta-analyses which focus on evaluating randomized controlled trials, although it can also be used for reporting reviews utilizing other forms of research, particularly evaluations of interventions. PRISMA is primarily designed to be used by the authors of systematic reviews and meta-analyses, journal peer reviewers, and editors. While not designed as an assessment instrument for the quality of a systematic review, it can be used for critical appraisal to determine how comprehensive the reviewers are in their reporting (Moher et al., 2009). There are now multiple extensions of the PRISMA Statement to facilitate the reporting of different types or aspects of systematic reviews, including PRISMA for Abstracts, PRISMA Equity, PRISMA Harms, PRISMA Individual Patient Data, PRISMA for Network Meta-Analyses, PRISMA for Protocols, PRISMA for Diagnostic Test Accuracy, PRISMA for Scoping Reviews, and PRISMA for Acupuncture. Links to supporting literature and checklists for each of the PRISMA extensions are available at www.prisma-statement.org/Extensions/.

For those who do not have advanced training in epidemiology but want to conduct a more rapid appraisal of a systematic review, the 11-question AMSTAR (Assessment of Multiple SysTemAtic Reviews) may be an appropriate tool. Scoring AMSTAR is estimated to take between 10 to 20 minutes, and several studies have shown the tool to be reliable and valid (Pieper et al., 2015). A revised version, AMSTAR 2, was recently published in response to critiques, feedback from users, and developments in the science of systematic reviews. AMSTAR 2 was consequently revised to: simplify the response categories; align the definition of research questions with the PICO (population, intervention, comparison, outcome) framework; seek justification for the selection of different study designs (randomized or nonrandomized) for inclusion in systematic reviews; seek more details on reasons for study exclusions; and determine whether the review authors had made a sufficiently detailed assessment of risk of bias for included studies; determine whether the risk of bias with included studies was considered adequately during statistical pooling of results and when interpreting and discussing the review findings (Shea et al., 2017). As more tools are developed and/or revised, a useful site for staying informed is the EQUATOR (Enhancing the QUAlity and Transparency Of health Research) Network, which provides current information and links to over 400 reporting guidelines and policy documents (equator-network.org/).

USE AND MANAGEMENT OF REFERENCE MANAGEMENT SOFTWARE

Knowing how to use reference management software effectively can be a game changer when it comes to managing information, as these tools can help to significantly save time when writing articles or books, conducting systematic reviews or meta-analyses, developing practice guidelines, or other activities that healthcare professionals may be involved with. When selecting a reference manager, the following functions should be supported (Gilmour & Cobus-Kuo, 2011, para. 2):

1. Import citations from bibliographic databases and websites
2. Gather metadata from PDF files
3. Allow organization of citations within the reference manager database
4. Allow annotation of citations
5. Allow sharing of the reference manager database or portions thereof with colleagues

6. Allow data interchange with other reference manager products through standard metadata formats (e.g., RIS, BibTeX)
7. Produce formatted citations in a variety of styles
8. Work with word processing software to facilitate in-text citation

While there are for fee and free versions of reference management software, the choice of which one to use really depends on the needs of the user. RefWorks, Zotero, Mendeley, EndNote Basic, and EndNote Desktop are some common examples of reference managers, but there are others available. Some important considerations when choosing a package should include computer/device compatibility, ability to search external databases, citation styles supported, ability to collaborate with others, and compatibility with other software systems such as word processors or those that support systematic review development.

The increasing emphasis by funding agencies and journals for transparency regarding research data is also driving several trends in information management, including the use of prespecified data management plans and making raw data accessible to other researchers and the public. Creating a data management plan prompts the researcher to consider the entire life cycle of data from creation through organization, accessibility, dissemination, and archiving. Each one of the life cycle steps prompts thoughtful analysis and planning that can strengthen the integrity and usefulness of the data. There are multiple versions of the data life cycle available, such as the DataONE data life cycle built upon a model proposed by the National Science Foundation. Composed of eight components, the DataOne data life cycle (DataOne, n.d.; Michener et al., 2012) specifies that researchers should:

1. Plan how the data will be compiled and how the data will be managed and made accessible throughout its lifespan.
2. Collect observations either by hand or with sensors or other instruments and the data are placed into digital form.
3. Assure the quality of the data is assured through checks and inspections.
4. Describe the data accurately and thoroughly using the appropriate metadata standards.
5. Preserve data by submitting it to an appropriate long-term archive (i.e., data center).
6. Discover, locate, and obtain potentially useful data, along with the relevant information about the data (metadata).
7. Integrate data from disparate sources to form one homogeneous set of data that can be readily analyzed.
8. Analyze data.

Not all research activities will require all of the steps, and different scenarios illustrating how users might progress through the data life cycle as well as best practices, publications and training materials can be found at the DataOne website (dataone .org/resources).

OPTIMIZING HEALTHCARE DELIVERY WITH DATA

As healthcare has increasingly adopted Electronic Health Records (EHRs), Health Information Systems (HIS) and handheld, wearable and smart devices, the amount of digital health-related information grows exponentially. This data is largely viewed as having great potential for optimizing healthcare delivery, primarily through the use of Big data analytics, which has the ability to analyze complex data and identify patterns to improve quality and reduce costs. Big data techniques such as natural language processing, cluster analysis, data mining, graph analytics, machine learning, neural networks, pattern recognition, and spatial analysis all have applicability to clinical and operational data in healthcare. The challenges to the adoption of big data analytics in healthcare are still quite formidable due to a variety of factors including inappropriate IT infrastructure, cost, data privacy and security, and fragmentation of data sources and types. However, there is evidence to show that the use of big fata analytics can enable delivery of care and reduce costs in clinical care (Mehta & Pandit, 2018). As Big Data analytics in healthcare is still in its infancy, the scope and impact of the changes to come have yet to be realized on a large scale. Correspondingly, the need for healthcare professionals who are savvy information managers who can successfully generate and use data as well as locate and critically appraise existing research evidence remains vital.

SUMMARY

- Evidence-based practice (EBP) is widely used to improve the quality of healthcare, patient outcomes, and organizational efficiency.
- Health science curricula introduce students to the concepts and models of EBP for implementation into practice.
- Various tools have been developed to assist with the creation and appraisal of preappraised resources, including clinical practice guidelines and systematic reviews.
- Understanding how to use reference management software effectively can be a game changer to managing information in healthcare.
- Funding agencies and journals for transparency is driving trends in information management and data sharing.
- Digital health-related information is growing exponentially and has implications to guide practice and operations.
- Big data have applicability to clinical and operational data in healthcare.
- Health professionals must be savvy information managers to be effective as healthcare continues to change.

REFLECTION QUESTIONS

1. What role can you assume to ensure that the timely implementation of evidence into practice occurs in a timely and continuous process?

2. Consider a recent improvement project and how you used information to guide the project. What information provided the most effective source(s) during the project development, implementation, and evaluation?

REFERENCES

Albarqouni, L., Hoffmann, T., Straus, S., Olsen, N. R., Young, T., Ilic, D., Shaneyfelt, T., Haynes, R. B., Guyatt, G., & Glasziou, P. (2018). Core competencies in evidence-based practice for health professionals: Consensus statement based on a systematic review and Delphi survey. *JAMA Network Open, 1*(2), e180281. https://doi.org/10.1001/jamanetworkopen.2018.0281

Alonso-Coello, P., Oxman, A. D., Moberg, J., Brignardello-Petersen, R., Akl, E. A., Davoli, M., Treweek, S., Mustafa, R. A., Vandvik, P. O., Meerpohl, J., Guyatt, G. H., Schünemann, H. J., & the GRADE Working Group. (2016). GRADE Evidence to Decision (EtD) frameworks: A systematic and transparent approach to making well informed healthcare choices. 2: Clinical practice guidelines. *BMJ, 353,* i2089. https://doi.org/10.1136/bmj.i2089

Andrew, T. J., & Theiss, M. (2015). Combining evidence-based practice, learner-guided education, and continuing education. *The Journal of Continuing Education in Nursing, 46*(12), 535–537. https://doi.org/10.3928/00220124-20151112-02

Brouwers, M. C., Kho, M. E., Browman, G. P., Burgers, J. S., Cluzeau, F., Feder, G., Fervers, B., Graham, I. D., Grimshaw, J., Hanna, S. E., Littlejohns, P., Makarski, J., Zitzelsberger, L., & AGREE Next Steps Consortium. (2010). AGREE II: Advancing guideline development, reporting and evaluation in health care. *CMAJ: Canadian Medical Association Journal = Journal de l'Association Medicale Canadienne, 182*(18), E839–E842. https://doi.org/10.1503/cmaj.090449

Copeland, D., Miller, K., & Clanton, C. (2020). The creation of an interprofessional evidence-based practice council. *The Journal of Nursing Administration, 50*(1), 12–15. https://doi.org/10.1097/NNA.0000000000000832

DataOne. (n.d.). *Data Life Cycle | DataONE.* https://www.dataone.org/data-life-cycle

Dicenso, A., Bayley, L., & Haynes, R. B. (2009). Accessing pre-appraised evidence: Fine-tuning the 5S model into a 6S model. *Evidence-Based Nursing, 12*(4), 99–101. https://doi.org/10.1136/ebn.12.4.99-b

Djulbegovic, B., & Guyatt, G. H. (2017). Progress in evidence-based medicine: A quarter century on. *The Lancet, 390*(10092), 415–423. https://doi.org/10.1016/S0140-6736(16)31592-6

Gilmour, R., & Cobus-Kuo, L. (2011). Reference management software: A comparative analysis of four products. *Issues in Science and Technology Librarianship.* https://doi.org/10.5062/F4Z60KZF

GRADE. (2019). *What is GRADE?* GRADE. https://www.gradeworkinggroup.org

Guyatt, G. H., Meade, M. O., Jaeschke, R. Z., Cook, D. J., & Haynes, R. B. (2000). Practitioners of evidence based care. Not all clinicians need to appraise evidence from scratch but all need some skills. *BMJ (Clinical Research Ed.), 320*(7240), 954–955. https://doi.org/10.1136/bmj.320.7240.954

Laibhen-Parkes, N., Brasch, J., & Gioncardi, L. (2015). Nursing grand rounds: A strategy for promoting evidence-based learning among pediatric nurses. *Journal of Pediatric Nursing, 30*(2), 338–345. https://doi.org/10.1016/j.pedn.2014.07.008

Mehta, N., & Pandit, A. (2018). Concurrence of big data analytics and healthcare: A systematic review. *International Journal of Medical Informatics, 114,* 57–65. https://doi.org/10.1016/j.ijmedinf.2018.03.013

Michener, W. K., Allard, S., Budden, A., Cook, R. B., Douglass, K., Frame, M., Kelling, S., Koskela, R., Tenopir, C., & Vieglais, D. A. (2012). Participatory design of DataONE—Enabling cyberinfrastructure for the biological and environmental sciences. *Ecological Informatics, 11*, 5–15. https://doi.org/10.1016/j.ecoinf.2011.08.007

Moher, D., Liberati, A., Tetzlaff, J., Altman, D. G., & PRISMA Group. (2009). Preferred reporting items for systematic reviews and meta-analyses: The PRISMA statement. *PLOS Medicine, 6*(7), e1000097. https://doi.org/10.1371/journal.pmed.1000097

Pieper, D., Buechter, R. B., Li, L., Prediger, B., & Eikermann, M. (2015). Systematic review found AMSTAR, but not R(evised)-AMSTAR, to have good measurement properties. *Journal of Clinical Epidemiology, 68*(5), 574–583. https://doi.org/10.1016/j.jclinepi.2014.12.009

Sackett, D. L., Rosenberg, W. M., Gray, J. A., Haynes, R. B., & Richardson, W. S. (1996). Evidence based medicine: What it is and what it isn't. *BMJ (Clinical Research Ed.), 312*(7023), 71–72. https://doi.org/10.1136/bmj.312.7023.71

Sadeghi-Bazargani, H., Tabrizi, J. S., & Azami-Aghdash, S. (2014). Barriers to evidence-based medicine: A systematic review. *Journal of Evaluation in Clinical Practice, 20*(6), 793–802. https://doi.org/10.1111/jep.12222

Saunders, H., Gallagher-Ford, L., Kvist, T., & Vehviläinen-Julkunen, K. (2019). Practicing healthcare professionals' evidence-based practice competencies: An overview of systematic reviews. *Worldviews on Evidence-Based Nursing, 16*(3), 176–185. Scopus. https://doi.org/10.1111/wvn.12363

Shea, B. J., Reeves, B. C., Wells, G., Thuku, M., Hamel, C., Moran, J., Moher, D., Tugwell, P., Welch, V., Kristjansson, E., & Henry, D. A. (2017). AMSTAR 2: A critical appraisal tool for systematic reviews that include randomised or non-randomised studies of healthcare interventions, or both. *BMJ (Clinical Research Ed.), 358*, j4008. https://doi.org/10.1136/bmj.j4008

Slawson, D. C., & Shaughnessy, A. F. (2005). Teaching evidence-based medicine: Should we be teaching information management instead? *Academic Medicine: Journal of the Association of American Medical Colleges, 80*(7), 685–689. https://doi.org/10.1097/00001888-200507000-00014

Straus, S. E., Glasziou, P., Richardson, W. S., & Haynes, R. B. H. (2018). *Evidence-based medicine: How to practice and teach EBM* (5th ed.). Elsevier.

Williams, B., Perillo, S., & Brown, T. (2015). What are the factors of organisational culture in health care settings that act as barriers to the implementation of evidence-based practice? A scoping review. *Nurse Education Today, 35*(2), e34–e41. https://doi.org/10.1016/j.nedt.2014.11.012

Zhang, Y., Akl, E. A., & Schünemann, H. J. (2019). Using systematic reviews in guideline development: The GRADE approach. *Research Synthesis Methods, 10*(3), 312–329. Scopus. https://doi.org/10.1002/jrsm.1313

CASE EXEMPLARS FOR APPLICATION

Research Initiatives Related to Hospital Respiratory Protection Practices

Debra Novak

DATA DEVELOPMENT, COLLECTION METHODS, AND TRANSLATION

Over 18 million healthcare workers are exposed to a variety of occupational hazards including exposures to aerosol transmitted diseases (ATDs) that require the use of respiratory protection (Centers for Disease Control [CDC], 2015). OSHA mandates that employers maintain a respiratory protection program (RPP) for employees in workplaces where respirators are necessary to protect the health of the worker. Beginning in 2009, during the influenza A (H1N1) pandemic, CDPH and CDC/NIOSH undertook a hospital-based evaluation, known as Respirator Evaluation in Acute Care Hospitals (REACH I), to better understand the extent to which respiratory protection programs and practices were being employed.

Sixteen California hospitals and 204 healthcare workers participated in the initial REACH I study with 15 to 21 onsite surveys conducted in each facility. To our knowledge, this was the first U.S. study of its kind to examine hospital respiratory protection programs and healthcare worker practices. Therefore all data collection instruments had to be developed (Beckman et al., 2013).

Three separate survey instruments were developed for each of the healthcare provider groups sampled: hospital managers (HMs), unit managers (UMs), and frontline healthcare workers (HCWs). In addition, a one-page checklist was developed to record observations of healthcare workers' actual use of respiratory protection. The hospital's written respiratory protection program was also assessed with a separate instrument. Given the necessity to obtain "real-time data" during the ongoing H1N1 outbreak, instrument development for REACH I was undertaken on a tight timeline. Prior to employing REACH I data collection each of the "newly minted instruments" were pilot tested and revisions were made based on feedback. The pilot testing of the instruments allowed for the beginning ofdevelopment of the data code book.

Beginning in January 2011, the REACH I study was expanded to include six states across five regions of the United States and referred to as REACH II (Peterson et al., 2015). This expanded data set included information obtained from 98 acute care hospitals and greater than 1,500 healthcare workers. REACH I field notes, maintained by the data collectors, provided rich information about "lessons learned" and informed REACH II instrument revisions to improve item(s) clarity while streamlining the redundancy of survey items to reduce participant and data collector time burden. For example, the observational instrument was revised to improve data collection regarding healthcare workers' competency with actual use of respiratory protection. Items to assess organizational safety climate and knowledge of infection control were also added to assess group differences among the provider groups (HM, UM, HCW) (Peterson et al., 2016).

Linking the database development to a conceptual model with targeted research questions provided a strong foundation for analysis. A conceptual model was used to guide the instrument development for REACH I (Mermel, 2009) and the REACH II organizational safety climate items were derived from (Gershon et al., 2000) and Turnberg (2006). All research activities were approved by the state health department or university and the NIOSH Humans Subject Review Board and facilities' institutional review. The complex levels of necessary review and approval for a multisite, multistate study required extra time to be built into the REACH II timeline. To ensure REACH II data quality an independent research analysis organization was utilized.

The REACH I and II initiatives were based on the belief that evidence-based practices are most likely to be employed and adopted when they are based on strong practice-based evidence (translational science). Selected translational outputs based on REACH II findings include:

- The Joint Commission Monograph: Implementing Hospital Respiratory Protection Programs (www.jointcommission.org/-/media/deprecated-unorganized/imported-assets/tjc/system-folders/topics-library/implementing_hospital_rpp_2-19-15pdf.pdf)
- AAOHN free, web-based training resources (aaohn.org/page/respiratory-protection-1278.)

The highlighted CDC/NIOSH research initiatives provide examples of how the government responded to respiratory protection HCW practice gaps, beginning with H1N1, to develop informed tools and resources. The best respiratory infectious disease preparedness strategy during outbreaks is based upon sound workplace evidence to reinforce HCWs proper daily use practices.

REFLECTION QUESTIONS

1. What steps are required by researchers to ensure ethical and legal standards are met before collecting data?
2. What is the difference between translational and data science? Provide examples of each.
3. What is the difference between qualitative and quantitative research methods?

REFERENCES

Beckman, S., Materna, B., Goldmacher, S., Zipprich, J., D'Alessandro, M., Novak, D., & Harrison, R. (2013). Evaluation of respiratory protection programs in California hospitals during the 2009-2010 H1N1 influenza pandemic. *American Journal of Infection Control, 41*(11), 1024–1031. https://doi.org/10.1016/j.ajic.2013.05.006

Centers for Disease Control and Occupational Safety Health Administration. (2015). *The CDC/OSHA hospital respiratory protection toolkit.* https://www.cdc.gov/niosh/docs/2015-117/default.html

Gershon, R. R. M., Karkashian, C. D., Grosch, J. W., Murphy, L. R., Escamilla-Cejudo, A., Flanagan, P. A., & Martin, L. (2000). Organizational climate and nurse health outcomes in the United States: A systematic review. *American Journal of Infection Control, 28,* 211–221. https://doi.org/10.1067/mic.2000.105288

Mermel, L. A. (2009). A global challenge, a global perspective. The Joint Commission. *Journal of Hospital Infection, 74*(4), 323–330.

Peterson, K., Novak, D., Stradtman, L., Wilson, D., & Couzens, L. (2015). Hospitals' respiratory protection programs and practices in six American states: A public health evaluation study. *American Journal of Infection Control, 43,* 63–71. https://doi.org/10.1016/j.ajic.2014.10.008

Peterson, K., Rogers, B., Brosseau, L., Payne, J., Cooney, J., Joe, L., & Novak, D. (2016). Differences in hospital managers', unit managers' and healthcare workers' perceptions of the safety climate for respiratory protection. *Workplace Health and Safety, 64*(7), 326–336. https://doi.org/10.1177/2165079916640550

Turnberg, W. L. (2006). *Respiratory infection control practices among healthcare workers in primary care and emergency department settings. Doctoral dissertation.* University of Washington Department of Environmental and Occupational Health Sciences.

Data and Clinical Decision-Making: The Link

Charlene M. Myers

The Electronic Health Record (EHR) advances in technology and daily team rounds provide evidence that the overall quality, safety, and efficiency in healthcare have improved (McGlynn et al., 2003). This data provides multiple opportunities for exchange of health information between all healthcare providers and guides clinical decisions in a coordinated and cyclical process.

Research supports that data from EHRs reduce medication, diagnostic tests, and procedure errors, and often overprescribing by medication reconciliation. Many EHRs have commercial or system-developed automatic alerts that display completed results from procedures, medication contraindications, and clinical guideline resources used for the management of disorders (Fadahunsi et.al., 2019). The data are available in real time and available to members of the clinical team.

Data utility requires accuracy in order to develop a plan of care. A strategy used to ensure data accuracy is to complete daily reports and attend rounds at the bedside where the patient is a central participant. Rounds should involve all team members and include attending physicians, medical residents, interns, nurse practitioners (NPs), registered nurses (RNs), respiratory therapists (RTs), PharmDs, physical therapists (PT), dietitians, social workers, others involved in the patient's care, and family members whenever possible.

This interprofessional approach is utilized in a Level I Trauma Center Intensive Care Unit (ICU) in the southern United States. Each morning, "the team" identified above, conduct bedside rounds for all patients assigned to the service. An important component of the rounds is an operable computer referred to as the Computer on Wheels (COW). The COW travels with the team and data are retrieved from each patient's EHR. The team reviews results from diagnostic procedures and tests, the medication administration record, and entries from physicians, RNs, PTs, OTs, RTs, etc. Reviewing and analyzing the data provides an opportunity to use the strengths and talents of each discipline culminating in clinically appropriate and evidence-based care decisions.

A common example is reviewing the medications with the PharmD. The team reviews any cultures, the antibiotics, dosages, and day number of the antibiotic in use. Often the team medications are omitted or changed with system-wide improvement methods focusing on antibiotic stewardship. Another example is reviewing the trends of the patient's vital signs and respiratory status. The RTs expertise assists in discussions related to Spontaneous Breathing Trial (SBT) results for ventilated patients, ventilator settings, and arterial blood gas results. The data assist providers to determine extubation options. The PT offers recommendations to identify if patients require an order or if the Early Mobility (EM) protocol has been initiated. Evidence supports that EM in the intensive care unit ICU) is associated with shorter length of stay (LOS), increased ventilator-free days, decreased incidence of ventilator associated pneumonia (VAP), and increased delirium-free days (Barr et al, 2013; Kayambu et al., 2013; Klompas et al., 2014). Improved quality of life and a reduction in pressure ulcers and falls are also benefits of EM (Fraser et al., 2015).

This approach utilizes data available from the EHR, interprofessional team rounds and input, and patient and family involvement is one example of an innovation approach to improve clinical practices, performance, and patient outcomes. Linking data to clinical decisions has provided overall expenditures. As care delivery and system operations rapidly advance and mandates to reduce costs while ensuring quality, safe, and value-based outcomes are employed, an approach such as described in this exemplar is timely.

REFLECTION QUESTIONS

1. What ways can you identify to ensure data and evidence guides clinical decisions.
2. How would you initiate interprofessional rounds on an identified unit and what performance indicators would be chosen to evaluate the outcome?

REFERENCES

Barr, J., Fraser, G. L., Puntillo, K., Ely, E. W., Gelinas, C., Dosta, J. F., Davidson, J. E., Devlin, J. W., Kress, J. P., Joffe, A. M., Coursin, D. B., Herr, D. L., . . . Jaeschke, R. (2013). Clinical practice guidelines for the management of pain, agitation, and delirium in adult patients in the intensive care unit. *Critical Care Medicine, 41,* 263–306. https://doi.org/10.1097/CCM.0b013e3182783b72

Fadahunsi, K. P., Akinlua, J. T, O'Connor, S., Wark, P. A, Gallagher, J., Carroll, C., Majeed, A., & O'Donoghue, J. (2019). Protocol for a systematic review and qualitative synthesis of information quality frameworks in eHealth. *British Medical Journal Open, 9*(3), eo24722. https://doi.org/10.1136/bmjopen-2018-024722

Fraser, D., Spiva, L., Forman, W., & Hallen, C. (2015). Original research: Implementation of an early mobility program in an ICU. *American Journal of Nursing, 115,* 49–58. https://doi.org/10.1097/01.NAJ.0000475292.27985.fc

Kayambu, G., Boots, R., & Paratz, J. (2013). Physical therapy for the critically ill in the ICU: A systematic review and meta-analysis. *Criiical Care Medicine, 41,* 1543–1554. https://doi.org/10.1097/CCM.0b013e31827ca637

Klompas, M., Branson, R., Eichenwald, E., Greene. L. R., Howell, M. D., Lee, G., Magill, S. S., Maragakis, L. L., Priebe, G. P., Speck, K., Yokoe, D. S., & Berenholtz, S. M. (2014). Strategies to prevent ventilator-associated pneumonia in acute care hospitals: update. *Infection Control and Hospital Epidemiology, 35,* 915–936. https://doi.org/10.1086/677144

McGlynn, E. A., Asch, S. M., Adams, J., Keesey, J., Hicks, J., DeCristofaro, A., & Kerr, E. A. (2003). The quality of health care delivered to adults in the United States. *New England Journal of Medicine, 348,* 2635–2645. https://doi.org/10.1056/NEJMsa022615

13

Leading Interprofessional Improvement Teams to Use Meaningful Data

Kathryn Sapnas and James L. Harris

OBJECTIVES

1. Identify key elements for leading interprofessional improvement teams to use evidence-based data and generate healthcare improvement.
2. Describe tools, strategies, and methods used to create synergy among interprofessional teams and customize meaningful data use and management.
3. Examine the importance of a common language shared by improvement teams and data managers.
4. Explore the value of sharing data, economics involved, and influence on improvement and team science in healthcare.

CORE COMPETENCIES

- Coordinate interprofessional team activities to ensure needs are assessed, improvement options are developed, and data are used to guide outcomes
- Collaborate with interprofessional teams to impact and inform change

- Effective communication with teams, organizations, and stakeholders to use and understand data and its value
- Exhibit interpersonal influence and a management style that transforms health and care delivery at various levels
- Knowledge of evaluation tools and models to identify gaps and opportunities in improvement processes
- Knowledge of systems thinking and application in healthcare

INTRODUCTION

Today's healthcare environments require team collaboration, idea sharing, and the use of evidence-base data for continuous improvement. Achieving optimal outcomes is a hallmark of any team effort. While there is no single formula to great teamwork, a leader who creates a climate and culture of inclusiveness is pivotal to success for any improvement team. Inclusiveness enables diverse thought and affects how teams function and communicate. A sense of belonging emerges, as team members understand the value of generational and cultural differences. New knowledge is possible from teamwork, collaboration, and a series of catalyzing changes that challenge others toward greater performance and improvements.

This chapter discusses key elements for leading improvement teams to use and create evidence-based data for improvements, methods that foster synergy among teams, the importance of language between and among disciplines, and how data informs decisions, transforms quality and safety, and influences improvement. The merits of improvement and team science are also discussed as well as how knowledge is leveraged across organizations.

LEADING INTERPROFESSIONAL TEAMS TO USE DATA AND GENERATE IMPROVEMENT IN HEALTHCARE

Transformation is central to improvement as leaders guide teams to use data and generate new ideas in healthcare. It is a social responsibility for leaders to direct teams to innovate, use data, and disseminate outcomes as excellence in healthcare is achieved. As a result, the innumerable opportunities available to improve the quality and safety of healthcare are cultivated. This responsibility offers improvement teams an opportunity to extract value from data when the leader nurtures its development, team cohesiveness, and exercises effective leadership. Data, therefore dramatizes the future for innovation and team accomplishments. Bieda (2017) supported this idea and suggested that improvement teams are able to acknowledge the crucial intersection where data, analytics, and access to new technology merge with effective leadership.

Irrespective of improvement team purpose, composition, or duration, there are key elements that must be considered by leaders in order for effective data use and improvement outcomes. Discovering what data works best under certain circumstances requires that leaders nurture teams to use data as a resource for continuous learning and the public good (Institute of Medicine [IOM], 2010). This may conflict with certain team values and biases. Therefore, it is imperative that the leader facilitates crucial conversations among team members and accepts that diversity of thought can guide and inform change, innovation, and the integration of data towards a common goal. Effective leaders that focus on team potential acknowledge that things are different today in healthcare. Leaders must share opportunities with others for mutual engagement in a journey where work is done differently. This requires emotional maturity, ability to exercise diplomacy, communicate effectively, and ready environments for change. When team leaders understand the value of communication, inputs will result in measureable outputs and all points of view are considered before an action occurs. Leader communication is accomplished in four ways: (a) conveying messages that are concise and direct, (b) viewing team members as a whole while respecting individuality, (c) demonstrating truth in what is said, and (d) seeking responses from team members and validating what is communicated both verbally and nonverbally (Maxwell, 1999).

Leaders who also understand the stages of team development contribute to a team's identity within an organization. If teams are allowed to progress through the stages, the potential gains will be continuous, add value, and sustainability of outcomes is intensified. In 1965, Tuckman proposed a model for group stages that proved valuable and remain relevant today in understanding team development. An additional stage was later identified that reinforced the value of team synergy (Tuckman, 2001). The five stages—forming, storming, norming, performing, and adjourning—are discussed below.

Forming is the initial stage in which a team meets for the explicit purpose of accomplishing an identified project goal. Throughout this stage, trust is foundational to the formation of relationships, communication, articulating and understanding the group's aim, and defining one's role and responsibilities.

Storming is the next stage where trust has not completely developed. Conflicts are common due to differing opinions, disciplines, and experiences. Communication and the leader's ability to directly manage conflict are essential in this stage; otherwise, emotions limit communication, productivity is reduced, morale among the team is diminished, and costs associated with a project will increase (Chinn, 2008; Feldman, 2008). The emotional intelligence (EI) of team members and the leader is extremely important in this stage. Emotions can become a barrier to a team's productivity, and if the leader does not proactively address them, team members are immobilized and project outcomes are jeopardized. According to Goleman (1998), EI is a valuable attribute and credited with team successes. EI often plays a more significant role than cognitive abilities as a team progresses in meeting an identified goal.

Norming is the stage where team identity is developing. Team members openly share ideas, opinions, and different insights are accepted. Leaders must be attuned to the possibility for groupthink and assure it does not inhibit progress in meeting the project aim.

In the *performing* stage, loyalty matures, flexibility ensues, and the assets of team members guide processes and outcomes toward achievement of the project goal. In the final stage, *adjourning*, progress and performance are evaluated based on outcomes that are linked to the project goal and modifications are made, as needed, to ensure their sustainability.

As previously discussed, successful leadership and progressing through the five group stages are pivotal to team success and group synergy. As teams progress through the stages, meaningful data will be used and created that foster healthcare improvement. However, barriers to team effectiveness and how data are used to achieve sustainable improvements cannot be dismissed. The inability to establish member trust, resolve conflicts, lack of member accountability, and an individual aim versus that of team members are common barriers that will alter group efforts and result in an unmet aim. Such barriers are avoidable with effective leader skills and direction (Ulrich & Crider, 2017). Leading teams toward healthcare improvements and using meaningful data effectively will result in new evidence. Evidence will further guide how others learn and create additional avenues that foster a culture of engagement and continuous improvement.

MEANINGFUL DATA, TOOLS, STRATEGIES, AND METHODS TO CREATE TEAM SYNERGY

Team synergy is fundamental to reducing fragmentation of care. Without team synergy, dissonance across disciplines occurs and preventable errors, inadequate communication, and failures in system processes persist. Strategies used to customize and manage data are strengthened when team synergy is present and healthcare issues will be reduced and ultimately eliminated. The Institute of Medicine's (IOM) report *To Err Is Human,* and the subsequent *Crossing the Quality Chasm,* offered valuable insights and direction for teams to synergistically align and use various tools, methods, and data as the tapestry for managing fragmented care is woven (IOM, 1999; 2001).

Without team synergy, improvement is sporadic and often absent. Despite efforts by leaders and team members, available data and tools are not fully utilized and the root cause of system disruptions is overlooked. Subsequently the momentum and vision for improvement and change are diminished. To avoid this scenario, strong team relationships must be developed. The potential for exchanging information will therefore determine the vision for quality, strength, and improvement longevity. Understanding the value of team synergy will continuously reinforce processes whereby a vision is spread and will leverage future improvements (Senge, 1990).

Team synergy does not occur in a vacuum and defining it can be difficult. As opportunities arise during team interactions, interprofessional collaboration, creativity, innovation, cultural differences, and appreciative inquiry offer clarity to define team synergy. Defining team synergy can be further clarified by examining how the forenamed concepts are linked to improvement initiatives (Joseph et al., 2019).

Interprofessional collaboration among improvement teams requires a transition where the expertise of other disciplines is respected and there is an understanding of what each individual brings to the discussion. This necessitates understanding other's education, scope of practice, areas of expertise, and language used by each discipline

(Jakubowski & Perron, 2018). In 2013, Day identified three elements that determine how collaboration develops and transitions into interprofessional team synergy. The first element focuses on systemic factors and includes influences outside an organization. These influences include the professional system and social system and will positively or negatively impact how teams function. Specifically, the professional system is influenced by individual socialization, language, conduct, and member acculturation. This requires effective communication and understanding among team members and stakeholders in order to accomplish an improvement initiative. The social system, on the other hand, is influenced by equality between different professional team members and requires equitable partnerships to be formed. Otherwise, collaborative relationships are compromised.

Organizational structure is the second element that impacts effective collaboration. Traditional hierarchical structures must be replaced with horizontal ones if teams share decision-making, communication, and collaboration in meeting an identified aim.

The third element is interactional factors. The most common influence is professional stereotyping. Various professionals hold numerous beliefs and perceptions. To avoid these distractions, teams must challenge each of the stereotypical beliefs if effective outcomes occur and are sustained.

Creativity is another concept heralded as pivotal to define team synergy and organizational success (West & Sacramento, 2012). Both individual and team creativity contribute to the development and effectiveness of organizations as team synergy matures. Ideas that are unique and relative to other ones are considered novel and valuable to an organization (Oldham & Baer, 2012). Organizations that foster creativity and team synergy prosper as new markets are created and offer creative services, improved work processes, innovative products, and state-of-the-art technology. As a result, organizations are positioned to influence future global challenges in health, education, and interdependencies between work units and complex systems (de Alencar, 2012; Kazanjian & Drazin, 2012).

As teams and organizations create and manage the canvas of creativity, innovation cannot be overlooked. The power of innovation may be more significant than previously envisioned. Innovation must be considered on a larger scale with the changes in healthcare technology, data utility, competition, and economic instability. However, planning for innovation requires flexibility. Organizations that encourage teams to be innovative create movement toward a strategic advantage over those who are risk averse and lag in development (Hunter et al., 2012). In 2016, Christensen and colleagues suggested that when individuals innovate, actions are directed at achieving solutions and advancing a position.

Isaacson (2014) suggested that innovation occurs from creators who can flourish when the arts intersect with the sciences and a rebellious sense of inquiry opens them to the beauty of both. If organizations and teams reject the interconnectedness of situations and opportunities, innovations in healthcare, research, and progressive team synergy become lost opportunities (Joseph et al., 2019).

In any organization, change is constant. As teams develop blueprints to manage change, they may sense a unique aligning effect such as sitting on a see saw, moving from past to future to present. The future movement creates tension and is motivation for collective actions by the team to extract the best of the past and positives for the future relative to the present organizational reality. Focusing on what is working versus the negatives offers teams opportunities to understand the value of appreciative inquiry.

Appreciative inquiry (AI) has its origin in the late 1980s as an adaptation of action research related to organizational development (Cooperrider & Srivastva, 1987). AI grew into an organizational development approach to change management recognized through organizational transformation (Cooperrider et al., 2008). Today, teams and organizations use AI to understand best practices, develop strategy, shift organization thinking from a problem-oriented mindset to a strength-based viewpoint, and build momentum for future directions (Whitney et al., 2010). As a result, performance is enhanced, team synergy and an organization culture of innovation are reinforced, and collective action becomes the norm.

If AI is achieved, a series of five stages provides a guidepost toward a desired outcome grounded by a positive nucleus (Priest et al., 2013). Defining is the first stage that asks, what is the focus of the inquiry? Discovery follows and gives purpose to a team necessary for discovery in identifying the positive core of an organization. Dream is the next stage where a desired future becomes transparent through the collective imagination and innovation of the team. Design ensues as the team identifies the elements that will bring the dream to reality. Destiny is the final stage where momentum is sustained and capacity for identifying opportunities versus problems coincides throughout the organization (Cooperrider et al., 2008; Donnan, 2005; Stratton-Berkessel, 2010).

Cultural differences also contribute to team synergy and how the accumulation of behaviors and interactions guide the development of organizations to accept change in the current diverse, dispersed, and digital environment. Diversity in knowledge, experiences, norms, age, and gender are drivers for team success. A balanced team mix provides opportunities for creativity and innovation while limiting groupthink (Haas & Mortensen, 2016). As teams coexist and focus their consciousness on a particular idea, it expands and a powerful momentum of knowledge and information evolves into a meaningful direction.

As discussed, a variety of factors intersect at different junctions to define team synergy. One factor does not supersede the other and they collectively merge to create innovative solutions to the challenges confronting healthcare organizations today. Success in healthcare has no prescribed formula, but as teams collectively use skills, data, and collective thought, the genius of attention to detail arises and victory is achieved.

MEANINGFUL DATA, TOOLS, STRATEGIES, AND METHODS TO SUPPORT TEAM SYNERGY

Data, tools, strategies, and methods are available to support and influence the development of team synergy. For purposes of this chapter, five separate, but closely aligned ones are presented in the following paragraphs.

Dating to 2009, the Interprofessional Education Collaborative (IPEC) recognized the value of individuals practicing team-based approaches to achieve patient-centered care as a fundamental component in synergistic learning and team practices. Based on this work, interprofessional collaboration was defined and four core competencies were identified: (a) values and ethics for interprofessional practice, (b) roles and responsibilities for collaborative practice, (c) interprofessional communication practices, and (d) interprofessional teams and teamwork. Further revisions followed in 2016 to include the addition of increased emphasis on population health (Interprofessional Education Collaborative [IPEC], 2016). With a renewed emphasis on population health, the social determinants of health were revisited. As such, active collaboration and team practice is shifting to the gold mark standard where care is provided to individuals, families, and communities at the right time for the right care (Brandt, 2015).

Design thinking is another tool that fosters team synergy. Design thinking is a framework useful in creating innovative solutions through creative problem solving. Teams understand the human needs involved and reframe identified problems through a five-stage process that are not always sequential and may occur in parallel.

The five stages of design thinking include empathize, define, ideate, prototype, and test. The initial stage, empathize, focuses on understanding the problem through a series of immersion experiences with individuals. Observation, engagement, and empathizing with individuals provide a clear understanding of the problem and needs while teams are able to separate personal assumptions. Define is the second stage where data gleaned from the empathize stage is assimilated to form a human-centered problem statement. As the problem statement is formed, the third stage begins. Ideas are identified in this stage enable alternative strategies to solve the problem. In the fourth stage, prototypes, products or features are tested in order to identify a possible solution to the identified problem. During this stage, prototypes and products may be acceptable, rejected, or modified based on the users' experiences. During the final stage, test, best solutions generated during the prototype phase are rigorously tested and includes refinement to culminate in an understanding of the product and users as the problem is solved (Dam & Siang, 2019). Each of the stages reinforces the value of team synergy using a different framework to solve a problem.

Evidence has evolved during the recent decades to create rigor, validity, and a balanced hierarchy for improvement teams to review its utility as insights are formulated to improve healthcare quality, safety, and sustainable approaches to care (Melnyk et al., 2016). Synergistic teams are able to use evidence to aggregate data using big data analytics and engage patients and providers toward collaborative decisions that advance care delivery and satisfaction. When disruptions occur in healthcare, leaders must use evidence generated by teams to identify whether and why change may be needed for administrative and clinical decisions. This allows new patterns for improvement to be recognized, tested, and implemented (Tucker & Melnyk, 2019; Weberg & Davidson, 2019).

Technology is another important consideration regarding the value of team synergy. Leading in a fluid world, where new technology is introduced daily, requires leaders to support teams as they quickly assimilate knowledge and create new boundaries that yield outcomes. This requires team members to be adaptive, understand the driving forces in political and economic environments, and transition quickly as they coordinate and facilitate efforts to a desired future state. New rules and actions will apply as technology advances and patients determine the parameters of the patient-provider relationship. Value will become the center of service delivery and will drive work processes that are disciplined and inform meaning for the development of technology and use by healthcare teams (Porter-O'Grady & Malloch, 2015a).

Never take any position as a team leader or member for granted or the power therein. Inherent in any team is the reality that as synergy develops, the power of the team can accomplish what an individual acting alone cannot (Craddock, 2011; Green, 1998). As teams identify improvement opportunities and use existing evidence and available technology, bold actions are possible and negative power forces resistant to change in an organization will be disarmed.

As team synergy develops, a spirit of trust attracts the best in any group. This allows the discovery of power styles within the team that benefit accomplishment of the identified improvement aim. Applying this lens to power styles offers opportunities to open doors in understanding the potential benefit to improvement and team function. Power holds influence over what resources are available, those that can be used, by what means they are dispersed when developing a project and desired outcomes. As a result, divergent outcomes are possible and the influence of power on team synergy is recognized (Greer et al., 2017; Zhao & Greer, 2017).

THE IMPORTANCE OF A COMMON LANGUAGE SHARED BY IMPROVEMENT TEAMS AND DATA MANAGERS

Healthcare systems are complex, adaptive systems requiring continuous communication and collaboration in order to maintain a competitive edge. During different programs of study, experiences and socialization processes occur that reinforce problem-solving techniques and a common language is developed for each profession. This requires teams and managers throughout any system to adopt a mutually agreed upon common language. In a technology-driven and virtual environment, the challenge of understanding a common language is pivotal to ongoing success, especially as improvement teams collaborate with each other. For example, a team comprised of different disciplines and an informatics specialist is tasked with developing a new medical admission form. As the team moves forward, different terms, techniques, and descriptors related to the medical admission assessment form may occur creating misunderstandings and impede progress. The value of developing a mutually agreeable language and process for documenting assessment findings is thus validated by this example.

Generational differences and preferences in the workplace must also be considered and used to the benefit of any improvement team (Harris & Ward-Presson, 2020). There are five currently recognized generations that encompass society and the workplace. The generations by birth year include according to the Center for GenerationalKinetics (2016):

- Gen Z, iGen, or Centennials: 1996-TBD
- Millennials or Gen Y: 1977-1995
- Generation X: 1965-1976
- Baby Boomers: 1946-1964
- Traditionalists or Silent Generation: Born 1945 or before

Each of the generations is an influential cue to improvement team effectiveness and influence in organizations. Current research has identified that there are more similarities than differences across the five generations and communication is a common denominator for success. More specifically, evidence suggests that differences in preferences and values are very small, and while various viewpoints exist, a common language is vital to meet any aim. Additionally, findings support that three key trends shape generations—parenting, technology, and economics (The Center for GenerationalKinetics, 2016). These findings are important to improvement team leaders and members in order to leverage the potential as project aims are accomplished and change occurs.

Additional important considerations for improvement team success include information about specific generations and geography. By 2025, millennials will comprise three-quarters of the global workforce and the largest customers in the marketplace. Millennials demand transparency and this is evident in team development, interactions, improvement activities, and leadership styles. Generation Zs, the latest generation, have an expectation of real-time communication and focus more on finances and social issues. Being knowledgeable of this information can benefit how improvement teams function as current information is communicated and linked to positive outcomes. Geography also is a consideration as birth years vary by global economics, characteristics, cultures, and languages. As events occur at different times around the world, various generations respond differently and this affects viewpoints, team interactions, and communication (The Center for GenerationalKinetics, 2016).

As healthcare organizations become more nimble, understanding and remaining proactive in managing different generational differences and similarities is a marker for success. This is extremely relevant for improvement team leaders as groups create new options where a common language and data drive quality, safety, and fiscal stewardship.

THE VALUE AND USE OF DATA SYSTEMS BY IMPROVEMENT TEAM PARTNERSHIPS

As information, globalization, and technology continue to expand and impact healthcare, teams must forge partnerships across disciplines where data are unrestricted and used to assess value while meeting the expectations and deliverables required in contemporary healthcare. Situations and conditions in healthcare environments are interconnected and as teams examine new ways to expand and use innovative data systems, high performance systems emerge. Likewise, interdependence is realized as improvement activities and new partnerships develop. Through partnerships, the centrality of information and its exchange will inform processes crucial to care delivery. Different prospects to examine the political-economic environment and impacts on population health are also possible through the improvement team partnership (Reid et al., 2005).

Healthcare is at a crisis and the obvious proximate causes must be addressed by improvement teams and leaders if a 21st century system meets the six aims: safe, effective, timely, patient-centered, efficient, and equitable healthcare—envisioned in *Crossing the Quality Chasm* (IOM, 2001). Advances and care complexities are continuously occurring. To address these opportunities, the historical underinvestment in information and communication systems, emerging information streams, and knowledge management systems must be addressed at the patient, provider, organizational, and environmental levels.

Systems engineering partnerships is a plausible answer to address previous and future healthcare advances, meet the intent of the six IOM aims, and capture the value of an integrated and information-rich healthcare culture. Cross-sector partnerships and collaboration offer combined talent in meeting the challenges linked to new technologies and quantum advances in bioengineering and genomics as they occur. The experience of systems and human factors engineers to use tools and methods to manage complex systems and interactions between systems and processes combined with expertise of healthcare providers, leaders, and researchers attest to the vitality this partnership. A convenient way to conceptualize the partnership is to develop a Venn diagram that illustrates the activities and relationship between systems engineers and the healthcare sector. A Venn diagram displays a representation of overlapping activities and interactions useful to document stakeholder needs, exploration of opportunities, and verifying and validating solutions throughout the life cycle of an improvement process (INCOSE, 2012; SEBok, 2019).

THE VALUE OF DATA SYSTEMS TO IMPROVEMENT TEAMS

Healthcare expenses continue to escalate irrespective of the organization or nation. In the United States alone, health-spending growth is projected to average 5.7 percent, from 4.8 percent in 2019, and will reach approximately $6 trillion by 2027. The health share of the gross national product from 2020-2027 will increase to 19.4 percent from the 17.8 in 2019. The key projected expenditure trends by payer will include Medicare, Medicaid, private health insurance, and out-of-pocket expenses, whereas, expenditures by section will comprise prescription drugs, hospital, and physical and clinical services (Centers for Medicare and Medicaid Services, 2019). This will require all healthcare organizations to achieve the highest value possible, understand the value and meaningful use of data systems, and apply the value equation posed by Lighter (2011) if they remain solvent. For purposes of discussion, the value equation posed by Lighter is communicated mathematically as Value = Quality/Cost.

Staging healthcare settings to understand and use data systems adds value and assists improvement teams to achieve positive outcomes as new ideas and shared thoughts converge to stabilize the value equation (Porter-O'Grady & Malloch, 2015b). Linking quality and financial data to decision-making, reducing data variability, and anticipating risks will contribute to continuous care improvements. Healthcare systems that use data systems to achieve value benefit all stakeholders and sustainability will be transparent in outcomes and actions (Porter, 2010). However, this does not spontaneously occur and requires several integrated components. For example, capturing value from data requires interdependencies of teams, their collective intelligence, and integration of business practices for ongoing data sharing. Informing the public about data, its use, and value offers opportunities for engagement, closing communication gaps, and activities to improve one's health and well-being. For data to be continuously collected and used to its full extent requires protection and regulations for access and use. Infrastructure compatibility is necessary if data quality is safeguarded and new data mining techniques emerge. The nexus of these components are only plausible when team skills and capabilities can connect with data. Otherwise, the data value will be underestimated and the benefits to individuals, healthcare systems, and the discovery of new products and models of care will be diminished. Lost opportunities for equitable distribution of care across populations will also occur (Marjanovic et al., 2017).

Uses of Data Systems

Data are continuously collected in healthcare and to have meaning to leaders and staff require an understanding of how maximum benefit from networks and available products may be achieved. This understanding will benefit patients and organizations in an era where practice changes occur daily and evidence-based information is promoting optimal benefits and health outcomes (McHaney, 2020).

Networks provide the infrastructure for data collection and sharing. Throughout this textbook various networks and types have been discussed and provided a framework for enterprise architecture consideration as transparency and innovation is promoted through accessible data. Open data portals for example provide tools, forums, and resources for data collection and dissemination. Corporate data warehouses are another example in use by the Department of Veterans Affairs that provides a business intelligence infrastructure by normalizing, combining, and streamlining clinical data systems. This infrastructure provides opportunities for organizations to become an industry benchmark for healthcare outcomes and leverage information technology investment (Health Services Research & Development, 2019).

As reimbursement has shifted from volume to quality relative to cost, health systems are focusing more on health maintenance. This shift offers conditions to effectively use digital information to effectively and efficiently improve population health. Various data are potentially available through social media, smart phones, and credit card statements and thorough analysis offer patterns of socioeconomic behaviors useful to customize community-based health maintenance programs (Mullangi et al., 2019).

HOW DATA SHARING ADVANCES QUALITY, SAFETY, EVIDENCE, AND ECONOMIES: IMPLICATIONS FOR IMPROVEMENT TEAMS

Healthcare organizations collect and document behaviors and outcomes during each admission and clinic visit and improvement teams use the data to improve outcomes. Some daunting questions remain unanswered: How, should, to whom, and where are data shared? The answer to these questions may lie in understanding the value of data sharing, the economic impact, and relation to improvement and team science. Being mindful of each of these areas will provide the answer to the question.

The lack of data sharing limits innovation and entrepreneurship. Cross-institutional data sharing is foundational to ongoing scientific development, testing of evidence-based interventions, and healthcare economics. As interventions are developed, tested, and shared, care coordination is increased, quality and safety enhanced, patients and families become partners in care, economic efficiency is achieved, and aggregated health registries offer robust information useful in community-based prevention (American Hospital Association, 2019). Economically, if the status quo of data sharing is unvalued, limited, and becomes optimal, poor health outcomes will persist and paralyze the development of new science, technology, precision medicine, and a healthy population evident economically (Hodson, 2016).

Shared data also promotes improvement and team science offer different insights that are spread beyond institutional data silos. As teams collaborate, science is supported and becomes the epicenter of any endeavor (Bennett & Gadlin, 2012; Tang et al., 2018).

Improvement and Team Science: The Data-Sharing Link

The intensity of quality, safety, and data value has created a call for action in healthcare that clusters around improvement and team science and sharing outcomes. While improvement teams are tasked daily with identifying the root causes of healthcare misadventures and developing corrective actions, rigorous approaches to determine which improvement efforts are effective are incomplete. Improvement research has great potential to improve healthcare as the "how" of interventions are identified, shared, and reliable evidence is formulated to support care delivery. Understanding the connection between critical appraisal of research, and the profiles of improvement innovations provides the underpinning necessary to evaluate what worked (Stevens, 2018).

The pervasive presence of technology in healthcare generates a myriad of large datasets and "big data" discussed in previous chapters. This reinforces the importance of team science in order to leverage change using the strengths and expertise of professionals from different disciplines. While single-investigator approaches may be best for many endeavors, a synergistic team approach to improvement is pivotal in today's healthcare environment. Combining expertise and differing opinions into an improvement endeavor provide promising approaches where the acceleration of evidence and translation through data sharing into policies and procedures are possible (Vogel et al., 2013).

Throughout this chapter, the importance of leading interprofessional teams and the processes toward synergistic maturity cannot be unrecognized as healthcare organizations manage the complexities of care, reduce costs whenever possible, and maintain economic sustainability. The iterative processes associated with data use and sharing, and the ongoing development of improvement and team science will offer the impetus for changing care inefficiencies and team development.

SUMMARY

- Team collaboration, idea sharing, and the use of evidence-based data are required for continuous improvement.
- Leaders who create a climate and culture of inclusiveness enable diverse thought and affect how teams communicate.
- Transformation is central to improvement in healthcare.
- Leaders have a social responsibility to guide teams to use data, innovate, and disseminate findings.
- Data dramatizes the future for innovation and team accomplishments.
- Crucial conversations and diversity of thought guide and inform innovation and change.
- Group stages include: forming, storming, norming, performing, and adjourning.
- Team synergy assists in reducing care fragmentation and dissonance across disciplines.
- Interprofessional collaboration requires a transition where experience of others is recognized and respected.
- Creativity is pivotal to team synergy and organizational success.
- Innovation occurs from creators who flourish when the arts intersect with the sciences and a rebellious sense of beauty opens them to the beauty of both.
- Appreciative inquiry is useful to teams to understand best practices, develop strategy, shift organization thinking to strength-based viewpoints, and formulate a future direction.
- Cultural differences affect team function and synergy development.
- Design thinking is a framework useful in creating innovative solutions through creative problem-solving where teams understand human needs and reframe identified problems toward resolution.
- Technology is a valuable asset to accomplish outcomes.
- Teams for ongoing success and communication must adopt a common language.
- Generational differences benefit team performance.
- Systems engineering partnerships are used in advancing healthcare, meeting aims, and capturing value.

- Healthcare expenditures continue to rise and will reach $6 trillion by 2027.
- The value equation is communicated mathematically as Value = Quality/Cost.
- Data systems add value to organizational function and decision-making processes.
- Networks provide infrastructures for data collection and sharing.
- Data sharing advances entrepreneurship and innovative thought and promotes improvement and team science.

REFLECTION QUESTIONS

1. Consider your current work environment and what leader attributes and qualities impact the success of improvement projects, practice change, and spread of evidence throughout the organization?
2. Identify what technology and data can assist you in leading and managing an improvement process. Which technology or data will assist you to evaluate the impact of the process within an organization?
3. What characteristics foster team synergy, creativity, innovation, and collaboration?
4. How does a common language and cultural differences assist or inhibit interprofessional team outcomes?
5. How can a team apply the value equation to an improvement project?
6. What ways can an improvement team meet the Institute of Medicine and the triple and quadruple aims?
7. How can understanding improvement and team science influence an improvement project in a healthcare organization?

REFERENCES

American Hospital Association. (2019). *Sharing data, saving lives infographic.* https://www.aha.org/2019-01-22-sharing-data-saving-lives-infographic

Bennett, M., & Gadlin, H. (2012). Collaboration and team science: From theory to practice. *Journal of Investigative Medicine, 60*(5), 768–775. https://doi.org/10.2310/JIM.0b013e318250871d

Bieda, L. C. (2017). *Leading analytics teams in changing times.* https://sloanreview.mit.edu/article/leading-analytics-teams-in-changing-times/

Brandt, B. F. (2015). Interprofessional education and collaborative practice: Welcome to the "new" forty-year-old field. *The Advisor, Journal of the National Association of Advisors for Health Professions, 35*(1), 9–17.

The Center for GenerationalKinetics. (2016). *Generational breakdown: Info about all the generations.* https://genhq.com/faq-info-about-generations/

Centers for Medicare and Medicaid Services. (2019). *National health expenditure projections 2018-2027. Forecast summary.* https://www.cms.gov/Research-Statistics-Data-and-Systems/Statistics-Trends-and-Reports/NationalHealthExpendData/Downloads/ForecastSummary.pdf

Chinn, P. (2008). *Peace and power.* Jones & Bartlett Publishers.

Cooperrider, D. L., & Srivastva, S. (1987). Appreciative inquiry in organizational life. *Research in Organizational Change and Development, 1*, 129–169.

Cooperrider, D. L., Whitney, D., Stavros, J. M. (2008). *Appreciative inquiry handbook: For leaders of change* (2nd ed.). Berrett-Koehler Publishers.

Craddock, M. (2011, September 26). The power of teamwork. *Harvard Business Review*. https://hbr.org/2011/09/the-power-of-teamwork

Dam, R., & Siang, T. (2019). *5 stages in the design thinking process*. https://www.interaction -design.org/literature/article/5-stages-in-the-design-thinking-process

Day, J. (2013). Challenges to effective interprofessional working. In J. Day (Eds.), *Interprofessional working: An essential guide for health & social care professionals 2/e nursing and health are practice series* (pp. 1–29). Cengage Learning EMEA.

de Alencar, E. M. L. S. (2012). Creativity in organizations: Facilitators and inhibitors. In M. D. Mumford (Ed.), *Handbook of organizational creativity* (pp. 87–111). Elsevier Inc.

Donnan, S. (2005). What is appreciative inquiry? *Metavolution*. http://www.metavolution .com/rsrc/articles/whatis_ai.htm

Feldman, H. (2008). *Nursing leadership: A concise encyclopedia*. Springer Publishing Company.

Goleman, D. (1998). *Working with emotional intelligence*. Bantam.

Green, R. (1998). *The 48 laws of power*. Penguin Group.

Greer, L. L., Bunderen, L. V., & Yu, S. (2017). The dysfunction of power in teams: A review and emergent conflict perspective. *Research in Organization Behavior, 37*, 103–124. https:// doi.org/10.1016/j.riob.2017.10.005

Haas, M., & Mortensen, M. (2016). *The secrets of great teamwork*. hbr.org/2016/06/ the-secrets-of-great-teamwork

Harris, J. L., & Ward-Presson, K. M. (2020). Managing the interprofessional project team. In J. L. Harris, L. Roussel, C. Dearman, & P. L. Thomas (Eds.), *Project planning and management. A guide for nurses and interprofessional teams* (pp. 121–132). Jones & Bartlett Learning.

Health Services Research & Development. (2019). *VA informatics and computing infrastructure*. https://www.hsrd.research.va.gov/for_researchers/vinci/

Hodson, R. (2016). Precision medicine. *Nature, 537*, S49. https://doi.org/10.1038/537S49a

Hunter, S. T., Cassidy, S. E., & Ligon, G. S. (2012). Planning for innovation: A process oriented perspective. In In M. D. Mumford (Ed.), *Handbook of organizational creativity* (pp. 515– 545). Elsevier Inc.

INCOSE. (2012). *Systems engineering handbook, version 3.2.2.* International Council on Systems Engineering (INCOSE).

Institute of Medicine. (1999). *To err is human: Building a safer health system*. National Academies Press.

Institute of Medicine. (2001). *Crossing the quality chasm: A new health system for the 21st century*. National Academies Press.

Institute of Medicine. (2010). *Clinical data as the basic staple of health learning. Creating and protecting a public good workshop summary*. National Academies Press.

Interprofessional Education Collaborative. (2016). *Core competencies for interprofessional collaborative practice: 2016 update*. Author.

Isaacson, W. (2014). *The innovators: How a group of hackers, geniuses, and geeks created the digital revolution*. Simon & Schuster Paperback.

Jakubowski, T. L., & Perron, T. J. (2018). *Interprofessional collaboration improves healthcare*. https://www.reflectionsonnursingleadership.org>interprofessional-collaboration -improves-healthcare

Joseph, M. L., Bair, H., Williams, M., Huber, D. L., Moorhead, S., Hanrahn, K., Butcher, H., & Chi, N. (2019). Health care innovations across practice and academia: A theoretical framework. *Nursing Outlook, 67,* 596–604. https://doi.org/10.1016/j.outlook.2019.05 .007

Kazanjian, R. K., & Drazin, R. (2012). Organizational learning, knowledge management and creativity. In M. D. Mumford (Ed.), *Handbook of organizational creativity* (pp. 547–568). Elsevier Inc.

Lighter, D. M. (2011). *Advanced performance improvement in health care.* Jones & Bartlett Learning.

Marjanovic, S., Ghiga, I., Yang. M., & Knack, A. (2017). *Understanding the value in health data ecosystems.* RAND Corporation.

Maxwell, J. C. (1999). *The 21 indispensible qualities of a leader.* Thomas Nelson, Inc.

McHaney, D. F. (2020). Information management and knowledge development as actions for leaders. In L. Roussel, P. L. Thomas, & J. L. Harris (Eds.), *Management and leadership for nurse administrators* (8th ed., pp.255–288). Jones & Bartlett Learning.

Melnyk, B. M., Gallagher-Ford, L., & Fineout-Overholt, E. (2016). *Implementing evidence-based practice in nursing and health care.* Jones & Bartlett Learning.

Mullangi, S., Pollack, J. P., & Ibrahim, S. (2019). *Harnessing digital information to improve population health.* digital-information-improve-population-health_article_hbr_corpmark .pdf

Oldham, G. R., & Baer, M. (2012). Creativity and the work context. In M. D. Mumford (Ed.), *Handbook of organizational creativity* (pp. 387–420). Elsevier Inc.

Porter, M. E. (2010). What is value in health care? *New England Journal of Medicine, 363,* 2477–2481. https://doi.org/10.1056/NEJMp1011024

Porter-O'Grady, T., & Malloch, K. (2015a). A new vessel for leadership: Changing the health landscape in an age of reform. In T. Porter-O'Grady & K. Malloch (Eds.), *Quantum leadership. Building better partnerships for sustainable health* (4th ed., pp. 1–39). Jones & Bartlett Learning.

Porter-O'Grady, T., & Malloch, K. (2015b). *Quantum leadership. Building better partnerships for sustainable health.* Jones & Bartlett Learning.

Priest, K. L., Kaufman, E. K., Brunton, K., & Seibel, M. (2013). Appreciative inquiry: A tool for organizational, programmatic, and project-focused change. *Journal of Leadership Education, 12*(1), 18–30. https://doi.org/10.12806/V12/I1/18

Reid, P. P., Compton, W. D., Crossman, J. H., & Fanjiang, G. (2005). *Building a better delivery system: A new engineering/health care partnership.* National Academies Press.

SEBoK. (2019). *Systems engineering overview.* https://www.sebokwiki.org/w/index.php ?title=Systems_Engineering_Overview&oldid=57360

Senge, P. M. (1990). *The fifth discipline. The art & practice of the learning Organization.* A Currency Book.

Stevens, K. R. (2018). Improvement science and team science: Links to innovation, effectiveness, and safety. In J. L. Harris, L. A. Roussel, & P. L. Thomas (Eds.), *Initiating and sustaining the clinical nurse leader role. A practical guide* (3rd ed., pp. 205–2011). Jones & Bartlett Learning.

Stratton-Berkessel, R. (2016). *Appreciative inquiry for collaborative solutions: 21 strength-based workshops.* Pfeiffer.

Tang, C., Plasek, J. M., & Bates, W. B. (2018). Rethinking data sharing and the dawn of a health data economy: A viewpoint. *Journal of Medical Internet Research, 20*(11), e11519. https:// doi.org/10.2196/11519

Tucker, S., & Melnyk, B. M. (2019). A leader's guide to implementing evidence-based practice. *American Nurse Today, 14*(6), 6–9.

Tuckman, B. W. (2001). Development sequence in small groups. *Group Facilitation: A Research and Applications Journal, 3,* 66–81.

Ulrich, B., & Crider, N. M. (2017). Using teams to improve outcomes and performance. *Nephrology Nursing Journal, 44*(2), 141–151.

Vogel, A. L., Hall, K. L., Fiore, S. M., Klein, J. T., Bennett, L. M., Gadin, H., Stokols, D., Nebeling, L. C., Wuchty, S., Patrick, K., Spotts, E. L., Pohl, C., Riley, W. T., Folk-Krzesinski, H. J. (2013). The team science toolkit. *American Journal of Preventive Medicine, 45*(6), 787–789. https://doi.org/10.1016/j.amepre.2013.09.001

Weberg, D., & Davidson, S. (2019). Future of evidence, innovation, and leadership in health care: A model for leading change. In D. Weberg, & S. Davidson (Eds.), *Leadership for evidence-based innovation in nursing and health professions* (2nd ed., pp.1–23). Jones & Bartlett Learning.

West, M. A., & Sacramento, C. A. (2012). Creativity and innovation: The role of team and organizational climate. In M. D. Mumford (Ed.), *Handbook of organizational creativity* (pp. 359–385). Elsevier Inc.

Whitney, D., Trosten-Bloom, A., & Rader, K. (2010). *Appreciative leadership: Focus on what works to drive winning performance and build a thriving organization.* McGraw-Hill.

Zhao, E. Y., & Greer, L. L. (2017). When the powerful is paranoid: Effects on power struggles and performance. *Academy of Management Proceedings, 2017*(1). https://doi.org/10.5465/AMBPP.2017.161

CASE EXEMPLARS FOR APPLICATION

Quality Improvement Guided by Data and Organizational Context in a Nurse-Managed Primary Care Clinic

Mark Contreras

Advancing expectations for cost-effective high-quality care perpetually challenges the healthcare system. Primary care is one sector of healthcare that has garnered significant consideration for the transformational change necessary to promote a paradigm shift towards reduced cost and improved patient care outcomes. Although primary care is a pragmatic area of focus, many primary care organizations are small or solo practices that lack the prerequisite structure to bring about change (Liaw et al., 2016). Often, these organizations also have unique characteristics that inherently challenge the capacity for quality improvement. To conduct quality improvement in an effective and sustainable way, considerable time and energy must be dedicated to developing an individualized approach for organizational change. This exemplar highlights activities and findings from a project that was completed at a small urban nurse-managed primary care clinic. The exemplar offers insight into the planning, implementation, and evaluation of quality improvement guided by data and organizational context.

The organization participating in this quality improvement initiative was motivated by ongoing changes with payer reimbursement that realign practice revenue with the delivery of quality care as opposed to the traditional fee-for-service model. This is a small independent practice with three nurse practitioners, two registered nurses, a practice manager, and a patient services specialist. To account for the inherent challenges associated with small practices exploring complex change initiatives, a systematic approach to quality improvement was adopted to provide structure and support to the process. This project was predicated on three core tenants: establishing meaning for the initiative, continuously engaging staff, and using data to drive change. These fundamental ideas used to guide the work of quality improvement were developed by the project facilitator following a comprehensive literature review examining exemplars of organizational change.

The work of quality improvement begins far before implementation. Efforts to instill meaning for the work at hand help to motivate staff and address preexisting concerns that may later manifest as change resistance among personnel. Explicitly defining the proposed change and exploring the internal and external motivators creates the opportunity for well-informed participants that share the vision for change. During this project, staff were educated on the patient-centered care delivery model, the opportunities for improved patient care and enhanced revenue, and the potential for process improvements to enhance efficiency. Guided by Donabedian's structure, process, and outcomes model and the application of the PARiHS framework, this information was communicated by formal presentations and consistently reinforced during informal interactions with staff. This unified sense of urgency and collective understanding of the achievable opportunities for improvement helped to set the foundation for sustainable change.

Staff were intentionally involved throughout the planning and implementation phases of this scholarly project. Efforts to foster continuous engagement from personnel included guided discussion forums and structured opportunities for routine feedback from staff. Engagement of personnel served to develop a communal environment of collective responsibility and accountability for the proposed practice change. When staff are involved in the development of quality improvement it fosters buy-in and communicates a model of shared leadership. During the planning stages, staff identified the quality measures of focus (breast cancer screening, cervical cancer screening, and tobacco cessation counseling) that were felt to be the most amenable to improvement with consideration to organizational context and the patient population.

Quality improvement initiatives need to be developed and driven by the analysis of practice performance indicators. For the organization participating in this project, data from the electronic health records were audited and interrogated to determine opportunities for improvement. Identified opportunities were further examined in the context of ongoing payment reform and organizational feasibility to adopt and maintain a proposed change. Alignment with performance-based reimbursement programs from insurance providers was a primary consideration for determining target improvement areas. Throughout the project, quality improvement data were continuously monitored to measure the impact of adopted changes and, if necessary, allow for informed redirection based upon lessons learned.

Following implementation, staff survey results from a validated questionnaire suggest that the organization successfully adopted a more comprehensive quality improvement strategy during the project period (see Table 13.1). Furthermore, review of quality data identified statistically significant increases in performance scores for cervical cancer screening for patients aged 21-29 ($+44\%$, $p < .001$) and 30-64 ($+24\%$, $p = .009$). Notable increases in breast cancer screening rates, 17% ($p = .021$),

TABLE 13.1 Aggregate Results for PCMH Assessment Survey on Quality Improvement

SURVEY ITEM	BASELINE AVERAGE NUMERICAL RESPONSE WITH CORRESPONDING DEVELOPMENTAL LEVEL	CURRENT AVERAGE NUMERICAL RESPONSE WITH CORRESPONDING DEVELOPMENTAL LEVEL
Quality improvement activities	3.5 - Level C ... are conducted on an ad hoc basis in reaction to specific problems	9.0 - Level B ... are based on a proven improvement strategy in reaction to specific problems
Performance measures	6.2 - Level C ... are available for the clinical site, but are limited in scope	9.2 - Level B ... are comprehensive, including clinical, operational and patient experience measures, and available for the practice, but not for individual providers
Quality improvement activities are conducted by	3.3 - Level D ... a centralized committee or department	6.5 - Level C ... topic specific QI committees
An electronic health record that supports meaningful use	7.7 - Level B ... is used routinely during patient encounters to provide clinical decision support and to share data with patients	10.2 - Level A ... is also used routinely to support population management and quality improvement efforts

Note: Level D, Level C, Level B, Level A: in ascending order from least comprehensive, and lowest degree of PCMH readiness, to most comprehensive, and highest degree of PCMH readiness.

PCMH, patient centered medical home; QI, quality improvement.

also occurred during the project period. Tobacco cessation counseling rates increased by 9%, but failed to achieve statistical significance ($p = .237$). Figure 13.1 and Table 13.2 display collated outcome measures based on the project findings. Through creating an environment of collective quality improvement, supplementary organizational benefits were realized during the project period. When reviewing quality data, an opportunity to identify and contact prospective patients led to the development of a novel process for increasing patient panels for providers. This practice change directly resulted in 39 new patients establishing care during the project period. Establishing an organizational culture that supports and acknowledges the value of continuous quality improvement has empowered this small health center to systematically identify and act upon opportunities to improve patient care and enhance practice revenue.

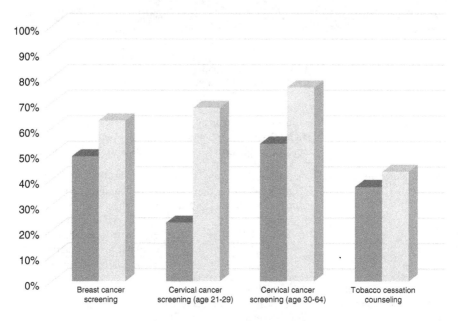

FIGURE 13.1 Project outcomes for pilot quality measures.

TABLE 13.2 Statistical Analysis of Pilot Quality Outcome Measures			
OUTCOME MEASURE	**BASELINE % SATISFIED (N)**	**CURRENT % SATISFIED (N)**	**PEARSON CHI-SQUARE P-VALUE**
Breast Cancer Screening Female patients 50–74 years of age during the reporting period who had a mammogram to screen for breast cancer within the past 24 months	50% (101)	67% (78)	.021*
Cervical Cancer Screening (21–29 years of age) Female patients 21–29 years of age who have had a cervical cancer screening within the last three years.	23% (602)	67% (206)	<.001*

(*continued*)

TABLE 13.2 Statistical Analysis of Pilot Quality Outcome Measures (continued)

OUTCOME MEASURE	BASELINE % SATISFIED (N)	CURRENT % SATISFIED (N)	PEARSON CHI-SQUARE P-VALUE
Cervical Cancer Screening (30–64 years of age) Female patients 30–64 years of age who have had a cervical cancer screening within the last three years or cervical cancer screening with concurrent HPV testing within the last 5 years.	54% (295)	78% (209)	.009*
Tobacco Cessation Counseling Patients 18 years of age and older who are identified as current tobacco users and received tobacco cessation counseling within the last 24 months.	37% (225)	46% (213)	.237

*Statistically significant at the $p < .05$ level.

REFLECTION QUESTIONS

1. How can quality improvement activities produce revenue in a nurse-managed clinic? Explain your rationale and provide supporting evidence.
2. Consider your current practice environment. How can you inform change using data? Provide a rationale for your answer.

REFERENCES

Liaw, W. R., Jetty, A., Petterson, S. M., Peterson, L. E., & Bazemore, A. W. (2016). Solo and small practices: A vital, diverse part of primary care. *The Annals of Family Medicine, 14*(1), 8–15. https://doi.org/10.1370/afm.1839

A Model to Improve Utilization of Community-Based Service Programs by Medicaid-Eligible Pregnant Women in an Urban Environment

Nancy J. Hauff

Pregnant women living in the Detroit area are estimated to be 80% Medicaid eligible. Although women received information on community-based services at their initial prenatal visit to one of our hospital clinics, they frequently expressed the need for assistance following the birth of their infants. It was timely to evaluate the current infrastructure for the referral of eligible infants to Michigan's Medicaid home visiting services: Maternal Infant Health Programs (MIHP) and Children's Special Health Care Services (CSHCS). The overall goal was to promote infant health and development through the provision of professional, quality, and consistent community support services during pregnancy and following hospital discharge. Furthermore, findings in gaps of services to Medicaid eligible pregnant women and young mothers in need were identified (Table 13.3).

BACKGROUND

MIHP is Michigan's largest evidence-based home visitation program for Medicaid eligible for pregnant mothers and their infants. Pregnant women enrolled in MIHP are eligible for transportation assistance to prenatal visits, Women, Infant, and Children's (WIC) food supplement program, and childbirth or parenting education classes. In addition, women can receive home visits from a healthcare professional such as a registered nurse or social worker to address educational needs such as self-care during pregnancy, preparation for childbirth, infant care, mental health, and domestic

TABLE 13.3 Project Objectives		
OBJECTIVES	**ACTIVITIES**	**OUTCOME MEASURE**
Create processes to improve the efficiency of Medicaid-eligible pregnant women into MIHP, CSHCS, and other community-based service programs.	Create a committee of hospital and community-based program representatives. Educate office and clinic staff on program objectives. Evaluate current processes for the referral of pregnant women into MIHP and CSHCS services.	Number of mothers referred for and enrollment into MIHP and CSHCS programs.
Develop a mechanism to evaluate the effectiveness of community service program utilization.	Survey mothers at postpartum discharge class for their knowledge and utilization of MIHP or other community service programs. Create arrangements with specific MIHP programs for hospital referrals. Track numbers of referrals made.	Improve utilization through: Collaborative private/public partnerships between hospital and community-based program staff. Postpartum survey results.
Develop a comprehensive hospital-community based model for the expansion of MIHP and CSHCS services for eligible Medicaid pregnant women.	Onsite MIHP enrollment at our prenatal clinics and postpartum units. Creation of unit-based posters and patient brochures on MIHP services.	Increase MIHP program enrollment. Identification of barriers to MIHP and CSHCS enrollment and underutilization of these programs. Future application to other communities or hospital systems.

MIHP, maternal infant health programs; CSHCS, Children's special health care services.

violence referrals. Children's Special Health Care Services (CSHCS) strives to enable infants and children with special healthcare needs to have improved health outcomes and an enhanced quality of life (MDHHS, 2019). Services include coverage and referral for specialty services based on the person's health problems, support for family caretakers of a special needs child, community-based programs to assist in the care of the child at home, and coordination of services.

The first step to the improvement of linking community-based service programs and our hospital system for Medicaid-eligible pregnant women was to develop an evaluation process. Our plan was to conduct an assessment of our hospital's current processes for MIHP and CSHCS referrals, meet with community leaders and staff from these programs, and to conduct a semi-structured survey of women who had birthed at our facility on their knowledge and utilization of these available community programs.

RESULTS

We learned that a solid process was in place at our institution for infant referral to CSHCS services through case managers working with families of babies in our NICU and Special Care Nurseries. All Medicaid-eligible babies in need of these services were referred to the Detroit Health Department CSHCS program and our neighboring Children's Hospital. Utilization of MIHP services were another matter. Despite numerous creative community ideas and recently developed initiatives, we have learned from the Medicaid-eligible mothers who had given birth at our facility:

- Forty-three percent of eligible mothers were aware of Maternal Infant Health Program services. 57% learned of their eligibility for MIHP services for the first time *after* the birth of their babies.
- Twenty-seven percent of the Medicaid eligible mothers were enrolled in a MIHP service; 73% were not. This finding was below the known State of Michigan utilization of 33% in 2015.
- Mothers receiving prenatal care at the hospital-based clinics were more likely to be enrolled in an MIHP service than mothers attending prenatal care at private practices.
- Twenty percent of the mothers (one out of five) requested more information on MIHP, mental health, and other community-based service programs.
- Eighteen percent of the mothers requested assistance with community program enrollment or wished to be transferred to another MIHP program.

There were barriers to Medicaid-eligible pregnant women receiving MIHP services in addition to their lack of knowledge of these programs. They included mothers:

- were not receptive to having someone come into the home
- were not finding the services beneficial
- found the transportation assistance burdensome
- did not like the MIHP program they were enrolled in and expressed frustration in their ability to transfer to another program
- who had received MIHP services were more likely not to enroll with a subsequent pregnancy.

RECOMMENDATIONS

Due to the lack of general knowledge of available services for Medicaid-eligible pregnant women, inservices were held for clinic and hospital staff. In addition to all clinic women receiving information about MIHP at their first prenatal visit, the hospital arranged for an MIHP program representative to enroll interested women onsite. This action facilitated prompt receipt of needed services to the family. In addition, two representatives from a Detroit Health department WIC program were placed on the hospital's postpartum unit to facilitate referrals for new mothers in need. Posters advertising MIHP services with pictures of new mothers and babies were created for the hospital clinics and postpartum units. In a one-year period, hospital MIHP enrollments increased from 27 % to 34%.

Collaborative efforts between hospitals and community-based service programs to improve the efficiency of healthcare service delivery can improve preventative care during pregnancy and birth and reduce adverse birth outcomes. Support of young mothers after birth through home visits and services can improve their transition to motherhood and investment in our city's future children. More research is needed to track MIHP enrollment with birth outcomes, eliminate programs that are substandard, and support programs with positive outcomes.

REFLECTION QUESTIONS

1. Consider health issues or health outcomes in the community that have been difficult to address. What recommendations would you make to service changes that might address the concern? What baseline data would be needed to make the case for change?
2. How might you gain insights from community members about reasons your existing programs or processes are ineffective?

14

A Kaleidoscope of Opportunities in a Data-Rich Biosphere: A Futuristic Perspective

James L. Harris

OBJECTIVES

1. Explore the influence of data in a futuristic society.
2. Identify how healthcare organizations will respond to future changes and opportunities.
3. Differentiate between cognitive mapping and concept mapping.
4. Provide responses to questions presented for managing data and relevant influences in a future healthcare environment transition from healthcare to wellness care.

CORE COMPETENCIES

- Knowledge of techniques such as concept and cognitive mapping
- Recognize future uses of data to shift priorities of care improvement, delivery, and value
- Recognize the relevance of cognitive mapping and concept mapping to healthcare
- Maintain a futuristic perspective to guide actionable outcomes related to health versus wellness

INTRODUCTION

When viewing the reflections and ever-changing symmetrical patterns produced by a kaleidoscope, one can easily become self-absorbed and distracted by the visual images. Similarly, one can become absorbed and distracted when analyzing large volumes of data and muse upon how to use and present the data that will benefit an organization, scholarship, developing and selling a business case, or reporting mandates. As discussed in the chapters throughout this textbook, data are constantly being produced, shared, and deliberately designed to achieve an outcome. The opportunities to collect, analyze, and use data for implicit purposes are endless in a global society. Individuals, groups, and improvement teams are well positioned to take advantage of the opportunities and utilize its richness in today's information-driven society. Data will continue to be produced and used for many advantageous outcomes. Data will be influenced by a variety of internal and external forces in the 21st century and beyond. New digital technology will be developed, market demands will dictate consumer desires, and healthcare advances will require quantifiable evidence designed to increase efficacy and efficiency. While the opportunities offered by data and its uses are boundless, one must not dismiss there are antecedents, consequences, and outcomes of data that necessitate deliberation and purposeful action.

This chapter presents a futuristic perspective to stimulate one's reasoning and prospective thought about data and its use. Questions are presented in respect to how data will determine and influence healthcare quality, improvement, innovation, and outcomes in an evolving data environment.

ANTECEDENTS, CONSEQUENCES, AND OUTCOMES OF DATA

During the past century, data collection, assimilation, and use have dramatically advanced due to the tireless efforts of clinicians, researchers, educators, leaders, and data scientists. One way to ensure that data remains central to improvement and evidence-based practice is to trace its history with a concentration toward the future. Two techniques, concept maps and cognitive mapping, are commonly cited in the literature and provide support for use when charting the course for a futuristic perspective of data and its crucial role in healthcare (Asadullh, Jaradat, & Hossini, 2014; Daley, Morgan, Black, 2016).

Concept maps were developed by Novak and Gowin (1984) and are "a schematic device for representing a set of concept meanings embedded in a framework of propositions" (p. 15). Kinchin (2015) identified that concept maps were developed through a process of three distinct, but interrelated stages that included emergence (introduction and testing), consolidation (effective to facilitate learning and thought), and transformation (activities occurring and challenging status quo). Daley, Morgan, and Black (2016) adapted Kinchin's work to nursing education to include three steps (emergence, expansion and adaption, and established).

Asadullah, Jaradat, and Hossini (2014) described the technique of cognitive mapping as a means to acquire, code or decode, assimilate, and recall attributes of a phenomenon related to a situation or the environment in actionable ways along a continuum. Three techniques are identified to include: (a) causal mapping (explores thought of decision-makers in business), (b) concept mapping (diagrammatic symbol where every idea and match characterizes idea relations, and (c) sematic mapping (map of ideas and thoughts). Regardless of the technique, one consistent component is an analysis of the cognitive content of a concept and the other is the implied or hidden meaning to guide actions and reflective thought (Huff, 1990).

For purposes of this chapter, data as a concept will be mapped as an example to illustrate how data, using a mental image, can have implications for a future reality in healthcare quality, improvement, innovation, and value. Three distinct, but interrelated domains are illustrated. The domains include: (a) antecedents, (b) consequences, and (c) outcomes as displayed in Table 14.1.

As presented in Table 14.1, concept mapping offers an avenue for exploration and explication of related processes and steps related to concept notions. The benefits associated with concept mapping provide visual displays and descriptors that create tangible links between antecedents, consequences, and outcomes.

TABLE 14.1 Antecedents, Consequences, and Outcomes of Data

ANTECEDENTS	CONSEQUENCES	OUTCOMES
Society requires rapid responses, continuous communication, and data to support decisions.	Communication excess and data are not supported by evidence and strategic foresight.	Communication and information flow are interrupted.
Big data are produced at exponential rates.	Data are not used to the range of possibilities.	Knowledge demands exceed capacity for change.
Funding decreases have reduced healthcare technology development and testing.	New technology is unavailable for use in health care.	Vision to advance care, spread evidence, and leverage learning opportunities foregone.
Mandates and reporting regulations for healthcare systems are constantly changing.	Increased labor costs for data development and inconsistent reporting occurs.	Sustainable fiscal stewardship questioned. Accreditation at risk and costly penalties possible when data are unreported.
Information needs are dynamic and static.	Staff productivity varies based upon need.	Inability to adapt to need and innovate.

(continued)

TABLE 14.1 Antecedents, Consequences, and Outcomes of Data (continued)		
ANTECEDENTS	**CONSEQUENCES**	**OUTCOMES**
Inadequate number of data scientists to meet demands.	Data rigor and utility are compromised.	Care advances, research, and practice inequity exist.
Information needs outweigh manpower to mine, analyze, and provide data.	Data mining, analysis, and dissemination are jeopardized.	Expectations and outcomes shift and decisions are made without evidence or vision.
Risks are associated with data reliability and validity.	Insufficient data to mitigate risks.	Current practices persist without new parameters.
Healthcare costs are escalating while care remains fragmented.	Fiscal instability and dissatisfaction of providers and stakeholders occurs.	Adaptation difficult and future growth at question. A culture of quality, safety, and value are endangered.
Time for innovation and reflective thought is limited.	Innovative initiatives are stagnant with a lack of direction. Decision-making is flawed and without boundaries.	Organizational chaos, dissatisfaction, and misguided decisions are consistent without design to course correct situations.

HOW DATA WILL INFLUENCE THE FUTURE FOR HEALTHCARE QUALITY, IMPROVEMENT, INNOVATION, AND OUTCOMES

Transformation and fluidity are cornerstones of contemporary healthcare. The pace of change is rapid and requires action by teams and leaders in order to ensure quality, continuous improvement, innovation, and sustainable outcomes. Otherwise, a competitive edge is lost. If a competitive edge is to be maintained and advanced, valid and reliable data are required to guide future actions that will revolutionize care. As new imperatives are introduced in health care, innovations will follow and technology will change how care is delivered. Evidence-based data of the future will underpin quality, safety, and efficiency. This will create opportunities to envision a new future for healthcare. To provide context for a future landscape of care, the following questions offer thoughts for leaders, providers, and stakeholders to contemplate.

What if the term healthcare became obsolete in a future society and wellness care became the norm? This novel idea would require a significant paradigm shift in care delivery, practice, operations, reimbursement, data collection, and analysis to name a few. Consider, what if data provided new information to identify individuals who engaged in wellness behaviors and were rewarded for their actions? The vision for a wellness-focused society would become reality and reshape care.

Also consider, what if additional data scientists were available to collect and analyze data and partner with researchers to use data that would ameliorate chronic diseases such as cancer and diabetes? Preventive strategies would become commonplace and greater possibilities would exist to present to future diseases. It is without question that care delivery, operations, and reimbursement would be disrupted and require change.

Challenged with climate change and its effect on wellness, what if new regulations were mandated to eliminate the deleterious effects of pollution and fossil fuel emissions to name two of many? Researchers could partner with providers, data scientists, legislators, and healthcare leaders to foster cutting-edge approaches to advance a global well-being. A social response to wellness would occur and spread globally.

While each of the aforementioned questions presents opportunities for thought and reflection, the realization of a future that utilizes data to the maximum level will advance quality, safety, and value. While healthcare pioneers are credited with modern care and wellness innovations, the time is now for a future that modernizes health care to wellness care reinforced by valid and reliable data. The kaleidoscope of opportunities provided by data is revolutionary and will provide leading-edge data and technological opportunities necessary for a future modicum of wellness care.

SUMMARY

- Data are constantly produced, shared, and deliberately designed to achieve outcomes.
- New digital technology will be developed, market demands will dictate consumer desires, and healthcare advances will require quantifiable evidence designed to increase efficacy and efficiency.
- Opportunities offered by data and its use are boundless, one must not dismiss there are antecedents, consequences, and outcomes of data that necessitate deliberation and purposeful action.
- Two techniques, concept maps and cognitive mapping, are commonly sited in the literature and provide support for use when charting the course for a futuristic perspective of data and its crucial role in health care.
- A concept map is a schematic device for representing a set of concept meanings embedded in a framework of propositions.
- A cognitive map is a means to acquire, code or decode, assimilate, and recall attributes of a phenomenon related to a situation or the environment in actionable ways along a continuum and includes causal mapping, concept mapping, and sematic mapping.
- Data as a concept is mapped in this chapter and includes antecedents, consequences, and outcomes.

- Transformation and fluidity are cornerstones of contemporary healthcare.
- If a competitive edge is to be maintained and advanced, valid and reliable data are required to guide future actions that will revolutionize care.
- New imperatives introduced in healthcare will drive innovations followed by technology that will change how care is delivered.
- Evidence-based data of the future will underpin quality, safety, and efficiency.
- A new future for healthcare will occur where a wellness care environment replaces a healthcare environment and innovation, dissemination, and partnerships flourish.

REFLECTION QUESTIONS

1. Consider each of the questions presented in this chapter. What role would you play in creating a society focused on wellness and why?
2. What different types of data can be collected to improve quality, safety, and value? Support your response with evidence.
3. What individuals should be key contributors in the movement toward wellness care and why?

REFERENCES

Asadullah, A., Jaradat, A., & Hossini, S. E. (2014). Utilization of cognitive mapping technique in information system development. *International Journal of Computer Trends and Technology, 11*(3), 105–108. https://doi.org/10.14445/22312803/IJCTT-V11P123

Daley, B. J., Morgan, S., & Black, S. B. (2016). Concept maps in nursing education: A historical literature review and research directions. *Journal of Nursing Education, 55*(11), 631–639. https://doi.org/10.3928/01484834-20161011-05

Huff, A. S. (1990). *Mapping strategic thought.* Wiley.

Kinchin, I. (2015). Novakian concept mapping in university and professional education. *Knowledge Management and E-Learning, 7*(1), 1–5. https://doi.org/10.34105/j.kmel.2015.07.001

Novak, J. D., & Gowin, B. (1984). *Learning how to learn.* Cambridge University Press.

CASE EXEMPLAR FOR APPLICATION

Future Innovation For Wellness

Lonnie K. Williams

You are the Director of Education in a hospital corporation with a 600-bed not-for-profit hospital in a large metropolitan area with three smaller hospitals, which have 200 beds or fewer, and three outpatient clinics located in rural areas. Members of the organization's Corporate Board have tasked you to develop, implement, and evaluate a feasibility study lasting over a period of one year (with monthly, in-person progress reports). An innovative and cutting-edge Wellness Care Program will be initiated in a pre-designated corporate-owned rural hospital and clinic. Once developed, the study must be submitted and approved through an expedited Institutional Review Boards (IRB) process. The study will include patient satisfaction, sustained overall patient health, cost-benefit analysis, and correlation between patient index admission and subsequent readmission benefits, including patient clinic visits. If the study renders positive conclusions based upon data driven outcomes, the Wellness Care Program will be implemented throughout existing hospitals and clinics.

REFLECTION QUESTIONS

1. What is your first priority in developing the constructs of this advanced study and the IRB approval process (in your literature review you discover a limited amount of existing complementary data concerning a Wellness Plan of Care)?
2. What additional hospital/clinical departments could assist in this inventive initiative?
3. What measuring tools will be needed/developed to collect/interpret data?

4. Once approved, how will you disseminate the information, role and degree of involvement and cooperation with identified hospital staff and clinic staff in this trail-blazing venture?
5. Through cognitive or conceptual mapping how will you be able present ongoing data collection to evidence outcomes?

Index

CPSIA information can be obtained
at www.ICGtesting.com
Printed in the USA
BVHW081927071220
595107BV00004B/20